HOW TO STAY HEALTHY

HOW TO STAY HEALTHY

Is your health at risk?
Recognize the symptoms
Find the remedy

———

Dr Michael Apple

BLOOMSBURY

This edition first published by Bloomsbury Publishing Plc, 38 Soho Square, London W1V 5DF

Copyright © 1996 by Dr Michael Apple

The moral right of the author has been asserted

A copy of the CIP entry for this book is available from the British Library

ISBN 0 7475 2671 0

10 9 8 7 6 5 4 3 2 1

Designed by Hugh Adams, AB3
Typeset by Hewer Text Composition Services, Edinburgh
Printed by Cox & Wyman Limited, Reading, Berkshire

ACKNOWLEDGMENTS

It has taken two years to bring this book from inspiration to publication. My thanks go to my agent Teresa Chris for having faith in the concept, to Rowena Gaunt and Isabelle Auden of Bloomsbury Publishing for editorial guidance and encouragement; to Karen Sullivan who copy-edited the book and added her knowledge to the sections on alternative therapy. Dr Rami Eliad checked the medical facts. I thank him and my other partner Dr Henrietta Antscherl for their tolerance of the many moments when my eyes glazed over as an apt turn of phrase came to mind.

Over the years innumerable patients have asked me for explanation and clarification of their medical conditions. They have been the stimulus for me to develop what I hope to be straightforward, honest and reassuring accounts of the endlessly fascinating subject of health.

CONTENTS

FOREWORD

One Wednesday lunchtime, many years ago, I gave a talk about medicine and the media to a group of general practitioners. I'd enthused about the power of television to get basic facts across in a striking and often entertaining way. I'd spoken at length about the high quality of medical information in womens' magazines. And I'd praised the press for putting crucial health issues on the agenda for public debate. All in all, by the end of my talk, I felt I'd presented a fairly robust case for the increased coverage of medical subjects in the media.

In the discussion afterwards, however, one of the GPs in the audience worked himself up into a state of considerable agitation, not to say anger. His blood pressure rose visibly. How could I, he fumed, let the medical profession down so badly by getting involved in the media? Television, he claimed, had done much more harm than good to the practice of medicine. A little knowledge was an incredibly dangerous thing. People would watch some half-baked, sensationalised or totally unbalanced TV programme and think they knew it all. His life was being ruined by partly informed patients who kept questioning his opinion and decisions. It would be a lot better for everyone if medical knowledge were restricted to health professionals. Doctors like me who persisted in trying to 'inform' the public should be drummed out of the NHS!

By the time I'd recovered from this onslaught, the perpetrator had left the room and his colleagues were muttering about stress and overwork. But his outburst had a profound effect on me. I was so shocked at his attitude, and so convinced he was utterly wrong, that I became even more determined to do what I could to dispel the view that a little knowledge is a dangerous thing, and that people should be kept in blissful ignorance of medical matters. I redoubled my efforts with the media and devoted a large chunk of my life to persuading doctors that giving people information about health and illness could often be more beneficial than dishing out pills.

I tell this story to illustrate how much things have changed over the past couple of decades. Medical programmes, articles and books are now very much part of everyday life and their contribution widely accepted – even by stressed-out GPs! People are now much better informed about medical matters and much more prepared to share responsibility for looking after their own health and that of their family.

One of the problems of all the medical information currently available to the general public, however, is the difficulty of knowing what's important and what isn't. What are the basics, the essentials? Do you know what you really *need* to know? This is why you'll find Michael Apple's excellent book so helpful. It does all the sorting and distilling for you, and gives you the essential information in a very clear and straightforward way. With a basic understanding of common illnesses, you'll have a much better idea of whether a particular problem will right itself or whether it needs to be checked and treated by your doctor. You'll know how common the illness is and what tests can help to diagnose it. You'll be aware of the various forms of treatment and their advantages and disadvantages. And you'll see whether there are ways of preventing it from happening again.

In short, I've no doubt that, armed with the 'little knowledge' in this book, you'll have enough of a grasp of what's going on, and why, to be able to ask the right questions, make better sense of the answers and, together with you doctor, come to the right decisions.

Dr Alan Maryon Davis
MB, BChir, MRCP, FPHM

INTRODUCTION

This book is about serious illnesses that are common; diseases that can occur in any one of us, given the right circumstances. It will also discuss some of the less common illnesses which can be prevented. There are plenty of things to worry about in our daily lives, without fearing things that may never happen. We are constantly assaulted by headlines warning of deadly viruses, frightening new strains of diseases that have been imported from other countries, or developed in our own. No one takes the time to tell us that these diseases are truly rare; the fact that they have hit the headlines at all is a mystery.

Remember the panic about mad cow disease? Or Gaucher's or Tay-Sach's diseases? These illnesses are genuinely serious and devastating for those they affect, but in most cases the publicity fails to make clear how uncommon they really are. Such diseases do not figure in these pages.

This book deals instead with those illnesses that pose a real risk to your health, and that of your family and friends. Many of these conditions can cause death or disability – such as a heart attack or breast cancer. It will also discuss some disorders which don't fall strictly into the category of diseases, like impotence, the menopause, or acne, but which trouble many of us from time to time. Anything which affects the quality of your life can be considered serious, and that's what will be discussed here.

This book is not a medical encyclopaedia; you won't encounter every disease you've heard mentioned on television, or seen flashing through the headlines. What you will find is a unique collection of up-to-the-minute information on diseases which could play an important role in many of our lives. It's been broken down into an accessible format, which begins with the 'three Rs'. After a brief introduction to each disease, we will discuss:

- **Risk**, which tells you how common the disease is and who is in danger.
- **Recognition**, which describes the warning signs, symptoms and the tests or investigative techniques undertaken to reach a diagnosis.
- **Remedy**, where treatment is discussed.

Additionally, there are, in appropriate entries, sections describing any further information which might be of some use. We've divided them into:

- **Ask your Doctor**, which outlines important questions about which you might want to enquire.
- **Alternative Treatment**, where we offer some advice about complementary treatments which work outside conventional medical practices. Many of these are unproved, but we have noted them here so you will know what is available.
- **Prevention**, where we'll discuss everything that is known about minimizing your risks of acquiring the illness.
- **Self-help**, in which useful contact addresses are supplied.

There is also a comprehensive listing of investigative, therapeutic and diagnostic techniques explained at the back of the book. If you want to know more about how your disease may be investigated, confirmed, or treated, this is the place to look.

HOW TO USE THE BOOK

First of all, consider which part of the body is most affected by your condition; obviously some illnesses may appear to affect more than one, but choose the one you think most likely. For example, a headache would be found under 'Brain and Nervous System'; diarrhoea under 'Digestive System', and asthma in the section entitled 'The Lungs and Breathing'. The illnesses are then listed alphabetically within these sections. If you can't find what you are looking for, try the index at the back of the book.

The risk and prevalence of every disease listed in this book are based on current findings in Great Britain, unless otherwise stated. There are certain conditions, like AIDS, where the figures change rapidly and may have done so between the research and the publication of this book.

Please remember that this book is not intended to be a substitute for seeing your own doctor. Self-diagnosis can be dangerous, and the scope of this book does not allow for a description covering every exception or variation of a disease to be included.

THE SKIN

• Acne • Eczema • Psoriasis • Skin Cancers

I T IS DIFFICULT to ignore any skin disorders, no matter what their severity. Fortunately most skin conditions are not dangerous, medically speaking. Their psychological importance is another matter.

In understanding skin disorders it is helpful to realize that the skin is one whole organ. This explains why a condition like eczema appears in one place, and then moves across the body. It's also important to realize that unblemished skin is rarely achievable; the skin is there to protect the body from the harsh world of ultraviolet light, water, heat, cold, infection and friction and it is bound to break down in places into minor infection and sore areas. The effects of ageing, in which the supporting structure of the skin becomes thinner as time goes by, also lead to wrinkles and colour changes.

The very visibility of the skin is an advantage because it means that potentially serious changes can be noticed at an early stage. Skin awareness has become a key health issue; we are all aware that we should restrict exposure to intense sunshine and bring to the attention of a medical practitioner any changes to the skin.

ACNE

The same hormones which turn sweet children into moody teenagers also cause acne. For some people the problem persists into adult life.

Surprisingly, for such a common condition, the exact reasons for acne are not certain. Partly it is to do with the increase in male hormones which begins at puberty and which affects girls as well as boys (we all have both male and female hormones circulating; it is the balance which keeps us feminine or masculine). Male hormones make the skin more greasy which in turn leads to colonization by bacteria. Bacteria appear to promote the pimples, probably by producing irritant waste products.

Whether through infection or through blockage by excess sebum (the oily secretions of the sebaceous glands, which act as a lubricant for the skin), sweat glands become inflamed and grow into the familiar spots. These are found especially on the face, back and chest, being areas of particular concentrations of fat-secreting (sebaceous) glands. Some individuals form cysts, large hollow infected lesions which leave scars.

A minority of people are affected by acne throughout their lives, women often noticing fresh lesions pre-menstrually. These women sometimes prove to have abnormal amounts of male hormone, for which there is effective drug treatment. There is no longer any reason to suffer severe and disfiguring acne. There is a wide range of treatment options which work for just about everyone. The first step is to accept that acne can be helped and to seek medical attention.

Risk

- Acne is extremely common during adolescence – few teenagers escape without having any at all.
- The condition clears in most people by their early twenties.

- Acne persists in about 6 per cent of individuals through their adult life.
- It's made worse by the use of oils which block pores, including cosmetics.
- Excess sweating can encourage acne.
- Acne in women is increasingly recognized as part of a poly-cystic ovary syndrome.
- Acne can be caused as a side-effect of steroid drugs taken for asthma or rheumatoid arthritis, among others.

Recognition

SYMPTOMS

The skin is usually greasy and there are many blackheads – these are the mouths of sweat glands blocked by the natural oils of the skin (sebum); the black is not from dirt but from the discoloration which occurs when the oil comes in contact with the air. Whiteheads also occur from blocked pores but they are not in direct contact with the air, so discolouration does not occur. Some of these lesions become inflamed and red; in bad cases they grow into large inflamed cysts which heal leaving a scar.

SIGNS

The appearance of acne is usually typical. A doctor might be suspicious if someone develops acne for the first time beyond their teens. Women with acne who are also unusually hairy and who have irregular periods may have the poly-cystic ovary syndrome.

INVESTIGATIONS

Are only necessary if a hormone disorder such as poly-cystic ovaries is suspected.

ASK YOUR DOCTOR

- **About your acne. Do not simply put up with it; it may not be entirely curable but it should be controllable in the vast majority of cases.**

Remedy

Treatment is based on the severity of the acne. Teenagers, who are expected to develop the condition at some point in their early adult years, may receive a less intensive treatment than a model, or a television personality, for whom one spot would make headlines. There is not, sadly, a cure-all for acne. A treatment which alleviates the worst of the outbreaks is a realistic expectation.

DIET AND CLEANLINESS

Particular foods may affect your acne; scientific trials fail to show any relationship between eating chocolate and acne, yet many people with acne both know and show that eating chocolate makes their acne worse within days. Similarly, a greasy diet will not necessarily cause acne, but many sufferers find their condition worsens after a fry-up. A good diet, with plenty of fresh water, will encourage healthy skin. Regular cleansing of the skin is recommended, but over-cleansing can strip the skin of its natural oils (sebum) and cause the glands to over-produce – another cause of acne. Be prudent.

SKIN APPLICATIONS

At the simplest level there are lotions which remove the hard keratin (surface) of the skin; these commonly contain benzoyl peroxide and cause a little redness and peeling; a more powerful medically prescribed substance is retinoic acid. Then there are antibiotic lotions – very useful for mild acne confined to a small area, like the chin or the forehead.

ANTIBIOTICS BY MOUTH

These have been a useful, safe mainstay of treatment for many years and are thought to work by controlling the bacteria which invade the blocked pores. Commonly used drugs are oxytetracycline, trimethoprim and minocycline. It can take up to six months for maximum effect and they often need to be taken for several years, changing the type of antibiotic as you become immune to its effect.

HORMONES

Women with acne who also want contraception will find it useful to take a birth control pill containing the drug cyproterone; this greatly relieves mild to moderate acne, again taking several months for full effect.

> **Severe Resistant Acne**
> *Acne that is still bad despite all these measures is unusual; the option here is to use a powerful drug called isotretinoin, available only from hospital dermatologists (skin specialists). It is highly effective, but there are many side-effects; in particular, it must not be taken by women who are pregnant or who are contemplating pregnancy. A four-month course of treatment works in 90 per cent of cases and the effect can last for two or more years.*

Alternative Treatment

Nutritional therapy might be useful if your acne is affected by what you eat; it might also suggest supplementation with zinc and other nutritional elements which may control the excess production of sebum. Many therapies will offer a cleansing diet, or a course of treatment aimed at expelling toxins from the skin. Some success has been indicated by homoeopathic, herbal and aromatherapeutic treatment.

Prevention

- Experiment with your diet; if you find something which affects your acne take note, even if your medical advisors scoff. Exposure to ultraviolet light is of undoubted benefit; many sufferers find that their acne improves in summer for this reason. However be aware of the danger of overexposure to ultraviolet light (see **skin cancer**, page 10).
- Avoid heavy make-up, or in the case of men, greasy hair preparations that can make acne worse by clogging the pores on the forehead.

- Hot atmospheres can make acne worse; see if you can change your working environment if this applies to you.

Self-Help

Acne Support Group
16 Dufour's Place, Broadwick Street, London W1V 1FE

ECZEMA

Coming from the Greek word meaning 'to boil over or break out', eczema is an extremely common skin condition affecting all ages. Eczema is classified as being either endogenous or exogenous. Endogenous means a constitutional tendency to eczema, that is eczema arising out of your own make-up. It might be due to some over-activity of the body's immune system. By contrast, exogenous eczema arises from some external stimulus – detergents, metals, etc. This type of eczema is commonly called dermatitis. In practice there is a bit of both in each case; anyone with endogenous eczema will have frequent outbreaks for no obvious reason and will also be more sensitive than average to a range of external stimulants.

Endogenous eczema is frequently associated with illnesses where allergy is an important trigger, namely **asthma** (see page 214) and **hay-fever** (see page 221). It does not mean that allergy causes the hay-fever or asthma or eczema in the first place, but that they can be made worse by allergic stimuli. Individuals who suffer from these types of allergies are called 'atopic'.

Eczema is not contagious; it can be unattractive in some instances, and the sufferer will certainly be made more uncomfortable by social isolation.

Risk

- Over 12 per cent of children are affected by atopic (endogenous) eczema.
- Cases of eczema have increased by two to five times over the last fifty years, presumably due to environmental factors.
- In 70 per cent of cases there is a family history of eczema, hay-fever or asthma.
- About 90 per cent of children grow out of the condition by adult life.
- Certain occupations are notorious for causing dermatitis, through the irritant chemicals used; these include hairdressing, engineering with oils, and work with constant exposure to water; e.g., bar work.

Recognition

Sufferers of all ages have patches of dry, itchy skin but the pattern can vary greatly at different times.

SYMPTOMS

Babies and Children
Within days of birth an atopic baby has a greasy, red rash over his or her cheeks and forehead. When they develop nappy rash, which is very common in atopic children, it is much redder than average and spreads over a wider area. As they grow older the eczema will look less greasy and tends to concentrate in skin folds behind the knees, in front of the elbows, and behind the ears, but it can involve much of the rest of the body.

The eczema will be itchy; the child might, if unlucky, also suffer from asthma or hay-fever by late childhood.

Adults

If they have had eczema all their lives adults will have dry, thickened and fissured skin. Other patterns include patches of eczema scattered over the body. The elderly are prone to a type of eczema where their skin becomes dry and irritable. Eczema confined to the hands or to one site of the body is highly suggestive of a dermatitis through some external irritant.

SIGNS

A first outbreak can look like infection but it soon becomes clear that the sufferer has a chronic (long-term) condition. Single patches of eczema in adults can look indistinguishable from fungal infection and often need investigation to establish a diagnosis.

INVESTIGATIONS

These are popular with patients but are less helpful than often thought, because they rarely influence treatment. The commonest is patch testing (see **allergy tests,** page 297). A series of possible allergens is painted on to the skin of the back and the response is gauged after a few days. This can identify an allergy to an individual chemical; e.g., a particular dye used in hairdressing or perfume. More often the patch testing shows up sensitivity to a range of allergens that cannot realistically be completely avoided; e.g., wool, detergents, paper or even sunlight (photo-dermatitis).

ASK YOUR DOCTOR

- **About general non-drug treatments that can make a difference to eczema. Many parents query diet or additives as the cause of their children's eczema. There are a few cases where this appears true; your doctor will be able to put you in touch with a sympathetic dermatologist or paediatrician if you wish to explore the possibility.**

Remedy

Most cases of eczema can be relieved by moisturizing the skin; often, steroid applications may be used to relieve the inflammation. Long-term use and use in children is no longer recommended for anyone who does not suffer severely.

EMOLLIENTS

Moisture is put into the skin using so-called emollients; there are several brands which are a skilful blend of creams that moisturize the skin without making it greasy – an important consideration when sufferers still have to deal with paper and use tools. They make the skin smooth and supple, so less likely to crack. Several are available as bath additives, a convenient way of dealing with widespread eczema. Emollients are harmless and even used alone can bring mild eczema under control. Their one drawback is that some people develop an allergy to one of their components.

Steroid Applications

The use of steroids transformed the treatment of eczema so that it is impossible to imagine skin care without their careful use. Over-liberal use many years ago has left a popular legacy of mistrust (this also applies to some doctors). We now know that prolonged use of potent steroid creams on the face can result in irreversible thinning of the skin and unsightly dilated veins. There is less of a risk elsewhere on the body. Another worry has been that enough steroid would be absorbed through the skin to have more widespread effects on the body – in particular, to restrict growth in children. Though this is possible in theory, it is only a serious risk if using more than 100 g per week of the most potent steroids for months on end.

Most doctors will bring eczema under control using a powerful steroid and then keep it under control with a far milder one.

Antibiotics

The cracked, weeping skin is an open invitation to infection; infection also causes flare-ups of eczema. For that reason doctors will commonly prescribe creams which contain an antibiotic as well as a steroid.

Intensive Treatment

This can include irradiation with ultraviolet light (see page 9), steroids taken by mouth and drugs which suppress the immune system; cyclosporin is the main one used.

Alternative Treatment

Oil of evening primrose taken in capsule form has been shown to help eczema. Less certain is the effect of diet on eczema. Some children improve if they avoid cow's milk or eggs. Allergy to wheat or food additives is another possibility, but many doctors refute the idea that eczema is caused by food allergy or intolerance.

There is no doubt that some sufferers become worse with stress and tension so any means of relieving that must be worth exploring; yoga, acupuncture, massage and aromatherapy.

There has been great interest in the effect of Chinese herbs on eczema, which is being taken seriously by orthodox dermatologists who are trying to work out scientifically what may be the active component. It's important to remember that although they are natural, herbs are potent and often powerful drugs. If you wish to try Chinese herbalism, you must do so through a registered practitioner. Homoeopathy has had remarkable success treating eczema; the rule of thumb is that it takes about as long to cure your eczema as the length of time you've had it.

Prevention

For children the best prevention is to ensure that the skin does not dry out and to treat flareups early and vigorously. Any infection needs similar aggressive handling. Ultraviolet light relieves eczema and exposure to sunlight is encouraged – but not to the point of burning. Adults may have to accept that certain occupations are closed to them, such as hairdressing, and the food industry.

ENVIRONMENT

Those severely affected should avoid common irritants such as biological detergents, perfumed products, woollen clothing (allergy to lanolin in wool is common). Being too hot increases itching, so wear loose clothing and try to not become overheated in bed. Wear gloves when your hands are in water and dry them carefully but beware of allergy to rubber gloves, which is again quite common.

By all means test out whether foods, additives or colorants affect you; do this one substance at a time, allowing at least two weeks before coming to any conclusions. In the case of babies or children we do not advise major dietary manipulation without taking medical advice.

DRUGS

Use the mildest steroid cream which keeps your eczema under control and combine this with liberal use of an emollient. Do not spurn using a potent cream for a brief period of time to control flare-ups. Very recently potent creams have become available which claim to be safe to use on the face and for prolonged use; they are still being evaluated.

Self-Help

British Allergy Foundation
St Bartholomew's Hospital, West Smithfield, London EC1A 7BE

The National Eczema Society
163 Eversholt Street, London NW1 1BU
Tel: 0171 388-4097

PSORIASIS

This is a chronic (long-term) skin condition which can be greatly disfiguring but which, for the majority of people, is not. The cause is an over-proliferation of the cells in the outermost layer of the skin. New skin cells are created at an accelerated rate, resulting in patches of pink, thickened new skin, covered with dead, flaking skin.

Risk

- Psoriasis affects 2 per cent of the population, and is less common in coloured races.
- The condition begins most often in the late teens/twenties but can occur for the first time in the elderly.
- Psoriasis is hereditary.
- In up to 10 per cent of cases there is accompanying arthritis of the fingers and the spine.
- It can occasionally begin abruptly in young people following a throat infection, but any more definite link with infection is unproved.
- There are genetic changes in most sufferers which overlap with the condition of ankylosing spondylitis.
- Stress can cause flare-ups of the disease.
- Psoriasis can be caused by drugs in rare instances, the commonest being the beta-blocker propranolol, used in treating high blood pressure, and lithium used to treat manic-depressive psychosis.

Recognition

SYMPTOMS

There are patches of thick, flaking skin over the knees, elbows and around the margins of the hair, but the rash can be much more widespread. The patches vary in size from coin-sized to several centimetres in diameter and there may be just a few or dozens. The flaky skin has a typical silvery appearance, while the underlying skin is a deep almost plummy red. The patches tend to be worse where the skin is most used; e.g., those in sedentary jobs find it worse around their lower back. Really severe disease leads to the constant shedding of scales from the skin, flying off whenever the sufferer undresses and can be a major embarrassment. Despite its appearance, the skin is not particularly itchy.

Another form of psoriasis affects the palms of the hands and the soles of the feet. Occasionally the finger- and toenails are affected, and the joints can become inflamed. Joint pain, if present, tends to involve the small joints of the fingers and the lower back. The diagnosis can be particularly puzzling if there are just isolated patches on the tip of the penis and around the anus, a not infrequent finding.

> *Very rarely, the whole of the skin suddenly becomes inflamed, known as erythroderma. It is like a widespread burn and, like extensive burns, is a medical emergency. If you think this is happening to you seek urgent help.*

SIGNS

The skin has a typical flaky appearance and sheds scales easily. Often there are small pits in the nails – this is especially the case in those with co-existing arthritis – and the nail can seem to be lifting off its nail bed.

INVESTIGATIONS

The skin lesions can be confused with eczema or fungal infections, so microscopic examination of scrapings is helpful; someone with joint pains needs investigation to exclude other causes for the pain, such as rheumatoid arthritis.

ASK YOUR DOCTOR
- **About seeing a dermatologist, if you have more than a few patches.**
- **About the most cosmetically acceptable forms of treatment for you.**

Remedy

Psoriasis is a chronic condition, so the sufferer has to learn to cope with lifelong daily treatment plus more intensive treatment during flare-ups.

SKIN PREPARATIONS

The treatment of any but the smallest degree of psoriasis is a real art. There are so many combinations of creams and lotions that have to be tailored to the individual. Dithranol and coal tar extracts have been found for years to be effective but used to be smelly and messy to apply. Modern preparations are far more cosmetically acceptable and are often combined with steroid creams. (see **eczema**, page 6, for further remarks about steroid creams). They are also available as scalp lotions.

Very recently a form of vitamin D has become available in a bland acceptable cream (calcipotriol) which can greatly reduce the thickness of individual patches.

ULTRA-VIOLET LIGHT THERAPY

This effective intensive therapy is reserved for severe cases. A drug is take by mouth which increases the sensitivity of the skin to ultra-violet light (similar to the medication found in tanning creams). Two hours later you are exposed to a few minutes of ultraviolet light; repeated two to three times a week for about four months. To keep the skin under control requires maintenance therapy every few weeks. This is specialized treatment with a risk of damage to the eyes and a long-term risk of skin cancer, so must be given only under the supervision of a dermatologist.

IMMUNO-SUPPRESSANT DRUGS

It may come as a surprise to learn that the same drugs used in the treatment of some cancers are also used in treating psoriasis. Severe psoriasis is a greatly disfiguring condition both in its appearance and by reason of the shower of shed skin that surrounds the sufferer; work and social activity can be non-existent. Powerful drugs may be necessary.

Methotrexate appears to be the most effective drug; others include cyclosporin, azathioprine. Of course these must be carefully monitored for any signs of damage to the bone marrow and liver.

Arthritis
Psoriatic arthritis is treated with standard pain-killers and anti-inflammatory drugs. The immuno-suppressants mentioned above may be needed for cases resistant to pain-killers.

Alternative Treatment

There are a variety of herbal baths and lotions prescribed, which may relieve scaling in individual cases. Acupuncture, homoeopathy and reflexology might prove useful; be sure to seek out a registered practitioner. Because psoriasis is exacerbated by stress, any relaxation therapies (yoga, massage, etc.) might be considered.

Prevention

Sufferers can reduce the frequency and severity of flare-ups by avoiding stress and emotional trauma in their lives wherever possible.

It is sensible to keep a record of the skin preparations which are most effective for you, so that you can treat yourself at the earliest sign of a flare-up. Try to build up a good relationship with your dermatologist; he or she will be seeing you through all the ups and downs of your condition and will advise on those minor adjustments to therapy which are the art of medicine and dermatology.

Self-Help

The Psoriasis Association
7 Milton Street, Northampton NN2 7JG
Tel: 01604 711129

SKIN CANCERS

Thanks to an increasing number of campaigns most people are aware of the risk of skin cancer and more and more people are taking steps to seek medical advice about changes in the skin. This is an excellent development, because early skin cancers are almost always curable. Most are due to malignant change in the outer layers of the skin and are slow growing. Malignant melanomas are an unusual exception; they arise in the pigment cells in the skin, are usually coloured and are far more aggressive in their spread and behaviour. However, these too are curable if diagnosed and treated early.

Risk

- The most common skin cancers are basal cell or squamous cell affecting mainly middle-aged and elderly people; there are an estimated 25,000 new cases per annum.
- Skin cancers are common in outdoor workers exposed to sunlight, especially if fair skinned.
- There is an increased risk in occupations with exposure to tar and other chemicals.
- Malignant melanomas are increasingly common but are still unusual; however, they do account for nearly 1200 deaths a year.
- You are two to four times more likely to develop a melanoma in your lifetime as a result of exposure to ultraviolet rays in sunlight; the greatest risk is after sunburn.
- There is a large genetic risk in melanoma.
- People with more than 100 moles have an eight to twenty times greater risk of developing a malignant melanoma.
- Melanomas can occur at any age.
- Melanomas and squamous cell tumours can spread elsewhere in the body; basal cell tumours virtually never do but will destroy local tissue if ignored (they are also called rodent ulcers).

Recognition

Skin cancers show themselves either as a lump, a persistent sore area or as an unusually coloured patch or mole.

SYMPTOMS

Most commonly you notice a small nodule on the face by the nostrils, over one eye or on the back of the hands (i.e., the areas most exposed to sunlight). The edges look lighter than the centre and often you can see a few small blood vessels. The centre is often crusted. Alternatively you may notice a scaly patch on the skin which does not heal and which may bleed.

In the case of a melanoma you may notice a dark spot that you have not seen before or you might notice that a pre-existing dark mole has become itchy, larger, looks darker and seems to be spreading into the surrounding skin. If neglected these may bleed. They can occur anywhere on the body.

SIGNS

Doctors look for the above features but in more detail; in particular basal cell tumours have a typical 'rolled edge' appearance under a hand lens. In deciding whether a pigmented lesion (a structural change in the fabric of the skin) might be a melanoma, the doctor takes into account how long it has been there, whether it is active in terms of itchiness or changes of colour.

INVESTIGATIONS

The diagnosis can often be made simply by examining the appearance of the skin; treatment is planned accordingly. Where there is doubt – and there frequently is – a **biopsy** (see page 298) is taken for microscopic analysis.

ASK YOUR DOCTOR

- **About any change in the appearance of your skin which worries you; you are not wasting your doctor's time.**
- **About changes in the size or texture of moles, or the growth of new ones.**

Remedy

Basal cell or squamous cell growths can be dealt with by freezing (cryotherapy), **X-irradiation** (see page 301), or by surgical excision depending on their size. Potential malignant melanomas must be completely cut out of the skin, together with a margin of skin sufficient to remove every trace of cancerous cells. This may mean cutting out a large patch which then has to be repaired with a skin graft.

Chemotherapy (see page 298) may be required if the tumour has spread.

Cure can be guaranteed in the case of virtually all basal cell tumours and in the majority of squamous cell tumours. Malignant melanomas are a special problem because it is such an aggressive tumour; if the tumour is up to 1 mm thick there is a better than 90 per cent, five-year survival rate; if it is thicker than 3.5–4 mm the chances of cure drop to 50 per cent. Death is caused when the aggressive malignant cells spread to other organs in the body but especially the liver.

Some people have inherently unstable skin and continue to develop tiny skin cancers. Others have a mass of pigmented patches or moles which increases the risk of a melanoma. Such people should have regular skin checks as well as being extra vigilant about excess exposure to sunlight.

Occasionally unusual skin lumps turn out to have spread from other malignancies elsewhere in the body; e.g., breast cancer, lung cancer. A particular form of skin cancer is associated with AIDS; the lesions in this case are called Kaposi's sarcoma and are rare except in those with immune disorders. In such cases the treatment is of the underlying disease.

Alternative Treatment

Any changes in the skin must be seen by an orthodox medical practitioner, as a matter of some urgency. Post-operatively, alternative medicine can be useful. There is some evidence that acupuncture can restore a battered system to normal; contact, too, a nutritional therapist, or a registered homoeopath or herbalist for advice.

Prevention

EXPOSURE TO SUN OR SUNBURN

It has been known for some time that ultraviolet light increases the risks of a range of skin cancers; the alarming finding has been that the risks of malignant melanoma seem to be doubling every ten to fifteen years. Given this evidence, it is advisable to limit exposure to the sun. That means avoiding sunburn because even a single episode of sunburn has been shown to increase the risk of developing malignant melanoma in that site.

CHILDREN

Should be kept out of constant strong sunlight, should wear hats and sunblocks to limit the amount of ultraviolet light they receive. A deep tan, especially if achieved after burning, should not be seen as a souvenir of a great holiday, but a needless precursor to later skin trouble.

ADULTS

Should follow similar guidelines, though probably the worst damage is done before adult life as far as the risks of melanoma are concerned. Adults should avoid sunburn and should think twice about using sun beds to maintain an all-year tan because excessive exposure to ultraviolet (UV) rays produced by sunbeds increases the risk of skin cancer.

You cannot and should not completely shield yourself from the sun; ultraviolet light is essential for our bodies to make vitamin D in the skin, without which there is a risk of **osteoporosis** (see page 174); the sense of well-being induced by a holiday in the sun will not need to be diminished by prudent sunbathing and the liberal use of sunscreens.

Workers in industries where skin is exposed to tar or chemicals should follow industry guidelines for skin care and have regular checks of their skin.

Skin Awareness
It should be easy to spot new and persistent skin changes on the face and hands. In the bath take the opportunity to notice skin blemishes. Take note of any area of skin which itches persistently. Ask your partner or a friend to examine anything you can't see. As you grow older, moles and patches of discoloured skin are inevitable, but size is absolutely no guide to malignancy. Learn to recognize what is normal for you.

The nail beds are a fairly common site for a malignant melanoma; look for any unusual blackness that is not the result of bruising. The soles of your feet are also possible sites, so check these from time to time.

If you have any doubt see your doctor; be vigilant in the case of a mole, coloured or otherwise, which grows, itches or bleeds.

INFECTIOUS ILLNESS

• AIDS • Colds • Influenza • Hepatitis
• Malaria • Meningitis • Sinusitis

WITHIN THIS SECTION you will find information about several infectious diseases which are either common or preventable. Elsewhere in this book there is information about infectious illnesses more appropriately covered in other sections: these include **pneumonia** (see page 226), **tuberculosis** (see page 229) and certain childhood illnesses (see pages 63 and 67).

You will come across the terms organisms, viruses and bacteria, and clarification seems sensible. Infections are caused by micro-organisms, living particles seen only under the microscope or, in the cases of viruses, only under high-power electronic magnification.

Bacteria are one-celled organisms that grow and reproduce in their own way. They cause disease by being in the wrong place, like the lungs or bloodstream, and through toxic chemicals that they release which cause fever and collapse of blood flow. Because they have their own metabolism, it is possible to tailor antibiotics against features of a bacteria unique to that organism, which is why these drugs are so effective.

Viruses are incapable of independent growth and reproduction. To achieve this they hijack the metabolism of a cell and force it into producing more viruses. They divert all available resources into their benefit, sustenance and reproduction. This makes it very hard to target them with anti-viral agents, because these would also be acting against the metabolism of the body's own cells. Only fairly recently have agents become available which are effective against some viruses; for example, acyclovir, which is effective against the herpes viruses. On the other hand, viruses can be hit by vaccination because they are a readily recognizable bundle of protein which the body can be 'taught' to recognize and so deal with by antibodies. It is most likely that AIDS will be controlled through such a means.

AIDS

In the late 1970s, infections once excessively rare began to occur with increasing and puzzling frequency in homosexual men. There were cases of pneumonia caused by bizarre organisms; unusual skin cancers and rare brain infections. Early cases were first seen as curiosities but by the early 1980s it was clear that a new, infectious and deadly disease had entered the world stage.

In 1981 the disease was named AIDS for Acquired Immune Deficiency Syndrome, the loss of natural immune defences being a central feature of the illness. By 1983 a causative virus was identified, this being the Human Immuno-deficiency Virus, or HIV. In 1985 a second HIV virus was identified in West Africa, where it infects many individuals and which is spread more easily by heterosexual contact.

In the brief period since AIDS has been recognized it has been realized that groups at risk are much wider than the homosexuals at first affected; within just a decade AIDS has become one of the major worldwide causes of death and debility. Fascinating studies suggest that the first documented case of AIDS actually occurred in a British sailor who died in 1959. At about the same time, the HIV virus was present in small numbers of people in Africa. What lead to the explosive spread in the 1970s is still a mystery.

HIV is transmitted by three routes: sexual contact, contaminated body fluids, especially blood and infected needles, and from mother to baby. The infected individual is then HIV positive but it may be several years before they actually show the features of AIDS.

Risk

POPULATION FACTS
- There have been an estimated 19.5 million cases of HIV infection worldwide.
- There are probably 4.4 million currently suffering from AIDS and an estimated 2.5 million who have died from AIDS.
- In the UK there have been in total approximately 10,000 cases of AIDS.
- The numbers infected with HIV in the USA are put at 600,000 to 1.2 million.
- In the USA there are an estimated 40,000 new cases of HIV per annum.

WHO IS INFECTED?
In Great Britain and North America, the following data applies.
- Over two-thirds of cases occur in homosexual or bisexual men, where 20 to 25 per cent are HIV positive.
- 21 per cent of cases are intravenous drug users.
- 25 per cent of drug users are HIV positive.
- 2 per cent of cases acquire the virus through infected blood products; haemophiliacs, for instance.
- 5 per cent appear to have acquired HIV through heterosexual contact (this is rapidly increasing).
- For 3 per cent of sufferers, the cause is unknown.
- 20 to 30 per cent of children born to HIV-positive women are in turn infected.
- The prevalence of HIV in heterosexual people without other risk factors, such as intravenous drug use, is put at just 1 in 5000, as against one in four or five for exclusively homosexual men.

RISKS OF HIV LEADING TO AIDS
- The annual risk of conversion from HIV infection to AIDS is estimated at 4 to 10 per cent.
- It may take ten or more years to progress from HIV infection to AIDS.
- It is not yet known whether every case of HIV progresses to AIDS but on present evidence it seems that eventually every case does.

FUTURE PATTERNS OF HIV
- Worldwide the majority of infections are by heterosexual contact. In the developed world this is still unusual, but is likely to become increasingly common over the next twenty to thirty years.
- A pin prick with an infected needle carries a 0.3 per cent risk of transmitting HIV as opposed to a 20 per cent risk of transmitting **Hepatitis B** (see page 21).

Recognition

In most cases of HIV infection the initial illness is vague and non-specific, with headaches, rashes, joint pains, fever. What happens next may take over ten years.

Symptoms of AIDS

The symptoms are a reflection of the decreased immunity; thus there is some combination of severe thrush in the mouth, pneumonia, ulcers, multiple warts, sweats, weight loss, chronic diarrhoea, recurrent shingles. While none alone may be diagnostic of AIDS, combinations point to a serious breakdown in the sufferer's immune system. Neurological features such as memory loss, confusion and odd sensations are common.

Signs

Certain tumours are diagnostic. Otherwise the diagnosis comes to mind when seeing an at-risk individual with features suggestive of breakdown of the immune system.

Investigations

Blood tests (see page 298) confirm the HIV virus and exclude other possible causes of immune breakdown such as **leukaemia** (see page 194).

ASK YOUR DOCTOR

- **About the latest views on risks.**
- **To discuss HIV testing if you may be at risk. Before doing so consider whether you wish this information to go on record, as it may adversely affect future insurance rates.**

Remedy

As AIDS develops the sufferer becomes increasingly at risk from infections; the major task of treatment is to identify those infections as early as possible and to treat them vigorously. Thus anything from chest infections to thrush have their specific treatments.

Anti-AIDS Drugs

These are the matter of intense research, driven not always by the strictest scientific desires but, understandably, pursued by sufferers well before any scientifically respectable evidence of efficacy. The best known drug is AZT. It appears to reduce symptoms and increase survival in people with active AIDS, but at the cost of toxic side-effects. There is no good evidence yet that AZT helps those with HIV before they develop AIDS. There are many other drugs being tried, but none has yet to show any real benefit.

Alternative Treatment

Any of the relaxation therapies, like yoga, vizualization or massage, among others, will help to relieve some of the tension caused by this illness. Most therapies offer one-to-one sessions with a trained practitioner and this can be invaluable as a support system. There are various therapies – homoeopathy, acupuncture and herbalism, in particular – which claim to have immune-boosting properties or remedies, and many can help with the symptoms of the condition. Such therapies may improve your general level of health and well-being, which can only help in the fight against this dreaded illness.

Prevention

There is well-publicized public health advice on prevention of AIDS, summarized here.

Blood and Blood Products

Blood products are now carefully screened for HIV and can be considered safe in the developed world. The same cannot be said for under-developed countries where blood transfusions and plasma, etc., may be contaminated. The same goes for needles and syringes. Some travellers to remote areas prefer to carry their own needles and drip sets in case of need, though how much protection this would offer in cases of emergency is questionable.

Sexual Practices

- Practices involving anal intercourse carry a high risk of transmission of the virus; this holds for men and women but is a higher risk in practising homosexual men.
- The risk of transmission by heterosexual intercourse, both from man to woman and from woman to man, is uncertain but is significant; there is evidence that this risk is increasing and it is likely to become the major method of spread of HIV in coming years.
- Prevention in all these categories calls for the use of condoms put on before sexual activity begins and combined with a spermicidal cream. This simple measure greatly reduces the chances of transmission of the virus.
- Any genital ulceration – for example, a herpes virus – will increase the chance of picking up HIV through the broken skin from an infected partner.

Intravenous Drug Users

Sharing needles is guaranteed to spread HIV, quite apart from its other risks. There are schemes in many parts of Britain for IV drug users to exchange clean needles.

Transmission from Infected Mother to Baby

The risk of transmission is estimated at 20 to 30 per cent. The only method of control is to offer abortion to HIV positive women, always supposing that they are identified as HIV positive early enough in their pregnancy. HIV can also be transmitted through breast milk in breastfeeding mothers.

Screening

The screening schemes that have been offered have had quite good uptake; in particular, those shown to be HIV positive do change their sexual practices. It is not known whether screening will be extended in the UK.

Know Your Partner

If you are in a stable, monogamous heterosexual relationship, and you and your partner have had a few similar relationships; if you do not visit prostitutes or if you do, you wear condoms; if you do not do intravenous drugs, be reassured that the chance of contracting HIV is still extremely low.

The Future

Very recently hope has emerged of a vaccine against AIDS. Even if this does prove possible its development is still years off.

AIDS is not the first and will not be the last disease to put mistrust and fear into human relationships. Syphilis and TB in their day were similarly lethal, untreatable, and unavoidable, without leading a hermit like existence. Yet there is something primevally awe-inspiring about a new disease arising within the developed world and killing so many young people.

In our present state of knowledge AIDS is invariably fatal; this puts a great onus on prevention as the only realistic means of control until drug therapy may become available. No one group in society can be complacent; although the risks are indeed still low for heterosexual couples every indication suggests that this will change over the next few years. Safe sex and avoidance of casual sex must become as natural to us as putting on a car seat belt.

Self-Help

National AIDS Line 0800-567-123

Scottish AIDS Monitor
26 Anderson Place, Edinburgh EH6 5NP
Tel: 0131 555-4850

Terrence Higgins Trust
52–54 Grays Inn Road, London WC1X 8JU
Tel: 0171 242-1010

This is just a selection of the many groups in existence.

COLDS

The medical term for a cold is upper respiratory tract infection, abbreviated to URTI. Many sufferers call the common cold 'flu', but flu is another beast all together (see **influenza**, page 19). The common cold is caused by any of over a hundred viruses. With each cold you develop immunity to that virus but not for long and as there are so many more, you can carry on catching colds all through your life.

Risk

- Children catch an average of four to eight colds a year, more perhaps in their first year at school.
- Adults catch perhaps two or three colds per year.
- Colds are spread through hand-to-hand contact and droplets in the air.
- The greatest infectivity is in the first two to three days.

Recognition

SYMPTOMS
The first symptom is a sore or ticklish throat followed by sneezing, a runny nose and a cough. The full picture can develop in one to five days. Often there is a mild temperature and muscle aches and pains. After a couple of days the nasal secretions become thicker, possibly yellow or green. In most cases the illness just fades away over the next week or two.

Only occasionally are there any complications. These might be pain over the sinuses (see **sinusitis**, page 28) or a worsening cough. Children are extremely prone to developing a painful ear infection.

SIGNS
There is really no mistaking the common cold but its very familiarity does lead doctors to hunt for other causes, maybe out of boredom or maybe out of true diagnostic zeal. Rhinitis is a possibility in anyone who keeps having sneezing and a runny nose; that is an allergic problem similar to hay fever. Rhinitis is not accompanied by temperatures or muscle aches. A persistently coloured nasal discharge raises the possibility of sinusitis or, in a child, a foreign object pushed up one nostril.

INVESTIGATIONS
These are only of use if chronic sinusitis or allergy is expected.

ASK YOUR DOCTOR
- **About the possibility of allergy if you or your child always seems to have a runny nose.**
- **If you or a child has a persistent discharge from one nostril only; this can be a symptom of a foreign body or, in adults, a growth in the nose or sinuses.**

Remedy

The principles of treatment are well known: rest, fluids and warmth. Paracetamol or aspirin (not to be given to children) relieve the aches and bring down the temperature. Thereafter, everyone has their own favourite remedy, as shown by the vast array of cold cures in pharmacists. Decongestants by mouth or as nasal sprays are helpful to relieve symptoms for a few hours but should not be overused.

Children are more difficult to treat, especially babies for whom no effective remedies are available. The best that can be done is to prop them up in their cots and to use decongestant nasal drops sparingly. There are some gentle inhalation preparations like Karvol, or decongestant rubs, which are useful for small children and babies.

ANTIBIOTICS
There are few circumstances where these are necessary; sinusitis will require antibiotics, and they can be used as a preventative measure in those with chronic chest problems or in children who frequently develop ear infections.

Alternative Treatment

Many alternative therapies are aimed at strengthening the immune system, in order to prevent infection altogether. An acupuncturist would aim treatment at the lungs, restoring balance to the energy there. Poor nutrition can make you more susceptible to colds, so nutritional therapy might be useful. Vitamin C has always been used to prevent colds and there is some evidence that it can, when taken in regular high doses, decrease the duration.

Prevention

- The cold viruses are highly contagious and are spread by coughs, sneezes and skin contact. So sneeze into tissues or handkerchiefs and wash your hands frequently.
- Infectivity is greatest just before the streaming nose stage and for the next two to three days, so it is a public-minded gesture to keep away from others if you can.
- There is some evidence that vitamin C increases the body's resistance to colds and infections. Ensure that you have a diet rich in this vitamin, especially in the winter months when colds abound.

INFLUENZA

True influenza is a most unpleasant and potentially serious illness, quite unlike the 'flu' that people claim to have all winter. Doctors having been trying to make this point for decades, to no avail, so that all but the most pedantic have given up and accept that people will call every sneeze flu. The real thing comes as a great shock.

There are three true influenza viruses, A, B and C, which have the slippery ability to alter their immune appearance. That is, they can change the way they look to the immune system, although deep down they are the same invaders that caused mayhem the last time. It means for all practical purposes that a totally new disease blows in from the East every year or two, even though the millions affected have met the virus before. This is why influenza epidemics are so serious; the population just does not have any immunity, so millions are at risk.

Risk

- Significant epidemics happen every ten to 15 years.
- Minor but still important epidemics happen every two to three years.
- Twice this century there have been major epidemics, such as in 1918, which killed 20 million.
- The elderly, those with chronic bronchitis or heart disease, and diabetics, are at greatest risk of complications; anyone of any age may contract the illness.
- Outbreaks begin in mid to late winter.

Recognition

SYMPTOMS
Symptoms begin suddenly, with high fever, muscle pains, backache and uncontrollable shaking. Accompanying this are headaches, a sore throat and a cough. The illness runs its course over about five days. Post-influenza debility is common and can last for weeks.

Pneumonia is the most serious complication. The symptoms are a rapid rate of breathing and continuing high fever (see page 226).

SIGNS
During an epidemic it is all too easy to label everyone with the above symptoms as having influenza. The cautious doctor will check for other features that could cause a similar picture, especially pneumonia.

INVESTIGATIONS

Investigations are unhelpful unless pneumonia is suspected.

ASK YOUR DOCTOR
● **About whether you should have a flu vaccination.**

Remedy

In most cases it is a matter of rest, aspirin or paracetamol and fluids. Those at greater risk of complications should go on to an antibiotic. The type of pneumonia that can complicate influenza is highly dangerous; if suspected, the individual should probably be in hospital for intensive antibiotic treatment and general nursing support.

Alternative Treatment

There are a variety of herbal and homoeopathic remedies, plus aromatherapy preparations which might help. Acupuncture might help to ease the symptoms.

Prevention

This needs to be addressed every year, as immunity from previous vaccination lasts for only six to twelve months.

VACCINATION

A tremendous amount of scientific effort goes into identifying the strains of virus that will cause the next season's influenza. On the basis of that, vaccines are available from late autumn onwards. Those who should consider having vaccination are the elderly, anyone with severe heart or lung problems, or diabetics. People working in large institutions should also consider being vaccinated.

The only people who should positively not have the vaccination are those who have a true allergy to eggs. The vaccine gives 60 to 90 per cent protection against that year's strain of influenza.

AMANTADINE

A drug mainly used to treat Parkinson's disease, amantadine reduces the severity of influenza if taken daily. It is under-used in treating influenza, perhaps out of fears about possible side-effects which include nausea, dizziness and insomnia.

ISOLATION

The influenza viruses are so aggressive that isolation makes little difference to the spread of the illness. Nevertheless it is sensible for those affected to avoid public places.

Self-Help

Your doctor will be able to advise about vaccination.

HEPATITIS

Hepatitis means inflammation of the liver and can be caused by a number of different viruses, as well as by drugs and alcohol. The two best known viruses causing hepatitis are Hepatitis A virus and Hepatitis B virus; scientists keep discovering new viruses that can cause hepatitis: as well as A and B there are now C, D and E.

Hepatitis is a common cause of ill-health and can lead to severe liver damage; it cannot be cured but it can be prevented.

Risk

HEPATITIS A
- This is the commonest cause of viral hepatitis.
- This condition spreads through sewage and wherever that contaminates seafood, such as shellfish, or water supplies.
- The risk is greatest in areas of poor hygiene.
- Hepatitis A affects up to 50 per cent of all adults at one time or other.
- There is a very small risk of causing liver failure; the risk of death through liver failure in the young is about one in 1000 cases, rising to 2 to 3 per cent in the elderly.

HEPATITIS B
- This is a very common infection worldwide with 350 million carriers.
- Hepatitis B is spread through blood; e.g., transfusions, tattooing.
- It is spread by sexual contact, especially through male homosexual practices.
- Infected mothers pass the virus on to their babies.
- Up to 10 per cent of people infected become carriers who can pass on the disease.
- Such chronic carriers number about one in every 1000 in the UK, but in Africa and Asia up to 15 per cent of the population are carriers.
- There is a 1 per cent risk of death through liver failure.
- Hepatitis B infection greatly increases the risk of contracting liver cancer.

Recognition

SYMPTOMS
Both forms have a similar set of symptoms; there is a one to two week period of feeling unwell, with nausea, headaches, a fever and some abdominal pains over the liver. Hepatitis B causes the same symptoms, but more severely. After one to two weeks jaundice appears: characterized by yellow eyes and skin. You may notice that your urine becomes darker and your bowel movements lighter. In some cases there is no jaundice; then the diagnosis relies on blood tests.

The incubation period of hepatitis A is two to six weeks. For Hepatitis B, the period of incubation can be from two weeks to six months.

SIGNS
The liver may feel tender; otherwise there are no specific features before jaundice appears.

INVESTIGATIONS

Once the diagnosis is suspected, liver tests show how badly the liver is affected and also identify the virus responsible.

ASK YOUR DOCTOR

- **If you are think you might have jaundice; its causes vary from the benign hepatitis A to severe forms of cancer.**

Be honest about your sexual conduct; if you are at risk from hepatitis B this should lead to special precautions whenever someone has to take your blood or give you an injection. If you have had hepatitis B and are a carrier, you are excluded from jobs where there is a risk to others of exposure to your blood; for example hepatitis B positive doctors must retire from performing surgery, though they can practise other forms of medicine.

Remedy

Being a viral illness there is no specific curative treatment. The treatment is general support; rest is important. Should liver failure threaten then highly specialized treatment is needed to reduce the risk to the liver. The illness lasts up to three months in all. You will be advised not to drink alcohol for up to six months afterwards. It is very common to feel tired after hepatitis, a condition which can last many months.

Alternative Treatment

There are no therapies to prevent or cure hepatitis in its various forms. Recuperatively, however, a number of the therapies may be useful to help strengthen the body and the liver itself. There are herbal and homoeopathic remedies available over the counter, but it is suggested that you see a registered practitioner for individual treatment. Acupressure or acupuncture may also help.

Prevention

HEPATITIS A

There is an effective vaccine recommended for people travelling to risky areas. This is replacing the older immunoglobulin injection which gave some protection but only lasted for three months. Avoid the foods that might pass on the virus. So insist on bottled or boiled water. Be wary of salads (which will have been washed in local water) and shellfish (which live in it). Avoid contact with anyone known to have the disease; they remain infectious for about a week after the start of the illness.

HEPATITIS B

In Britain blood and blood products are scrupulously screened for hepatitis B (and C since 1991) and should be safe. Such standards may not apply elsewhere. Do not share needles with drug users and check on the standards of hygiene of tattooists and acupuncture clinics.

Homosexuals are at especial risk through their sexual practices but there is a risk to the sexual partners of anyone carrying hepatitis B, through the transmission of the virus in saliva and in semen. Anyone at risk of exposure to blood products or other infected material should consider vaccination against hepatitis B. This involves three injections over six months and needs to be repeated every few years. This is recommended for doctors, dentists, nurses and workers in related jobs. It is also recommended for babies born to Hepatitis B positive mothers.

If you have been exposed to possible infection, there is an excellent immunoglobulin which should be given immediately.

Self-Help

Group B Hepatitis
Basement Flat, 7a Fielding Road, London W14 0LL
Tel: 0171 244-6514

MALARIA

It is misleading to think of malaria as a disease confined to the tropics. It is only a century ago that malaria was commonplace in England and in theory the warm wet conditions could recur for malaria to become more common again. The main current risk is that with the growth in rapid international travel, carriers of malaria can find themselves back in England while still incubating the illness.

Malaria is caused by one of four related micro-organisms spread by the bite of the anopheles mosquito. The parasites live, grow and reproduce in a complex life cycle within the human host's liver and red blood cells; the parasites complete their life cycle within a mosquito which has sucked blood from an infected human. The mosquito then in turn injects the parasites into another human victim.

The symptoms of malaria are the result of the release of a fresh lot of parasites into the bloodstream; this happens at periods varying from every two days to months or even years. The parasites cause red blood cells to burst open; in addition, the parasites can lodge in the brain, kidneys and elsewhere, where their toxic effects can cause widespread damage.

Malaria is one of the most important international causes of chronic illness resulting in one to three million deaths per annum, most of which are in children.

Risk

- The disease affects about 270 million people per annum.
- The overall death rate is 1 per cent, mainly in children.
- There are about 2000 cases per annum in the UK, with five to ten deaths each year.
- Anti-malarial drugs reduce the chances by 80 per cent but do not guarantee prevention.
- Carriers of sickle-cell disease (West Africans, Black Americans) enjoy a degree of protection against malaria.

Recognition

The incubation period of the parasites can be up to six weeks; therefore, anyone who has returned from a malaria zone must consider themselves at risk for several weeks after return.

> *As a rule of thumb anyone who develops a feverish illness within a short period of return from an at-risk area should seek medical attention.*

SYMPTOMS

Fever is the earliest symptom, rising over several days. Then there begins a series of rigors, when fever suddenly increases and the sufferer is shaken by uncontrollable shivering for an hour or two followed by several hours of heavy sweating. Depending on the type of malaria these bouts of fever and shivering return every two or three days.

Ironically the most serious type of malaria actually causes less serious symptoms initially. So-called falciparum malaria begins as a vague fever plus headache. It can progress within days to coma, liver failure and death.

SIGNS

In an acute attack the doctor can go on little other than suspicion in an at-risk individual. As the illness develops over the next few days it may be possible to feel an enlarged spleen and there may be signs of anaemia due to rupture of red blood cells.

INVESTIGATIONS

The essential investigation is examination of a blood sample (see page 298) under the microscope, looking for the typical parasites in the bloodstream. It may be necessary to take several samples.

ASK YOUR DOCTOR

- **About any feverish illness that you develop soon after returning from a tropical zone. Do not assume that you are immune because you took your anti-malarial tablets.**
- **If you are contemplating a trip to the tropics seek advice on vaccinations and anti-malarial treatment well in advance of travel.**

Remedy

Treatment of the acute attack is with chloroquine, quinine or one of the newer variations on these drugs. Sufferers from falciparum malaria will need intensive therapy with intravenous drips, blood transfusions and infusion of quinine by drip.

To eliminate chronic disease, combinations of drugs are taken for several weeks. Treatment should be given by specialists in infectious diseases, who are familiar with the subtleties of the disease.

Alternative Treatment

It is folly to travel into tropical zones without taking conventional medical advice on vaccinations and malaria prophylaxis. If you do acquire the parasite, alternative treatments may help you to recover more swiftly, but these should complement, and not replace, conventional treatment.

Prevention

Travellers to malaria zones should take early advice about anti-malarial medication. Remember to take account of stop-overs in malaria zones even though your final destination may be malaria-free. There is widespread resistance of the parasites to the older drugs so up-to-date advice about the currently recommended drugs is essential even if you are returning within just a few months to the same country.

Drugs should be taken before you depart and continued for six weeks after returning. However drugs are just one aspect of prevention; the whole aim is not to be bitten by mosquitoes in the first place. So use mosquito repellents, cover arms and legs in the evenings, which are high risk periods, and use mosquito netting or window screens if these are available.

Once back home be cautious about any feverish illness for a few weeks, especially one with progressive fever or rigors. Of course many travellers do develop a cough or cold on return, but if you have a feeling that you are more ill than you might expect seek medical advice, being sure to tell your doctor that you have recently returned from a malaria zone.

In the long run malaria eradication may be possible by programmes of marsh drainage and drug treatment; but realistically war, famine, cost and lack of political will mean that it will be with us for the foreseeable future.

There is intense research to develop an anti-malaria vaccination. There is an experimental vaccine but it is still in a trial stage only.

Self-Help

Advice for Travellers: 0891 600350 (these calls are charged)

MENINGITIS

The brain is a soft structure which is enclosed by delicate membranes called the meninges. Meningitis refers to infection of those meninges. Infection can result from viruses and from bacteria – it is the bacterial infections which are the most serious. Meningitis is a much feared diagnosis; there is good reason for this because even with the best of treatment there is a significant risk of disability or death. This is all the more upsetting because it is so often children who are affected; therefore, it is right to keep a high index of suspicion of the illness. However, remember that many viral illnesses are accompanied by headache and mild neck stiffness so that these features alone do not confirm a diagnosis of meningitis.

Risk

- Overall, there are 15 cases per 100,000 population per annum; that is, about 8,100 a year; this includes both viral and bacterial forms.
- The risk of bacterial meningitis for children below one year is about 150 per 100,000 each year.
- 50 per cent of cases of bacterial meningitis are caused by the one germ Haemophilus Influenzae; there are many other germs that cause all the other cases.
- Bacterial meningitis carries a 10 to 15 per cent risk of death despite treatment.
- The mortality in viral meningitis is less than 1 per cent and complete recovery can be expected even without treatment.

Recognition

The diagnosis of meningitis can be straightforward, or it can be impossible without tests. It may be best to admit an ill child with suspected meningitis for tests rather than take a chance.

SYMPTOMS

Babies

There may be vomiting, irritability, a high-pitched cry and drowsiness. The child feels floppy and unresponsive; it jerks when touched and may look pale, with cold hands and feet.

Older children and adults

Sufferers usually complain of a severe headache, that bright light irritates their eyes and that their neck hurts when bent, called neck stiffness.

● Confusion

In severe cases at any age the sufferer lapses into confusion or coma but in the early stages they may be relatively alert.

● Purple Rash

At any age you may see a fine purple rash on the limbs or, in babies, around the face. This ominous symptom is caused by small blood clots within the skin and is a particular feature of the blood poisoning (septicaemia) that accompanies meningococcal meningitis (bacterial).

> *All cases of meningitis need urgent treatment, but if you see this characteristic rash, treatment is required within minutes.*

SIGNS

Babies

In dealing with babies the doctor will feel the soft spots (fontanelles) of the baby's skull. These bulge in many cases of meningitis because of swelling of the brain due to the infection. However, a normal fontanelle does not exclude the diagnosis. Neck stiffness is not found in babies.

● Neck stiffness

In older children or adults, the doctor will check for neck stiffness, bending the head forward with the patient lying flat. Another test is the Kernig test; the doctor raises one of the patient's legs and asks him or her to bend their head forward. This is a more sensitive test for neck stiffness that is caused by irritation of the meninges by the infection. At any age the doctor looks for the characteristic rash of meningococcal meningitis.

INVESTIGATIONS

These are needed to confirm the diagnosis and to differentiate from other illnesses which can mimic meningitis; for example, a **subarachnoid haemorrhage** (see page 266). Secondly, they detect what sort of meningitis is involved. The fundamental test is a lumbar puncture; a needle is guided into the fluid which circulates around the brain and spinal cord, the easiest spot to sample is low down in the back, in the lumbar region. This sounds alarming but in skilled hands takes just a few minutes, in babies even less. The sample is immediately examined looking for the white cells which signal infection, blood which accompanies a subarachnoid haemorrhage and any bacteria which can be seen under the microscope.

ASK YOUR DOCTOR

- **For an urgent assessment if your baby or child becomes unusually drowsy or irritable.**

Remedy

Viral meningitis follows a benign if uncomfortable course; treatment consists of monitoring of the condition; only occasionally is the person ill enough to be on a drip.

Bacterial meningitis is a medical emergency. Once the diagnosis is suspected the sufferer is put on to high doses of the antibiotics which cover the likely germs. These may be altered as the laboratory tests come in. Other drugs reduce swelling of the brain and it may be necessary to give sedatives to reduce the risk of epileptic fits caused by the brain irritation.

In suspected cases of meningococcal meningitis, it can be lifesaving to give an immediate injection of penicillin on suspicion and even before starting tests.

It is common for survivors from bacterial meningitis to have some neurological damage but this generally recovers over the next few months or years. The main long-term risks are of deafness, blindness, paralysis, epilepsy and impaired intellectual development. Babies are at the greatest risk of such long-term damage, which affects up to 50 per cent after meningitis.

Alternative Treatment

Alternative remedies are never appropriate in the case of a medical emergency, which meningitis is. Some of the therapies may, however, be helpful in the recovery stages of the illness. A registered practitioner will provide details of treatment that will help you to recuperate.

Prevention

Prevention falls into 3 categories: early recognition of meningitis; preventing spread to contacts; and long-term prevention.

EARLY RECOGNITION

Parents and doctors worry endlessly about meningitis. It can begin in a totally innocuous way with symptoms indistinguishable from those of a common cold, a mild viral illness or just being off-colour. The younger the child the more misleading the initial symptoms may be. Therefore, most doctors approach an ill baby with that thought in mind. Doctors will often follow an instinct that something out of the ordinary is going on. They will listen to the parents who may equally have a feeling that their baby is not quite right and that this seems more than a simple cold or virus. Paediatric departments in hospitals are well used to babies being referred for assessment on such vague, seemingly non-scientific suspicions.

Fortunately it does become easier to recognise meningitis in older children and adults, so there are fewer chances of missing the diagnosis.

Dealing with Contacts

In cases of meningococcal meningitis there is a greatly increased risk to close family or work contacts. These should treated with a short course of an antibiotic called rifampicin which is a highly effective preventative. Sometimes vaccination is also advised. There are no specific measures to take for contacts of meningitis caused by other organisms but it is sensible to be alert for warning symptoms in the week after contact.

Long-Term Prevention

● Hib vaccination

A vaccine to give immunity against bacterial meningitis in childhood was introduced in the UK in 1992 and already there has been a significant fall in the number of cases (87 per cent in one study). This is an important public health advance; the first injection of the vaccine is given when your baby is two months old.

● Meningococcal vaccination

At present this is used only for travellers to countries where there are outbreaks of the disease or others at high risk. Trials are just beginning of a new vaccine for babies which can protect against meningococcal meningitis.

Self-Help

National Meningitis Trust
Fern House, Bath Road, Stroud, Glos GL5 3TJ
Tel: 01453 751738
  Your doctor or health visitor can advise on Hib vaccination.

SINUSITIS

The sinuses are a number of connecting hollow areas around the front of the skull. There is the maxillary sinus, which is underneath each eye in the cheekbone, the frontal sinuses found above each eye and the ethmoid sinuses near the inner part of each eye. Another sinus, the sphenoidal sinus, is located deeper inside the skull. The sinuses have a drainage system that should sweep secretions into the nose or the back of the throat; it is not terribly good, which is why sinusitis is so common.

During a common cold secretions increase and build up. It takes only a small blockage to cause a build up of secretions within the sinuses and that easily becomes infected. Added to that is the problem that pollutants hit the nose first, and the lining of the nose and sinuses reacts to this in many people, giving an allergic element to chronic sinusitis.

Risk

● Sinusitis is an ordinary complication of the common cold.
● Chronic sinusitis is one of the commonest diagnoses referred to ENT surgeons.
● Dental problems can contribute to sinusitis, because the roots of the upper molar teeth lie very close to the floor of the maxillary sinuses.
● Chronic sinus problems are made worse by dust, smoke, emotion and alcohol.

Recognition

SYMPTOMS

After a few days of a common cold, a feeling of pressure builds up across the front of the face. This is worse if you lean forward. You are aware of an unpleasant smell and a thick discharge down the nose or at the back of the throat. Often there is pain near or behind the eyes or deeper in the skull. You can see how this links up with the position of the various sinuses. In chronic sinusitis there is a persistent feeling of discomfort over the sinuses, a constant mucous drip and interference with taste or smell.

SIGNS

Tenderness is often found above and below the eyes.

INVESTIGATIONS

These are rarely done but can now extend to **CT** (see page 298) or **ultrasound** (see page 301) scanning of the sinuses. The plain **X-ray** (see page 301) of the sinuses may show a fluid level from a build-up of pus; it is otherwise not very helpful in making the diagnosis.

Allergy testing (see page 297) is sensible if the history suggests that allergy plays a part.

ASK YOUR DOCTOR

- **Whether dental problems might contribute; these are quite common.**
- **If you notice blood in the nasal discharge; this is an important warning symptom.**
- **If your child has symptoms of sinusitis; it is impossible below five because the sinuses are undeveloped, and unusual below twelve. Therefore, other diagnoses must be considered.**

Remedy

ACUTE SINUSITIS

In many cases cure comes over a week or two by the body's own systems. There are all manner of drops and sprays for the nose, which work by shrinking down the lining of the nose and sinuses. This both reduces the flow of mucus and opens up the drainage channels. Aromatic inhalations work by making the mucus more liquid and free flowing, thereby aiding drainage.

Do not use decongestant preparations for long periods, because they will eventually alter the lining of the nose in such a way that the symptoms come back much worse when you stop the medication. You then fall into a vicious circle of treating symptoms caused by the very medication you used to treat the symptoms.

Antibiotics are very helpful; they must be taken in high doses and for up to ten days to penetrate the sinuses. Thanks to the widespread use of antibiotics, complications from sinusitis are extremely unusual.

CHRONIC SINUSITIS

Sinusitis where there is an allergic element can be treated with one of a range of excellent steroid sprays, which reduce the amount of secretion from the lining of the nose (these treatments are covered in more detail in *Hay-fever*, see page 221). They can be taken in combination with antihistamine tablets.

As a last resort there are operations to improve the drainage from the sinuses. The operations are not done frequently, the reason being that they do not have a high cure rate. However recently improved techniques have appeared which allow much more accurate treatment using **endoscopic** (see page 299) devices to look inside the sinuses.

Alternative Treatment

There are herbal and homoeopathic remedies, many of which are inhalations in one form or another and are as likely to work as anything else commercially available. Any chronic condition may be worth a visit to a registered and trained alternative practitioner, who will endeavour to get to the root of the problem instead of just treating the symptoms.

Prevention

Presumably the sinuses do have a function, but they seem very much to be a design fault in the skull with unhappy consequences. If you know you are prone to sinusitis with a cold, use decongestants and inhalations early; try not to sniff (this may force mucus up into the sinuses). For similar reasons do not swim underwater and avoid flights if possible during an episode of sinusitis.

Allergic, pollutant and emotional factors may be controllable or you may need to use one of the medical nasal sprays mentioned earlier.

Surgery is a preventative measure to be considered in resistant cases and preferably by a surgeon who spells out all the drawbacks rather than one who is overkeen to operate.

THE EYES

• Blindness • Cataracts
• Retinal Detachment • Glaucoma

T HE IMPORTANCE OF vision in our culture cannot be overstated. People are, accordingly, very sensitive to minor problems with their eyes and usually seek early medical advice about blurred vision, itchy eyes and visual disturbances. It is ironic that the greatest threats to sight, namely glaucoma and diabetic complications, are just those which can progress without causing much in the way of symptoms. This section provides advice about recognition and screening for such disorders.

Complete blindness is uncommon; often some vision can be saved, which makes it possible to live quite independently and enjoy life nearly as much as anyone with full vision might.

BLINDNESS

Blindness can be complete or, far more often, partial. It can be the end result of a number of diseases or it may occur suddenly after injury or a stroke. Blindness in adult life cuts people off from our visually oriented culture but not from social interaction through speech and to that extent blindness, though serious enough, is probably less harrowing for an adult than becoming deaf.

Those blind for many years say they develop greater acuity in their other senses, such as smell and touch and this can sometimes compensate for their blindness and open other work possibilities (like piano tuning).

Risk

- There are nearly 140,000 people registered blind in the UK.
- There are nearly 100,000 registered partially sighted in the UK.
- Diabetic complications are the commonest cause of blindness up to age sixty.
- Beyond the age of sixty, glaucoma, cataracts and macular degeneration are the commonest causes of blindness.
- Other risks to sight are from blockage of the blood supply to the retina, strokes and detachment of the retina.
- **Multiple sclerosis** can cause temporary blindness in one eye (see page 255).
- Rare causes of blindness include poisoning by methylated spirits, tobacco, vitamin B12 deficiency, infection and congenital reasons (those you are born with).
- In parts of Africa and South America, the most common cause is infection by a worm spread through the blackfly (onchocerciasis). In the worst affected areas as many as 40 per cent of adults become blind for this reason.
- Lack of vitamin A is another common cause of blindness in the developing world, affecting an estimated 250,000 children a year.

Recognition

Sudden visual loss will be immediately noticed yet it is remarkable that people can lose a staggering amount of vision and not realize a problem exists, as long as it happens gradually. In these cases eyes tests are necessary to detect early problems.

SYMPTOMS

People speak of blurring of vision, of difficulty focusing, of a haze over their vision. They may have a series of falls or other accidents before suspicion arises. Complete visual loss speaks for itself.

SIGNS

Complete and sudden loss of vision is obvious. Yet if just one eye is affected it may only be by covering the good eye that the extent of blindness becomes clear.

Pupil reactions to bright light give some idea of where the problem lies; for example a completely unresponsive pupil means a problem affecting the optic nerve to the eye on that side.

Following a serious stroke people commonly lose a complete section of their field of vision; e.g., the right half of the field of vision in both eyes. In the drama of the rest of the stroke this is easily missed unless specifically tested. People with advanced **glaucoma** develop tunnel vision; they become unable to see outside of a central area of focus (see page 35). Conversely, people with degeneration of the most sensitive part of the retina – the macula – cannot focus clearly but can see things outside of that central area of vision. **Cataracts** cause a white opacity visible in the pupil (see page 33).

INVESTIGATIONS

Inspecting the back of the eye reveals the damage caused by diabetes; there is a typical appearance when the blood flow to the eye has been affected. Eyes tests map out where and how badly vision is lost. Glaucoma is detected by measuring the pressure within the eyeball.

ASK YOUR DOCTOR
- **About having specialist eye checks if you are diabetic.**
- **About treatment for cataracts.**
- **About any persistent distortion of vision because some causes can be treated early.**

Remedy

Glaucoma, diabetes, cataracts, detached retina (see pages 35, 204, 33 and 37) have their specific treatments. If the blood supply to the eye has become blocked, emergency treatment with anticoagulant drugs may restore sight, but probably not completely.

Macular degeneration is due to deterioration of blood supply to the most light-sensitive part of the retina and cannot generally be cured, though sometimes laser treatment can arrest its spread. Sufferers have to learn to look slightly to one side in order to make use of the remaining peripheral vision; good illumination is important and magnifying glasses help.

Alternative Treatment

No specific therapy is recommended as treatment, but some might help in easing the stress involved with increasing blindness.

Prevention

- **Diabetes, glaucoma, detached retina** and **strokes** have specific preventative treatments (see pages 204, 35, 37 and 262 respectively). The importance of good diabetic control and regular eye checks cannot be overstated. If you are having difficulty seeing at night or notice poor peripheral vision, check out the possibility of glaucoma. Headaches plus tenderness of the temples may mean poly-arteritis; again, see your doctor. Seeing showers of flashing lights is a detached retina till proven otherwise. People over 40 years of age with a family history of glaucoma are entitled to free eye tests.
- Giving vitamin A supplements is widely undertaken in the developing world. A normal Western diet should contain adequate vitamin A; it occurs naturally in liver, fish, dairy products and in green vegetables. Pregnant women must not take supplementary vitamin A and it is not recommended that liver be eaten as a source of the vitamin.
- Onchocerciasis is effectively treated by drugs and there are programmes to eradicate the black fly; unfortunately established blindness cannot be improved.
- Accidents are an important cause of eye damage and blindness; prevent them by wearing eye protection during any hazardous procedure such as working with corrosive liquids (at home or in a laboratory) or while drilling or hammering. Certain sports carry an inherent risk of damaging the eye because the balls used exactly fit the eye socket. Squash is the classical example; consider wearing reinforced glasses when playing.

Self-Help

Royal National Institute for the Blind
224–228 Great Portland Street, London W1N 6AA
Tel: 0171 388-1266

Macular Disease Society
PO Box 268, Weybridge, Surrey, KT13 OYW
Tel: 01932 829331

CATARACTS

A cataract occurs when the lens of the eye becomes opaque. Since all light has to pass through and be focused by the lens, any interference to its transparency will cause deterioration in vision, in much the same way that dirt on a car windscreen reduces visibility and produces glare. Cataracts form as a result of a build-up of water and calcium within the lens; this is mainly a natural part of ageing.

In the developed world we are fortunate to have access to relatively simple surgery to relieve cataracts but elsewhere in the world untreated cataracts are a common cause of blindness.

Risk

- Cataracts affect probably 10 to 20 per cent of 60 year olds, and most people by 90 years of age.
- Cataracts are usually a natural part of the ageing process.
- They are more common in diabetics and smokers.
- The risk is greatly increased if taking steroid tablets for long periods of time; 75 per cent of cases are likely to develop cataracts after a few years.
- There is possibly an increased risk in adults whose mothers had poor nutrition during pregnancy.
- The ultraviolet light in bright sunshine probably causes many cataracts; the exact risk is disputed.

Recognition

SYMPTOMS
In the early stages there are no symptoms. As the cataract becomes more dense so vision becomes more and more indistinct; bright lights become a glare; fine work or reading becomes difficult.

SIGNS
The lens, normally clear, shows as a white opacity in the eye; shining a bright light at it makes this more obvious.

INVESTIGATIONS
These usually just confirm the loss of vision and are a way of measuring deterioration in order to judge when to perform surgery.

ASK YOUR DOCTOR
- **About eye trouble sooner rather than later if you think you might have a cataract, because the waiting times for surgery are long.**

Remedy

Treatment is by surgical removal of the lens. The technique has become safe enough to be called routine, though the skill of the surgeon is still paramount. The opaque lens is replaced by an artificial lens. If for some uncommon technical reasons this is impossible there is a choice of having contact lenses or special glasses with thick lenses.

As well as having sight restored, people often comment about how colourful things seem, after having had this distorted by the cataract (think of how colourless things look through frosted glass).

There are risks from surgery, mainly infection or bleeding; for that reason surgeons operate on one eye at a time.

Alternative Treatment

Some practitioners of nutritional therapies recommend dietary changes, increasing vitamin C and vitamin A in the diet. There are homoeopathic and herbal remedies which will decrease the rate of cataract growth. Post-operatively, many alternative therapies are excellent for convalescence.

Prevention

- The major avoidable risk factors are smoking and over-exposure to ultraviolet light (though not all eye specialists agree on the latter). It is sensible to wear good sunglasses if you are going to have exposure to intense ultraviolet light; especially when skiing and sailing.
- Anyone unavoidably on steroids runs a serious risk of cataracts and should discuss alternatives with their doctor or aim for the minimum dose.
- Diabetics must ensure that they have regular eye checks, so cataracts should be detected early.
- The concept that poor nutrition during pregnancy may increase the risk of cataracts in adult life is relatively recent, but is in line with similar suspicions concerning obesity, high blood pressure, heart disease and diabetes. Ante-natal care in the developed world should reduce this risk but it could be an explanation for cataracts in the under-developed world.

GLAUCOMA

The globe of the eye contains jelly-like material – the vitreous humour – through which light passes. Fluid circulates within the front of the eye, between the cornea and the lens; that fluid – the aqueous humour – drains through tiny channels. The fluid within the eye should remain at a modest pressure; in glaucoma that pressure increases, because of blockage to the drainage channels.

Slowly that increased pressure interferes with and, if untreated, destroys the visual acuity of much of the retina. This results in so-called tunnel vision; central vision remains sharp and focused but the more peripheral vision is lost. Caught early, this process can be controlled, but first the condition must be detected.

Risk

- Glaucoma is rare below middle age.
- The condition affects 1 per cent of the adult population, 5 per cent of those over sixty-five.
- Glaucoma often runs in families.
- Acute (of sudden, intense onset) glaucoma can be provoked by drugs such as propantheline, and certain drugs for Parkinson's disease (anti-cholinergics), but only in susceptible individuals.

Recognition

Without specific tests it is unlikely that someone would detect any early features of the condition. As it becomes more serious certain symptoms occur.

Symptoms

Night vision becomes worse and lights have a halo around them. Observant individuals might notice that they fail to see things which happen 'at the corner of the eye'; e.g., seeing other cars on the road.

In acute glaucoma, by contrast, there is a sudden blockage to the drainage of fluid leading to sudden excruciating pain in the eye, which becomes temporarily blind.

Signs

Careful inspection of the back of the eye through an ophthalmoscope can reveal subtle signs of increased pressure. Simple sight tests suggest loss of peripheral vision, confirmed by investigation. Acute glaucoma is likely in someone with a painful, hazy-looking red eye which feels hard to the touch.

Investigations

There are special eye charts to map out the field of vision. The pressure within the eye can be estimated by an ingenious device which blows a puff of air against the eyeball. For more accuracy there are devices that are placed on the anaesthetized eye. An **ophthalmoscope** (see page 301) will reveal signs of pressure.

ASK YOUR DOCTOR

● **Where you can go for screening of pressure in your eyes. Do not ignore pains in the eye. Though many are innocent, in the elderly they may be a warning sign of increased pressure.**

Remedy

Eye drops are the usual first line treatment; common drugs are timolol, pilocarpine. They work by keeping the pupil constricted; this aids drainage of fluid. There are a number of different operations, all of which aim to improve the drainage of fluid by making a tiny nick or a laser guided cut in the iris (coloured part of the eye).

Acute glaucoma is treated in a similar way but treatment to reduce pressure must be given within one to two days, in order to preserve sight. Surgery (see above) will follow.

Alternative Treatment

Acute glaucoma is a medical emergency and must be seen immediately by a medical doctor. Alternative therapies provide a variety of options for long-term (chronic) glaucoma, but must only be used alongside conventional treatment. Some nutritional therapy may help or perhaps cranial osteopathy.

Prevention

Screening for Glaucoma

Anyone who has a close relative with glaucoma such as a sibling or a parent should have regular eye checks from age forty onwards. In recognition of the importance of these tests, they are still available free in the NHS. Even allowing for a family history 1 per cent of the elderly will have glaucoma and will suspect nothing until either too late or an eye test brings it to their attention. Over sixties should have an eye test every two years.

EXISTING GLAUCOMA

If you do have glaucoma in one eye ask about preventative treatment for the other eye. It should be examined as part of your regular specialist review.

If you have had the misfortune of acute glaucoma in one eye, there is a high chance that acute glaucoma will affect the other eye within ten years. For this reason specialists will normally advise you to have surgery on both eyes.

DRUG INTERACTIONS

Always let doctors know you have glaucoma so that they can avoid drugs which might trigger an acute attack.

RETINAL DETACHMENT

The retina is a wonderfully complex array of light receptors, and is the mechanism by which we see. It lies like a web of electronic circuitry against the back of the eye. Vital though it is, it is held in place by a peculiarly risky arrangement; only the pressure of fluid within the eye ball keeps the retina pressed in place. If the pressure is removed (e.g., in the case of trauma), the retina can literally drift off the back of the eye; this is what is meant by retinal detachment.

Risk

- There are nine to twenty-four cases of retinal detachment per 100,000 people every year.
- There is an increased risk in the very short-sighted, whose retina is thinner.
- A blow to the head can detach the retina, by causing a small tear.
- Someone who has had a detachment in one eye has an increased chance of detachment in the other eye.

Recognition

SYMPTOMS

You may see a series of flashing lights in the affected eye as light receptors are torn from their blood supply. There is an increase in floaters; that is, cells drifting around in the fluid of the eye and seen as spindly objects floating across the field of vision. These symptoms can happen either days before detachment or immediately beforehand, there is no way of telling which. As the retina detaches people describe it as being like a curtain coming across their field of vision. All of this is painless.

SIGNS

Using the right equipment a specialist can look through the lens of the eye and see the retina lying in folds and behind it the site of the original tear. The specialist has to consider other possible causes of sudden loss of vision in one eye, of which blockage of the blood supply is likeliest.

INVESTIGATIONS

If there is doubt about a detachment despite inspecting the eye, it can be confirmed by an **ultrasound** scan or **CT scan** (see pages 301 and 298).

ASK YOUR DOCTOR
- **If you experience spontaneous flashing lights; this is the most significant warning symptom.**

Remedy

A retinal detachment is an emergency for there are just a few hours to try to reposition the retina before parts of it die through lack of blood supply. The operation aims to stick back the retina by a freezing probe or by a laser beam and is successful in most cases.

Alternative Treatment

A detached retina is a medical emergency and should always be seen immediately by a doctor. Post-operatively, various alternative therapies may encourage healing.

Prevention

Always take visual disturbances seriously, especially if you are short-sighted. Floaters are common and are not as good a symptom of detachment as flashing lights, but even so if you experience an unusual increase in floaters you should have your eyes checked. This advice is extremely important for anyone who has had a detachment before.

THE EARS

• Deafness • Tinnitus • Vertigo and Dizziness

THE MOST COMMON problems with ears are excess wax and minor infections. These are rarely of any long-term importance, except in children where it is important to screen for deafness after infection (see page 42). The topics covered in this section are those which pose the greatest long-term risk to health and well-being.

DEAFNESS

Fortunately, few people are completely deaf; most retain enough hearing to manage on a day-to-day basis, and modern hearing aids help many.

Hearing relies on the complexities of the inner ear, a marvel of electro-mechanical engineering. Sound waves cause the eardrum to vibrate; that vibration is picked up by a series of tiny bones and transmitted to a fluid-filled structure, the cochlea, which turns those vibrations (as little as one-millionth of a millimetre) into electrical discharges. These in turn are interpreted by the brain as pitch and loudness. The cochlea is a coiled tube about 3.5 cm long and lined with 3500 cells whose vibrations are the key to hearing.

Like many other complex bodily functions it is astonishing not that things go wrong but that they ever go right. Deafness occurs for two main reasons. One is a problem with the mechanical parts of hearing, called conduction deafness. Most common is a progressive stiffness of the bones conducting sound (the condition of otosclerosis). Then there is perceptive deafness, which is deafness arising from problems on the electrical and nerve side of hearing. The commonest form of this is presbyacusis, which is loss of ability to hear high-pitched sound due to age.

Risk

- One child in 10,000 is born deaf; some for genetic reasons.
- Rubella in pregnancy and rhesus incompatibility were serious causes of congenital deafness, but are now rare.
- Oxygen deprivation and drugs used to treat serious infections around the time of birth can cause deafness.
- The cause is unknown in the majority of cases of congenital deafness.
- Many children become temporarily deaf through glue ear (see below).
- About 7 per cent of adults have significant hearing loss and about two per 1000 are profoundly deaf.
- Wax, ageing, infections, injury, and sound trauma account for the majority of cases, though many other conditions can cause deafness, such as strokes and tumours.
- Ageing causes a gradual loss of the ability to hear high-pitched sounds; this interferes with the ability to hear conversation.
- One in 200 are affected by otosclerosis, a familial condition in which the tiny bones of hearing stiffen up; otosclerosis is more common in women.

Recognition

It is most difficult to recognize deafness in babies and children. Adults can be expected to distinguish poor hearing (even if they are reluctant to accept it).

SYMPTOMS

Babies

- Babies and young children should look startled in response to a loud noise.
- By three to four months they should react to a noise near one or other ear and try to turn to it.
- From six to eight months the child should be showing some sort of response to being called.
- Both deaf babies and normal babies babble from about nine months and even babies known to be deaf may seem to be trying to say dada or mama; the difference is that the babbling increases and becomes more complex in normal babies; in deaf babies it gradually diminishes. Some babies with perfectly good hearing don't babble until after a year; check with your health visitor. It may not be anything to worry about.

Children

- Normal children say their first words around one year and have a useful vocabulary by three years.
- Older children who become deaf may start to perform badly at school, perhaps ask to sit near the front of the class.
- An older child will also complain if their hearing is indistinct.
- It is unusual for a child not to be speaking at all by about two and a half years of age.

Adults

- Adults often genuinely fail to realize the gradual decline in hearing which is a feature of ageing. This is especially so if they spend much of their time in the company of other elderly people. It takes someone with younger ears to notice how loud they have set the TV or that they fail to hear a ring at the doorbell. Eventually the individual becomes aware that they are missing conversations.

SIGNS

The doctor checks the ears in the event that a wax build-up is to blame or, in the case of children, that they might have an accumulation of fluid behind the eardrums called a glue ear, because the fluid is thick and sticky.

INVESTIGATIONS

The standard audiogram plots how well someone can hear across the whole range of sounds, from very deep low-frequency sounds to high-pitched high-frequency sounds. This technique can be used from childhood onwards. It is more difficult to assess babies, but the technology now exists to test hearing right down to a few weeks of age by demonstrating the electrical responses in the brain to sounds. Additional tests gauge whether hearing loss is due to mechanical problems or due to deterioration on the electrical/perceptive side of hearing.

ASK YOUR DOCTOR
- If you have any doubts about a child's hearing; the sooner the better.
- If your child has been unfortunate enough to contract meningitis (see page 25). Deafness is a definite risk after a serious episode and is one you should discuss with the doctor.
- About any changes in hearing. A degree of deafness is to be expected in late adult life but your doctor can check to see whether wax is a simple factor making things worse.

Remedy

This will vary according to the underlying cause. Wax can be easily and safely removed by syringing. Some people have to have wax removed every few months. Many children and adults experience a temporary deafness during a cold due to congestion of the inner ear by fluid. Most cases settle with simple remedies such as inhalations, decongestant tablets.

MIDDLE EAR FLUID
Is an important cause of acquired deafness in children, less frequently in adults. Cases resistant to decongestants may need to be drained, followed by the insertion of grommets. At times it seems every child is awaiting, having, or recovering from the insertion of grommets. They are tiny plastic tubes fitted in the eardrum with the aim of allowing fluid to drain away. After an era of unbridled enthusiasm the insertion of grommets is becoming a little less routine, with ENT surgeons increasingly prepared to wait for nature to cure the condition.

SURGERY
Surgical procedures can help where the problem is stiffening of the tiny bones of hearing (otosclerosis). The stiffened bone is replaced with an artificial bone. This operation works in the majority of cases.

HEARING AIDS
Children born deaf and adults who go deaf through natural degeneration should have a hearing aid. The selection of aids is an art, the most important thing being to ensure that the aid does not irritate the ear canal while fitting snugly enough to avoid irritating feedback amplification, which is the cause of the high-pitched squeals they sometimes make.

COCHLEAR IMPLANTATION
This is a state-of-the-art technology involving implanting an electrical device in the skull; this helps where the cochlear is damaged but where the nerve pathways to the brain are still working. It aims to reproduce the output of the cochlear cells which normally respond to sound and is a most exciting development. Although it does not yet restore normal hearing it can help adults and children to cope much better with speech recognition and with lip reading. Its use is certain to become more widespread, limited by cost.

Alternative Treatment

Acupuncture and herbal remedies are described, the value of which is unproved but which adults might like to try. Orthodox medical treatment should always be sought, for any kind of deafness, but the plethora of alternative therapies around can sometimes make a difference where conventional medicine cannot.

Prevention

AVOIDANCE OF LOUD NOISE

There is no doubt that exposure to loud noise for long periods of time, or very loud noise for short periods of time, will cause deafness. At first this may be reversible; we have all experienced temporary deafness after going to a loud party or concert. Pity the disc jockey or musicians exposed to such noise levels regularly. Workers in noisy industries must use ear protection; e.g., road repairmen should be protected when using compressed air tools. There is a rising tide of litigation which will no doubt change attitudes on this question.

AVOIDING BABY/CHILDHOOD RISKS TO HEARING

Rubella (German measles): all women hoping to conceive should endeavour to find out whether they are immune to rubella and if they are not, to be vaccinated well before conception. If you catch rubella during the first four months of pregnancy your child has a high risk of being born with deafness, heart disease and brain damage.

Measles and mumps are two other infectious diseases carrying a small risk of deafness, avoidable as long as your child (or you) is vaccinated.

Rhesus incompatibility is a technical problem to do with blood groups, which should be picked up as part of the routine investigations of pregnancy. Rhesus–negative mothers (those with a negative blood type, like A or B negative) can be given an injection called 'Anti-D', which prevents the body from rejecting a fetus of a positive blood group. Speak to your doctor if you are concerned about this.

Premature babies or those born in emergency situations risk infection and lack of oxygen, one consequence of which can be deafness. The doctors dealing with these babies will be well aware of the risks, including the hazards of some of the drugs used to treat infection, but parents should be extra vigilant about identifying signs of deafness as well as signs of poor vision and delay in development.

> **Regular baby checks by doctors and health visitors aim to detect deafness at the earliest possible stage. If you feel that a problem has not been identified, it is essential to bring it up with your medical practitioner.**

RECOGNIZING HEARING PROBLEMS

Trust your instincts; if you feel there is a hearing problem in your baby, seek a medical assessment. The earlier it is recognized the earlier a programme can be implemented to facilitate the acquisition of language skills, and maximize what hearing does exist. In older children it's important to realize that a cold will leave them slightly deaf for a week or two, but anything longer should be assessed. Be more attentive where deafness runs in the family.

For deafness that is the result of accidents or strokes: see pages 50 and 265 for discussion on prevention.

Self-Help

British Deaf Association
38 Victoria Place, Carlisle, CA1 1HU
Tel: 01228 48844 (televisual links available)

National Association of Deafened People
103 Heath Road, Widnes, Cheshire WA8 7NU
Tel: 0151 420-7316

National Deaf Children's Society Family Services Centre
43 Hereford Road, London W2 5AH
Tel: 0171 229-9272

Royal National Institute For the Deaf
105 Gower Street, London WC1E 6AH
Tel: 0171 387-8033

TINNITUS

Most of us have experienced ringing in the ears after a blow to the head or after a sudden loud noise. This is tinnitus; imagine that same ringing carrying on and on, day and night. Truly this is a form of torture and sufferers from the condition are desperate for help. In the great majority of cases there is no definite cause and the condition is thought to be due to general deterioration in the complex structure of the inner ear and its blood supply.

Risk

- There are an estimated one million sufferers from persistent tinnitus of some degree or other.
- There is commonly no cause found and it is considered to be part of the general deterioration of hearing that accompanies age (presbyacusis).
- Wax build-up may make it worse.
- Menière's disease (tinnitus plus deafness and vertigo) is less common, but nonetheless a cause of tinnitus.
- Rare causes include drugs such as aspirin, quinine.

Recognition

SYMPTOMS

The noise may be low or high pitched, but it is always ringing or rushing in nature. Anything more organized by way of actual speech or a musical or rhythmic sound suggests some other diagnosis. Usually one ear is affected more than another. Menière's disease consists of the three symptoms of tinnitus, vertigo and deafness all together.

Signs

The doctor has to rely on the patient's reports of their sensation. The possibility of ear disease must be considered and various tests will rule this out. Deafness and tinnitus in one ear is unusual enough to provoke a search for a tumour, even though these are rare.

Sounds other than ringing may be a feature of psychiatric illness, especially if the sufferer describes hearing speech or music. In such cases **schizophrenia** is a rare possibility (see page 290).

Investigations

Probably all cases merit a specialist opinion to exclude the rare alternative diagnoses.

ASK YOUR DOCTOR

- **How to relieve your condition. Although tinnitus cannot usually be cured, it can often be alleviated. Your doctor will know which local ENT specialists take an interest in tinnitus.**

Remedy

The basic defect is believed to be an increase in the pressure of the fluid inside the ear. So treatment aims at reducing the pressure. Commonly used drugs are betahistine, prochlorperazine and cinnarizine. With similar aims doctors prescribe diuretics, to stimulate the kidneys to excrete excess water, and a diet low in salt would be suggested. In extreme cases surgeons have actually destroyed the inner ear on one side; this may be a realistic option in someone with severe symptoms who is also deaf in the offending ear.

Masking Devices

This is a growing field; the idea is to use a sound generator that produces sounds which cancel out the tinnitus. Though this is not a cure it can render life bearable.

Despite the best efforts of the medical profession, many sufferers are left with symptoms requiring psychological support.

Alternative Treatment

Strategies include yoga, a diet high in potassium, manganese and magnesium (see a good nutritional therapist for details), and acupuncture. As orthodox medicine has no cure to offer, these may be a worthwhile alternative.

Prevention

- Avoid drugs which cause tinnitus as a side-effect, such as quinine, aspirin, alcohol and excess tobacco.
- A low-salt diet may help in established cases and in any case helps to reduce blood pressure.

- Have excess wax removed regularly from your ears and have infections treated promptly.
- Atherosclerosis probably accounts for most cases; a diet low in saturated fats and rich in fibre reduces the possibility of it occurring. Antioxidant vitamins A, C and E may have a role in preventing atherosclerosis; these are found in bright-coloured vegetables and fruit.

Self-Help

British Tinnitus Association
14–18 West Bargreen, Sheffield S1 2DA
Tel: 0114 279-6600

Royal National Institute for the Deaf Tinnitus Helpline
105 Gower Street, London WCIE 6AH
Tel: 01345 090210

VERTIGO AND DIZZINESS

These are conditions in which there is an overwhelming sense of being rotated; as if the room is spinning round. It does not mean a feeling of pressure in the head or the kind of light-headedness that elderly people often experience when they stand up. This condition has much in common with **tinnitus** (see page 43). Vertigo is to do with malfunction in the semi-circular canals; these are three fluid-filled tubes deep within each ear, which respond to movements in each direction; think of them as a sort of gyroscope. Vertigo results from interference with their functioning or damage to the nerves that run from them to the brain.

Risk

- This condition is extremely common; precise figures are unavailable.
- Vertigo and its associated dizziness are caused mainly by infections of the ear (vestibulitis, labyrinthitis) or injury to the ear.
- It is often associated with Menière's disease (which is characterized by vertigo, deafness and tinnitus).
- Unusual causes include multiple sclerosis, brain tumours and certain drugs, especially aspirin in overdose.

Recognition

SYMPTOMS
Every time the head is moved, the room spins; in severe cases this happens from the first moment you attempt to raise your head upon waking. There is nausea or vomiting. The attacks can last for just a few seconds or several days and are often recurrent over several months.

SIGNS
While watching the movements of the eyes, the doctor will request that the head be moved. He or she will be looking for flicking movements called nystagmus. The type of

nystagmus gives an indication of the cause of the vertigo. There are other tests of balance; e.g., standing with eyes closed and hands held in front. Although causes other than injury or infection are rare, it is normal to check blood pressure and, if symptoms persist, to test for unusual neurological disease such as multiple sclerosis.

INVESTIGATIONS

These will be required only if symptoms persist. They aim to reproduce the vertigo by tests such as running cold water into the ear or by tilting the sufferer in a special chair and measuring response. If neurological disease is suspected a CT **brain scan** (see page 298) will be necessary.

ASK YOUR DOCTOR
- **About persistent vertigo, especially if it is combined with tinnitus** or **deafness** (see pages 43 and 39).

Remedy

The great majority of cases are caused by ear infections which will settle with a course of antibiotics or, if viral, on their own. There are several anti-nauseant drugs helpful in the acute attack; prochlorperazine is often used. Because of the associated nausea these may need to be given by injection, by suppository or by a tablet stuck on the inside of the cheek.

The rare tumours which can cause vertigo and deafness require delicate surgery.

Alternative Treatment

Some people find that manipulation of the spine relieves recurrent dizziness. There are herbal, homoeopathic and Chinese remedies which can help in recurrent vertigo but it is always necessary to see your doctor first, to rule out any more sinister implications. Ginger, grated in hot water, is a traditional remedy for nausea. There are many homoeopathic remedies, depending on the cause. See a registered practitioner for details.

Prevention

Common causes of vertigo include aspirin, alcohol, quinine, but only if taken in excess. Do not neglect recurrent ear infections as these can lead to long-term damage of the balancing mechanisms of the inner ear.

Self-Help

Menière's Society
98 Maybury Road, Woking, Surrey GU21 5HX
Tel: 01483 740597

CHILDREN

- Accidents • Cerebral Palsy • Childhood Cancers
- Cot Death • Heart Disease • Infectious Diseases
  - Vaccinations and Reactions

I N THE DEVELOPED world parenting has become in the main a matter of safely bringing up healthy children. Antenatal care, good living conditions and good nutrition have combined to see infant mortality rates fall to extremely low levels in comparison to underdeveloped countries, where death and serious disease in childhood are common. This has the effect of making it appear that diseases such as leukaemia or meningitis are major killers of children. This is true only insofar as other causes of death (apart from accidents) have become so unusual, that these devastating but rare conditions stand out by comparison. So it is easy to form a distorted view about the true health hazards to children, at least in the developed world. This section will give you a more balanced view of the real risks to your children.

ACCIDENTS

Now that the risk of infectious disease is so low, accidents are the single biggest threat to children's health and indeed are the commonest cause of death in people up to age thirty. Many are preventable; awareness of simple precautions can reduce the toll of accidents. Much of the following can be applied to people of all ages.

Risk

- Accidents account for over 10,000 deaths per annum.
- 6.7 deaths per 100,000 population (of children) are accidentally caused.
- Forty-seven children under the age of one die accidentally each year.
- Accidents account for 224 deaths in one- to four-year-olds per annum.
- Vehicle accidents, pedestrian accidents, fires and drownings are the commonest causes of accidental death.
- Road traffic accidents account for 40 per cent of all deaths through accidents.
- 35 per cent of accidental deaths occur in the home.
- In boys, injury and poisoning account for 25 per cent of all deaths between ages one and four; and 50 per cent of all deaths between ages of ten and 14. In girls these figures are 20 per cent and 33 per cent.
- At least 1 per cent of children are admitted to hospital per annum as a result of accident and about 25 per cent of all young children will each year have a more than trivial accident.

Recognition

Cuts, bruising, abrasions are evident. Blows to the head may require specialist attention; fractures are also not always obvious to the untrained eye.

SIGNS

Non-accidental injury is a possibility that anyone working with children has to bear in mind. Suspicious features include injury inconsistent with the circumstances described, repeated minor injury, burns and cuts in unusual places (e.g., the buttocks), multiple bruises of varying ages, and unexplained delay in obtaining help. An abused child may seem either withdrawn or disturbed. This is but a summary of suspicious features, which could, but does not definitely, point to child abuse.

INVESTIGATIONS

Will be undertaken according to the type of accident. If non-accidental injury is suspected a number of **X-rays** (see page 301) may be taken looking for fractures, where the accident described may not necessarily point in that direction. Palpation (examination by feeling), and checking for bruising, bleeding, signs of trauma, shock or internal bleeding may all be appropriate.

ASK YOUR DOCTOR

- **About guidelines on accident prevention in childhood.**
- **What to do if you think a child is being abused. There are sensitive, discreet procedures for dealing with such suspicions.**
- **About any unusual behaviour following an accident; abnormal sleepiness, hyperactivity and pain can all indicate that something is wrong.**

Remedy

Treatment will of course be appropriate to the accident but there are some general principles (these apply as much to adults as to children).

THE UNCONSCIOUS CHILD

Three vital checks in anyone unconscious are ABC: Airway, Breathing, Circulation.

- **Airway** – *Try to clear the mouth of any obstruction such as vomit or the tongue itself. The airway should be clear.*

- **Breathing** – *If breathing has stopped, give artificial respiration.*

- **Circulation** – *If the heart has stopped, give external cardiac compression. Never do this if there is any suggestion that the heart has not stopped.*

Keep artificial respiration going in cases of drowning, suffocation or head injury until a full medical assessment has been made because recovery is possible even after prolonged unconsciousness.

FRACTURES

Splint the limb to prevent further movement and damage. Move the child as little as possible, especially if there is any possibility of a neck or spinal injury.

BURNS

Cool the burn with cold water; for example, by putting a burnt hand into cold water. Continue to cool it for ten to fifteen minutes, or until help arrives. Large or inaccessible burns should be covered with absorbent material, placed very gently on burnt skin, after cutting away any hot or smouldering substances.

POISONING

Find out what and how much the child has swallowed. Do not make the child vomit if there is any possibility that they have drunk an oily or corrosive material. Seek emergency medical attention.

HEAD INJURIES

Children who have had a head injury need special observation (see page 246). The younger the child the more easily a head injury can occur; with babies even moderate shaking can cause internal bleeding.

CUTS

Apply firm pressure over the cut with an absorbent pad; most will stop bleeding in a couple of minutes unless an artery has been cut, which will need more intensive treatment. Any bleeding which continues for more than ten minutes, and defies staunching, must receive emergency medical attention.

CHOKING

Try to dislodge the obstruction by hitting the child on the back or hooking it out with your fingers. Familiarize yourself with the Heimlich manoeuvre, a simple lifesaving device to eject an obstruction of the airways in adults or children. Younger children should not be treated too energetically. A toddler can be held upside down and gently patted on the upper back.

The detailed treatment of accidents is beyond the scope of this book, except to say that even a modest first-aid knowledge can make all the difference.

Alternative Treatment

Minor bruises where the skin is not broken are helped by applying arnica cream. Homoeopathic arnica tablet will reduce bruising and pain and facilitate healing. Witch hazel is a traditional remedy for bruising. Honey and aloe are soothing for burns (but treat with caution, for aloe is a common allergen), applied externally. A gentle herbal wash with calendula can help. Bach Rescue Remedy is excellent for shock; in small children it can be applied to the temples and pulse points instead of taken internally.

Prevention

Preventing accidents is a matter of identifying potential risks and taking steps to reduce their possibility. The problem with children is that they cannot be expected to recognize hazards that adults automatically notice; e.g., sharp corners to tables, the slippery footpath by a pond, the danger of dashing across a road.

ROAD TRAFFIC ACCIDENTS (INCLUDING PEDESTRIANS)

- There are well known national strategies on speed limits, alcohol, child restraints in cars and encouraging safer car design.
- Programmes to teach children traffic sense come and go and must be reinforced by parental teaching and example. These programmes become so familiar that they lose their edge yet as long as we have cars we must remain vigilant about undertaking preventative measures.
- Until parents are absolutely certain of their children's sense of responsibility, all children should be accompanied when playing or walking near roads. The lower age limit for this is probably nine to ten years of age, a limit woefully unobserved by many parents.

WATER

- A child can drown in just a couple of inches of water, so the risk is not just one for families with swimming pools but extends to ornamental pools and, of course, baths.
- No child should be left unattended by water; fence off obvious hazards.
- Don't ever leave a child alone in the bath. Even sturdy toddlers and younger children can slip, fall and drown in very little water.
- Whenever possible, teach children to swim.

FIRE

- No child should be left with access to a naked flame; there are all manner of guards available.
- Some families often rely on heating by oil stoves, or open gas fires, which puts an even greater responsibility on those parents to supervise their children.
- Smoke detectors are cheap and can be fitted in a few minutes; test them regularly!
- In the kitchen where risks are especially high consider buying a fire extinguisher.

ACCIDENTAL FALLS

- It can be revealing to look at your home from the viewpoint (and height) of a child to see the major avoidable risks.
- While it is not necessary to make your household a fortress, ensure that loose carpets are tacked down, floorboards are nailed securely, the mattress is lowered on a baby's cot when he or she can sit, the ladder is removed from the bunkbeds in a toddler's bedroom, stairs are gated (even attractively decorated and furnished houses can successfully integrate these!), and a child is never left alone on a work surface, table or high chair.

Self-Help

Child Accident Prevention Trust
4th Floor, Clerk's Court, 18–20 Farringdon Lane, London EC1R 3AU
Tel: 0171 608-3828

Royal Society for the Prevention of Accidents
Cannon House, The Priory, Queensway, Birmingham B4 6BS
Tel: 0121 200-2461

CEREBRAL PALSY

Cerebral palsy is a condition in children characterized by muscle weakness and paralysis, and attributed to brain damage. Brain damage can occur during pregnancy or about the time of birth. Cerebral palsy is a very general term, including as it does children with barely detectable problems to children who require complete care. The basic defect is brain damage, whether through infection, through bleeding into the brain or from oxygen deprivation; in many cases no definite cause can be found and it is assumed there is some congenital malformation of the brain.

Cerebral palsy is commonly associated with mental handicap or epilepsy but this is by no means inevitable and it is possible to have quite severe cerebral palsy but normal or above normal intelligence. It remains a fact, however, that once a child is diagnosed as having cerebral palsy his or her mental development over the next few years will be questionable.

Children with cerebral palsy used to be called spastic. The term 'spastic' has a precise medical meaning, referring to the increased tension or 'tone' in muscle, which is a consequence of certain forms of brain damage and which leads to the deformities associated with cerebral palsy. It has become a term of abuse and is rightly dropped from general use.

Risk

- Cerebral palsy affects one to two children per 1000 births in the developed world, many more in the Third World.
- About 40 per cent of cases are due to problems around birth including prematurity; the active management of birth including Caesarean section has greatly reduced the incidence by preventing the possibility of oxygen starvation during delivery.
- 55 per cent of cases occur intra-uterinely; e.g., malformation, or infections such as rubella.
- 5 per cent of cases happen after birth, following meningitis and similar illnesses.

Recognition

The more severe the brain damage the earlier the condition is recognized. In many milder cases it may be one or two years before a suspicion is confirmed and longer than that before the full extent of the child's disability is established.

SIGNS

In Newborn Babies

- High-risk factors include jaundice, oxygen starvation at birth and an obviously small head.
- The child often feels floppy, feeds poorly and is irritable.
- There may be weakness or paralysis of a limb or one half of the body.

Up to Two Years

- The child fails to meet milestones of development; i.e., walking or crawling at appropriate ages.
- The child may not use the arm and leg on one side (hemiparesis) or all four limbs may be weak and stiff (quadraparesis).
- The child may have fits.
- It may become clear that the child is not seeing or hearing properly, by not responding to sound or to familiar faces, though this can be difficult to judge.

Over Two Years

- The child appears clumsy, is slow to learn, and perhaps unable to feed him or herself.
- In severe cases the child cannot walk and the limbs become deformed. (This is because of unbalanced muscular groups).
- The child fails to become continent of urine or faeces.
- It becomes obvious that the child's movements are either very stiff (spasticity), tremorous (ataxic palsy) or involve curious writhing movements (athetoid palsy). These types carry different outlooks, complications and treatment.

INVESTIGATIONS

CT scans (see page 298) can reveal severe brain damage; blood tests can show the effects of infection in the womb. An **EEG** (see page 299) might show abnormal brain activity and it is usual to do **chromosomal studies** (see page 298) looking for a congenital defect.

ASK YOUR DOCTOR

- **About testing of your child's development if you have any doubts about progress. Parents are extremely sensitive to abnormalities in development; it is an unwise doctor who fails to take note of a mother's concerns.**
- **About the range of normal development milestones; just because your child is not walking at eighteen months does not mean that he or she is brain damaged.**

Remedy

Treatment is based on the knowledge that the developing brain of a child can overcome damage which would be permanent in an adult. Thus, every effort is put into encouraging children to use their limbs and minds to the fullest extent.

FULL ASSESSMENT

It may not be clear what the child's disabilities are without careful and repeated testing; this is especially the case in trying to detect hearing problems.

THERAPY

Speech therapists encourage the child to talk and can help them overcome difficulties posed by poor hearing or by poor coordination of the muscles of speech.

Physiotherapy is very important. Because the child's muscles are unbalanced in strength, one group of muscles will pull the limb more strongly than the others. Typically this will lead to a child whose arms are pulled tight against the body, while the legs twist across each other and are contracted at the hips and knees. Physiotherapy aims to counter this imbalance by forcing the limbs through a full range of movements and by teaching parents what to do.

SURGERY

Can correct the worst excess of poor posture, awkwardly shaped feet, and severely contracted hands.

EDUCATION

There is no reason why children with mild disability should not go to an ordinary school; as well as being in their best interests it shows their fellows that disability is not something extraordinary, to be shut away. Those children with severe mental and physical disability often do need to go special schools, geared to coping with their special demands.

SUPPORT

It is difficult to overstate the demands made on the family by a child with cerebral palsy; normal children may feel they lose out on attention, the parents must be constantly available, holidays are difficult, the house may need to be adapted for a wheelchair, etc. There is often an underlying worry about what will happen to the child when the parents can no longer provide care. Family breakdown is common, but equally many families cope with quiet dedication.

Alternative Treatment

Programmes providing intensive therapy have been widely publicized in recent years. The theory that increased stimulation improves development has now been accepted. It is likely that osteopathy and chiropractic would be useful for working the tissues. All members of the family could benefit from the relaxing effects of aromatherapy or soothing herbal preparations.

Prevention

IMMUNIZATION

Rubella (German measles) and childhood illness such as mumps, measles and haemophilus meningitis can all be avoided by vaccination. Every woman contemplating pregnancy owes it to her unborn child to check that she is immune to German measles. The childhood **vaccination** programme is discussed on page 67.

Management of Pregnancy

With modern ultrasound scans a fetus failing to grow normally can be investigated before birth; serious congenital defects of the brain can be detected early enough for termination to be an option. Caesarean sections are increasingly offered whenever vaginal delivery is considered to carry a risk of brain damage to the baby. Fetal monitoring during delivery can display early signs of distress so the baby can be delivered more quickly, or delivered by emergency Caesarean.

Spina Bifida

The incidence of this condition is greatly reduced by taking folic acid 0.4 mg a day before pregnancy and during the first twelve weeks of pregnancy. A spina bifida child risks having weak legs and brain damage through hydrocephalus (water on the brain), though in themselves such children have perfectly normal intelligence.

Alcohol and Smoking in Pregnancy

Babies born to heavy drinkers are about twice as likely to have a congenital abnormality. This can include heart and brain defects leading to lifelong disability. There is no safe lower limit of alcohol; the less you drink the less the risk; there will always be some risk compared to mothers who do not drink at all during pregnancy. The safest advice is to abstain.

Babies born to mothers who smoke during pregnancy are on average half a pound lighter at birth; whether this implies long-term mental damage is uncertain but as a general rule light for date babies risk poor growth. There is also evidence that smoking during pregnancy can contribute to the risk of cot death (see page 58), and to problems with the baby's heart and circulatory system.

Chromosome Analysis

It is possible to sample the tissue of the fetus to see whether it is carrying a known chromosomal defect. This technique (which carries a risk of causing miscarriage) is used where a mother has a known genetic disease in the family or has had a child with a genetic defect. Genetic screening is likely to become more common; it does in turn raise the moral dilemma about terminating a pregnancy (see page 298).

Premature Babies

It is now technically possible to keep babies alive who are born before thirty weeks' gestation. These tiny scraps of life are at high risk of infection and brain damage. Though many will grow up to be normal, a large proportion, perhaps 40 per cent, will have serious brain damage despite the best efforts. This is a dilemma which has yet to be resolved, for it is a natural reaction to put all efforts into saving the premature baby's life and to worry about the baby's long-term prospects later.

Despite attention to all the above factors, babies will continue to be born with cerebral palsy. It remains a huge personal and social problem and the biggest single cause of disability in children.

Self-Help

Cerebral Palsy Help Line.
PO Box 833, Neath Hill, Milton Keynes, Bucks MK14 6DR
Tel: 01800 626216

Scope (was Spastics Society)
12 Park Crescent, London W1N 4EQ
Tel: 01800 626216

Foundation for Conductive Education
University of Birmingham, Edgbaston, Birmingham B15 2TT
Tel: 0121 414-4947

CHILDHOOD CANCERS

It seems unimaginable that children should suffer from cancer. Because of its nature, we tend to see cancer as a disease of the elderly, and in many instances it is. It's important to begin by recognizing that childhood cancer is rare. In children cancers usually involve some rapidly growing part of the body – the marrow of the bones, or the bones themselves – or they occur in a remnant of foetal tissue. In adults cancers arise in previously stable tissue.

Cancer is rare in children yet deaths from other causes are also so unusual that cancer is the second commonest reason for death in children below the age of fifteen (the main cause is accidents). In the past children died as a result of illnesses like diarrhoea, chest infections, measles and most of the conditions that we now immunize against. In many parts of the world children are as likely to die from these things as they were in this country a hundred years ago; in under-developed countries cancer is hardly considered as a cause of death in children and it is no less common there than it is here. Because we have found ways in which to treat illnesses that were once fatal, and cancer has remained one of the few illnesses that can still be deadly, its prevalence among the fatal illnesses appears much more significant than the actual number of cases.

As it is in adults the treatment of childhood cancers is a matter of gradual innovation and refinement of techniques rather than dramatic breakthroughs. Certain cancers are now considered curable; these include forms of **leukaemia** and **Hodgkin's disease** (see pages 194 and 192). The other most frequent cancers are tumours of the kidney, bone tumours and tumours of the brain or spinal cord. In general, cancers of this type are more aggressive in children than their counterparts in adults. This makes early diagnosis even more of a priority in children than it is in adults.

Overall there has been a steady improvement in the survival of children with cancer; currently an average of 63 per cent of children with cancer survive for at least ten years.

Risk

- There are 130 to 160 cases per million children per annum: this includes all forms of **leukaemia** and **Hodgkin's disease** (see pages 194 and 192).
- Leukaemia and Hodgkin's disease account for about one-third of childhood malignancies; brain and nervous system tumours for about another third.

- Bone and kidney tumours each account for about nine cases per million children per annum.
- The overall death rate (over five years) is 33 per cent, but this masks wide variation between different cancers; e.g., Hodgkin's disease is virtually always cured, bone tumours carry a 50 to 65 per cent, five-year survival, whereas advanced brain tumours carry a very high mortality, and kidney tumours are now usually curable.

Recognition

Cancer can affect as many different organs of the body in children as it can in adults, so the presenting symptoms can be many and varied. Below we list some symptoms of the commonest tumours.

SYMPTOMS
- Brain Tumours

A mixture of unsteadiness, headache and poor coordination, plus effortless vomiting, due to the increased pressure within the brain. More unusual symptoms are fits, failure to grow, a bulging head. Drowsiness or coma are late symptoms.

- Kidney Tumours (Wilms' Tumour) and Neuroblastomas

These generally cause a swelling in the child's abdomen. There is occasionally pain and blood in the urine.

- Bone Tumours

There is pain in a bone; eventually a visible swelling.

- Eye Tumour (Retinoblastoma)

Instead of a reddish reflection of light the affected eye reflects white light, because of the mass of tumour. There is also commonly a squint and a bulging eye.

- Leukaemia

Spontaneous bruising, pallor, severe persistent sore throat (see page 194).

- Hodgkin's Disease

Affects mainly teenagers, causing rubbery swollen glands in the neck, malaise and night sweats (see page 192).

SIGNS AND INVESTIGATIONS

The child may look completely well in cases of kidney tumours, or clearly unwell in cases of leukaemia, with all grades in between. **X-rays** and **blood tests** (see pages 301 and 298) establish the diagnosis of leukaemia and Hodgkin's disease; **CT scans** (see page 298) confirm the extent of abdominal masses and brain tumours while in other cases a **biopsy** (see page 298) is needed to establish the exact diagnosis.

ASK YOUR DOCTOR
- **About unusual or persistent symptoms in your child. This sounds vague, as indeed it is, but it is always the first step towards medical attention. Be especially suspicious of a change in behaviour; e.g., a normal child who becomes clumsy.**
- **About persistent bone pain.**

Remedy

Treatment depends of course on the precise nature of the tumour. It will include some element of **radiotherapy**, **chemotherapy** and surgical removal of the tumour (see pages 301 and 298). This could mean removal of the kidney, amputation of a limb in some (though not all) cases of bone cancer, removal of the eye in cases of retinoblastoma. Brain tumours pose particular problems; many cannot be removed – some can be, if they extend down the back of the brain or along the spinal cord. Removal of this sort of tumour calls for immensely skilled surgery.

There follows a long period, checking for regrowth of the tumour which can be as worrying as the initial diagnosis and treatment. Childhood cancer is so rare that only a few specialized centres treat the condition. It is to those centres that every child should be sent.

Alternative Treatment

Alternative therapies offer a holistic view of medical care which can be very beneficial for cancer patients. Most therapies will address every aspect of lifestyle, including diet, hobbies, sleep patterns and exercise. Ensuring that these are undertaken in a healthy and satisfying manner increases the overall health of the child, as well as their sense of well-being. Many therapies are excellent for recuperation following surgery or chemotherapy. In particular, homoeopathy, aromatherapy, acupuncture (or acupressure) and nutritional therapy can be useful.

Prevention

It is difficult enough to prove any environmental influences on common adult cancers, let alone rare childhood cancers. One recent example is the supposed clustering of cases of leukaemia near nuclear power stations; the occurrence of just one or two extra cases may represent a doubling of the expected frequency, but is actually explained entirely by chance fluctuations, so this particular suspicion remains unproved.

Early detection is the most important means by which cancer can be beaten. This is important because the earlier the diagnosis the better the chances of cure in most forms of childhood cancer. This does not mean becoming paranoid about every persistent symptom; there are only one or two new cases of cancer per 10,000 children per annum, so it's likely that persistent leg pain is, in fact, a sports injury, or vomiting the result of a tummy bug. Use your instincts. If you are alarmed by any symptoms in your child do not hesitate to seek medical advice.

SCREENING

Some neurological tumours called neuroblastomas produce a by-product in urine which can be detected. From every 100,000 children screened, there would be about one case.

Most doctors will agree that the best pointer to serious childhood illness is a parent's suspicion of an abnormality, all the more so in the cases of infants unable to report symptoms themselves. Mothers who spend hours touching, prodding, calling, holding babies are sensitive to subtle changes in their baby's behaviour, detect swellings in the belly, suspect an inability to see or hear, and have a feeling when a child is not using its limbs properly. It is a foolhardy doctor who ignores a parent's suspicions in such cases.

Self-Help

Childhood Cancer and Leukaemia Link
20 Haywood, Bracknell, Berks RG12 7WG
Tel: 01344 750319

Cancer and Leukaemia in Childhood (CLIC)
11–12 Freemantle Square, Cotham, Bristol BS6 5TL
Tel: 0117 924-4333

Rainbow Centre (Especially complementary therapies)
PO Box 604, Bristol, BS99 1SW
Tel: 0117 985-3343
See also **leukaemia** and **Hodgkin's Disease** (pages 194 and 192).

COT DEATH

The more precise term for cot death is Sudden Infant Death Syndrome (SIDS), reflecting the fact that babies can and do die unexpectedly, not just in their cots but anywhere. It has even been known to happen to babies while being carried by their mothers. Until very recently SIDS was one of the most common causes of death in babies up to one year of age. There has, however, been a dramatic fall in SIDS since new evidence has changed the way in which babies are put down to sleep. Cot death is much less common in babies who sleep on their backs, and who are not over-wrapped, which can lead to overheating.

It is probable that several different conditions can result in sudden infant death.

Risk

- In 1993 there were 442 deaths. This compares with 1469 in 1988 in the UK when SIDS accounted for one-fifth of all infant deaths (deaths in children below one year of age).
- Worldwide, one in 500 babies dies in its first year from SIDS.
- Three months is the age of greatest risk.
- There is a higher risk in babies who sleep face down.
- There is evidence that overheating can cause cot death.
- The death by cot death of one child in a family increases the risk for other siblings by five times.
- Babies born to women who smoked during pregnancy are at greater risk – possibly 6 times greater if mother smoked more than 20 cigarettes a day.

Recognition

The diagnosis is suggested when a baby or small child in previous good health is found dead. All such deaths are investigated for evidence of any other cause, such as sudden overwhelming infection or unsuspected internal malformations. By definition SIDS is the diagnosis where no other cause is found.

INVESTIGATIONS

Though there are many theories it has not proved possible to link up SIDS with clear causes.

ASK YOUR DOCTOR
- If you worried about your child's breathing.
- If your are alarmed about your child's colour.
- What to do if there is a familial history of cot death.

Remedy

If a baby appears to have had a near-miss, it will be investigated to detect previously unsuspected abnormalities in the heart, lung or metabolism.

Many parents wish to have a heart/breathing monitor, but there are great problems with these (see below).

The greatest challenge is to provide psychological relief for the parents and siblings after a SID. Parents often have a huge feeling of guilt at the thought that they might have ignored some significant symptom, some oddness about the child's behaviour of which they feel they should have taken note. There may be gossip that the death was not accidental but deliberate. Fortunately there are excellent charities which provide sympathetic counselling at these times, though no one suggests that such a terrible event can ever be forgotten, only come to terms with.

As theories come and go there may be fashionable things to avoid. One current suspicion is to do with antimony in cot mattresses, put there as a fire retardant. There is nothing to support theories of food or other allergies being responsible. There is very good evidence that smoking by either parent can increase the likelihood of the disease.

Alternative Treatment

None is applicable.

Prevention

BACK TO SLEEP

This brilliantly simple and successful campaign has reduced by nearly two-thirds the number of cot deaths. Instead of placing your baby face down to sleep, place it on its back or side. There were fears that babies on their backs risked choking on vomit but the figures show otherwise. The research reaching this lifesaving conclusion comes from New Zealand.

DON'T OVER-WRAP

Babies need to be kept warm but not hot. Do not pile clothes on to the baby; avoid heating its room above a comfortable sixty-eight or seventy degrees. It is particularly important to avoid overdressing a baby if there is fever present.

Heart/Breathing Monitors

There is no good case for widespread use of these. They give rise to many false alarms and are therefore a source of great anxiety. Where a family has suffered a previous cot death it will be an understandable wish to have an alarm but evidence suggests this is more comfort to the parents than an actual preventative measure; other parents swear by them.

Give up Smoking

Don't smoke in the vicinity of any child; it has been proved that even diffused passive smoking can present a risk to babies and young children. There is a distinct link between smoking and cot death. Avoid it.

Self-Help

Cot Death Society
1 Browning Close, Thatcham, Berks RG18 3EF
Tel: 0163 586-1771
Foundation for the Study of Infant Deaths
35 Belgrave Square, London SW1X 8QB
Tel: 0171 235-1721

HEART DISEASE

Heart disease is one of the more common congenital problems (conditions that they are born with) in children, but it is usually treatable or at least controllable in childhood. During embryonic life the heart is formed by an intricate sequence of events which transform a primitive heart tube into the beating heart by a process rather like Origami; bending and twisting the tube and then pulling out a completely unexpected final structure. The primitive heart starts to beat from about three weeks when the embryo is just over 2 mm in length, but the heart is not recognizably complete until about nine weeks when the embryo is still just 16 mm long.

In the normal heart the right side of the heart receives venous blood from the body, then pumps that blood around the lungs where it picks up oxygen. The blood returns to the left side of the heart to be pumped off to the body again.

The main congenital problems are abnormal development of one side of the heart, abnormal 'holes', which allow leakage between the two sides of the heart, and abnormal formation of blood vessels. So-called 'blue babies' are those in whom there is a malformation which lets 'blue' venous blood (low in oxygen) leak from the right side of the heart to mix with arterial blood from the lungs, thereby reducing the overall oxygen supply to the body and resulting in a dusky blue appearance of the baby's lips and tongue.

Risk

- Heart disease affects 1 per cent of babies.
- A familial history of congenital disease increases that risk to 2 to 4 per cent.
- Only about a third of affected babies display symptoms in the first year.
- Two-thirds of heart disease diagnoses in children are detected by examination or as a result of symptoms in later life.

- Many children suffer from minor leakages which may produce a heart murmur but are of no more significance.
- Serious malformations can be fatal without urgent surgery.
- Rubella in pregnancy is the commonest avoidable cause of congenital heart disease.
- Rheumatic fever is still the greatest worldwide cause of acquired heart disease in children but is now a negligible risk in the developed world.

Recognition

Most serious abnormalities are picked up at birth or soon after, usually through routine health checks.

SYMPTOMS
In serious cases the baby seems constantly irritable and becomes agitated when feeding because of breathlessness; its lips or tongue may look blue. Older children turn blue on exertion and are small for their age. In one very serious form of disease (Fallot's tetralogy) the child finds that squatting improves blood flow to the brain.

Many other forms of heart disease produce no symptoms in childhood and are detected only by examination, but they increase a risk of infections of the heart (see Subacute bacterial **endocarditis**, page 141) or **heart failure** (see page 147), the exact risk depending on the nature of the abnormality.

Rheumatic fever presents with joint pains, unusual rashes and fever. The damage to the heart becomes apparent by the appearance of heart murmurs. It's important to note, however, that heart murmurs are not always sinister. Many children have innocent murmurs which disappear as they grow older and which pose no threat to their quality of life.

SIGNS
The cardinal features are a blue baby, breathlessness while feeding and poor growth. By listening to the heart it is possible to hear murmurs produced by abnormal blood flow and this is often the first clue that there may be something wrong.

INVESTIGATIONS
Echocardiography (see page 299) uses sound waves to create images of the beating heart and allows rapid diagnosis of abnormal valves and blood flow. If surgery is planned it is necessary to inject a dye into the heart to demonstrate the precise abnormality. Rheumatic fever is confirmed by **blood tests** (see page 298).

ASK YOUR DOCTOR
- **About unusual breathlessness in your baby or the sudden or prolonged appearance of blue lips and tongue. This is of more significance than blue hands and feet which are usually perfectly normal.**
- **About surgical options, if your child is diagnosed with heart disease.**
- **About antibiotic protection for surgery or dental care (see below), if your child has heart disease.**

Remedy

Many minor defects need no treatment and will rectify themselves over a period of years. Of course the child is kept under regular review. Other defects are not immediately life-threatening and can be surgically repaired when the child is a little older, perhaps two to four years of age. Until that time medical means are used to control heart infections and to prevent heart failure.

The serious major malformations are either treated soon after birth in what is hoped to be a life-saving operation or major surgery is delayed till the child is one or two, but medication keeps the child stable through what will often be a series of operations. In rare cases, the fetus can be operated on while still in the womb.

Heart transplantation offers an increasing successful chance of survival to children with otherwise untreatable and certainly fatal defects and will probably be used more and more to deal with the most serious abnormalities.

> *The outlook for the great majority of children with heart disease is good. Many can forget about their abnormalities, except for regular courses of antibiotics during dental or operative procedures.*

Rheumatic fever is now extremely rare in the developed world. It is due to infection by the streptococcus bacterium, a common cause of pharyngitis (inflammation of the pharynx, in the throat). This is eliminated by the use of antibiotics and it is this plus improved living standards which has, with the increased standard of living, reduced the incidence of this previously greatly feared disease.

Alternative Treatment

None is recommended, although post-operatively many therapies can offer restorative treatment. Some therapies may encourage rehabilitation following invasive treatment like surgery.

Prevention

PRE-CONCEPTUAL CARE

- Check that you are immune to Rubella (German measles) well before you plan to conceive. Rubella that is caught before four months of pregnancy presents a 30 per cent chance of having a child with heart defects, cataracts, mental deficiency and deafness. Immunization is a matter of a single injection followed by a blood test to confirm immunity.
- Drinking alcohol in high quantities during pregnancy increases the chance of heart defects as well as carrying a risk of brain damage. Drink in moderation; some would say do not drink at all in pregnancy. Smoking (see above) carries the same risk.
- Children with Down's syndrome are at risk of heart disease. The chances of having such a child greatly increase in mothers above the age of thirty-five, for whom screening tests are offered. Termination is an option in these cases.
- Take medication only if necessary, checking with your doctor that what you are taking is safe. Especially avoid aspirin in late pregnancy; it can cause changes in the blood circulation in the unborn child.

ULTRASOUND SCANS

These can pick up gross abnormalities in the heart and are a valuable screening test where there is a family history of congenital heart disease.

ANTIBIOTIC COVER

Antibiotic cover is generally a safeguard against heart infection, taken in the event of dental treatment or any surgery, no matter how minor. Some doctors will err on the side of caution and prescribe a course of antibiotics for what appear to be simple surface wounds, burns or abrasions. If you or your child has been advised to take this cover, it is essential that you follow the advice. There is a risk in even modest dental procedures and from invasive surgery because such procedures can allow bacteria to enter the bloodstream and be carried to the heart where they can lodge on any malformed structure (see Sub-acute bacterial **endocarditis**, page 141).

LIVE!
For the great majority, congenital heart disease is a relatively minor problem and should not affect your child's life or lifestyle.

Self-Help

Association for Children with Heart Disorders
26 Elizabeth Drive, Helmshore, Rossendale, Lancs BB4 4JB
Tel: 01706 213 632
British Cardiac Patients Association
c/o Mrs N. Jackson
6 Rampton End, Willingham, Cambs CB4 5JF

INFECTIOUS DISEASES

Asked to name an infectious disease, you may think of a cough, a cold or perhaps an ear infection – something inconvenient but of no great long-term concern. It was not that many years ago when childhood infection was enormously feared; fevers were cause for legitimate alarm. Nights were spent anxiously treating an ailing child, to see whether the fever would be the prelude to a common cold, or the beginning of something much more serious – a deadly disease, like rheumatic fever, scarlet fever, pneumonia or measles.

It is difficult for us who enjoy easy access to antibiotics and intensive care even to begin to understand the sense of sheer helplessness inspired by infectious illness, but this remains the case across great swathes of the undeveloped world. The international statistics speak for themselves: simple gastro-enteritis alone is believed to kill 10,000,000 a year; measles 1,000,000; whooping cough 400,000; and neonatal tetanus 150,000. This is quite apart from chronic (long-term) infections such as tuberculosis, malaria, schistosomiasis and hepatitis B.

Medicine alone cannot take the credit for the dramatic fall in infectious disease in the developed world. Improved living standards, simple hygiene, pure food and water are the real heroes and antibiotics play a relatively minor role.

Risk

- Polio, measles, mumps, diphtheria, German measles (rubella), tetanus and whooping cough are all now unusual in childhood, thanks to immunization.
- There are several thousand cases a year of chicken-pox.
- Haemophilus meningitis (bacterial meningitis) is rapidly becoming less common since the introduction of the specific vaccination (Hib) a few years ago (see **meningitis**, page 25).
- An average child will suffer from four to eight colds each year and a chest infection every couple of years.
- There are innumerable episodes of damaged/infected skin (like cuts), any of which could progress to generalized infection.
- Babies, in particular those who are bottlefed, can be expected to have about three episodes of gastro-enteritis in their first year of life.
- Poor food handling accounts for the greatest number of cases of gastro-enteritis.

Recognition

SYMPTOMS

The child becomes feverish, with a warm forehead, a hot dry skin and a flushed appearance. He or she loses their appetite and, in the case of babies, may vomit feeds. Older children can tell you that they are feeling ill, or complain of a sore throat, aching joints or headache. Babies just become irritable and sleepy. Young children can become badly behaved, sometimes irrational, for no apparent reason.

Usually fever lasts only a day or two before more specific symptoms emerge, such as sneezing and a runny nose, a cough, earache, diarrhoea or a rash. Fever lasting more than a week without other symptoms is unusual and calls for investigation.

SIGNS

At the onset of a feverish illness a doctor often cannot make a diagnosis; the doctor's concern at that early stage is to exclude serious, rapidly progressing illness such as meningitis and abdominal infection from an appendix. So the doctor looks for neck stiffness, an aversion to light, a purple rash (see **meningitis**, page 25). The ears, nose and throat are checked, looking for early tonsillitis or an ear infection. The doctor listens to the chest to detect the wheezes or crackles of a chest infection and feels the abdomen for the tenderness that may signify an abdominal infection.

Most doctors will take into consideration the overall appearance of the child and their instinctive sense of the seriousness of the child's condition. Doctors prefer not to admit this, because it sounds non-scientific, but it is actually the perfectly respectable warning sense that comes from years of experience of dealing with children who are ordinarily ill as opposed to dangerously so. It can be based on a child's paleness, degree of drowsiness or confusion, whether a baby feels floppy and cold; in an older child rapid breathing, the hint of a rash or just something less articulated may be sources for alarm in the diagnosing doctor. Parents will often share this feeling and it is a mark of wisdom in a doctor to hear and respond to parental instinct.

INVESTIGATIONS

Investigations are rarely needed in brief feverish illnesses; the results of any tests would come back after the illness has gone. One exception is glandular fever, often suspected on clinical grounds and easily checked by a **blood test** (see page 298). A urine infection is one illness which can give rise to no other symptoms in children and so, if appropriate, a urine culture is often sent for analysis. If there is cause for concern, a full paediatric examination can be arranged at a local hospital.

Persistent fevers – i.e., those lasting more than a week – can be caused by many illnesses other than those which are infectious; e.g., rheumatic conditions, chronic infection such as an abscess or TB (tuberculosis), and even, rarely, cancers.

ASK YOUR DOCTOR

- **About dealing with fever in a child and when to become concerned. Often a quick word with the doctor will allay your fears. Do not be hesitant about drawing attention to your concerns. Point out any relevant information – for example, a friend who has gone down with meningitis or a neighbour who has TB. The doctor can then focus in on these valid worries.**
- **About reducing fever in your child. Fever is a good sign, in that it indicates the body is working to fight off invaders, but high temperatures in children can cause convulsions and must be controlled – usually by paracetamol (Calpol, etc., see below), and, when necessary, sponging with lukewarm water.**

Remedy

GENERAL MEASURES

Whatever the cause you should cool your child's fever by giving an antipyretic (fever-reducing medication). The two best ones are paracetamol or ibuprofen.

Other tricks for lowering temperature are directing a fan over the child or bathing the child in a lukewarm bath. Give plenty of cool, clear drinks to replace the fluid lost by sweating; but do not worry if the child is not eating for a few days.

Aspirin should never be given to children under twelve years except on medical advice (it can cause a rare brain disease called Reye's Syndrome).

SPECIFIC MEASURES

Where the doctor finds a definite infection; e.g., a red ear, inflamed tonsils or signs of chest infection, they will often give an antibiotic; many doctors will advise giving nature a chance to help the body heal itself rather than always giving antibiotics. So be prepared for your doctor to advise against an antibiotic where the child is otherwise well.

Diarrhoea is common in babies and can be treated by giving small regular sips of a salt and glucose solution (available at chemists or on prescription) instead of milk. This does not stop the diarrhoea but it replaces the fluid loss during the 24 to 72 hour period the illness takes to settle.

> *If your baby stops passing urine, dehydration is a possibility and medical attention should be sought immediately.*

The combination of vomiting and diarrhoea is common, but any baby or small child who suffers from this for more than a few hours should be assessed.

ISOLATION
With the disappearance of the serious infectious illnesses, strict isolation is rarely necessary. If your child suffers from rubella, it is wise to keep him out of contact with anyone who may be pregnant. Anyone with a bad cough or cold should not visit people in hospital and should stay away from others with serious heart or chest trouble. Chicken-pox can be dangerous for people with leukaemia, and in older people or those with immune system weaknesses. It's sensible to avoid contact with other ill children as well.

INTENSIVE THERAPY
This is rarely necessary but is reserved for children with overwhelming infections such as meningitis, osteomyelitis (infection of the bone) or as part of the investigation of prolonged fever.

Alternative Treatment

There are herbal and homoeopathic remedies for bringing down fever; homoeopathic treatment includes aconite or belladonna. Herbal remedies embrace everything from aromatherapeutic baths or massages (lavender, eucalyptus and tea tree are both good by the bedside) to aromatic infusions like eucalyptus oil in steaming water. Catmint can be drunk, as can elderflower. Vitamin C is widely used to prevent colds, and there is some evidence that large doses (1000 mg per day) can facilitate faster recovery. Young children should always receive conventional medical attention before seeking alternative treatment.

Prevention

SOCIAL INFRASTRUCTURE
The great preventative measures are those which we in the developed world take for granted: clean abundant water supplies; good sewage arrangements; a varied diet with adequate vitamins and minerals; access to fresh air; and uncrowded and sanitary living conditions. These provisions in any country will reduce infectious illness significantly.

IMMUNIZATION
The value of immunization cannot be overstated; polio, tetanus and measles, to name but three, are diseases which continue to kill and to maim children all round the world but which are almost entirely preventable with vaccination. In the UK your child will be automatically invited for immunization against disease in a programme which begins at age three months and finishes after secondary education (see also page 67).

COMMON SENSE MEASURES

The old phrase 'coughs and sneezes spread diseases' holds true; viruses are spread in the droplets that explode around you after a cough or sneeze. So cough or sneeze into a handkerchief. It is a lesser known fact that cold viruses most often pass hand to hand so it is a preventative measure to wash your hands frequently and to avoid contact. Viruses are usually spread by touching a hand to nose or mouth; if you are in contact with an ill child, avoid touching your face.

As serious infections become rarer, there is a stigma developing around them. Try to overcome this; you are doing no one in your family any favours if you conceal from them that you have measles or chicken-pox, let alone meningitis, tuberculosis or hepatitis. Illness is not a sign of poor hygiene, or habits. Many infectious diseases are 'notifiable', meaning that your doctor must notify the public health authorities so that outbreaks can be controlled. There are recognized problems of confidentiality in the cases of diseases such as **AIDS, hepatitis B**, or venereal disease. See relevant sections.

TRAVELLERS

Exotic diseases such as malaria, rabies, diphtheria are real hazards both for adults and children. Take advice about the recommended injections and tablets for your itinerary and be sure to mention recent travel if you become ill soon after your return. Consider carefully whether you wish to expose your children to the health risks of the Third World and what were once Eastern bloc nations.

Self-Help

Your health visitor is a mine of information about vaccination, infant care and general practical advice on childhood ailments.

VACCINATIONS AND REACTIONS

It is the dilemma facing all parents: whether to leave their child exposed to the known risks of infectious diseases or to have them immunized, thereby exposing them to the rare but possible reactions to the vaccines. It is a question which people in many parts of the world would regard as meaningless; when measles or tetanus are daily killers in a community, a risk from vaccination measured below one in hundreds of thousands is negligible. In the developed world it is a valid question, because childhood has become so safe that there is an illusion that every childhood would be perfect if left alone. This is far from true, but it is difficult to avoid experiencing some concern when contemplating the best course of action for your own baby.

The recommended schedules for vaccination are always under review and gradually change as new vaccines are developed. The current schedule is as follows:

- *Two, three and four months of age: diphtheria, tetanus, whooping cough (pertussis) Haemophilus influenzae (Hib) polio*

- *Around fifteen months of age: measles, mumps, rubella (MMR)*

- *Pre-School (three to five years old): diphtheria, tetanus, polio, measles, mumps, rubella*

- *Around ten years old: BCG, rubella in girls*

There are very few children who should not have a vaccination on medical grounds.

Risk

- If a child has a true sensitivity to egg then vaccines grown on egg cannot be given; these are measles, mumps, rubella.
- Some children have a proven allergy to the antibiotics in the vaccine; i.e., neomycin, polymyxin.
- There is an increased risk of reaction in children with poor immune systems; e.g., those with AIDS or who are having chemotherapy for cancer.
- Any child who is unwell or feverish should have vaccination delayed.
- Polio vaccine is excreted by the child in its faeces so there is a theoretical risk to anyone handling the child who is not themselves immune to polio. This occurs in about one case per two million vaccinations. One child per two million vaccinated contracts polio as a result of the vaccination.
- Women who have been vaccinated against rubella should avoid pregnancy for one month after immunization (this is the current advice even though there has been no reported case of a fetus being affected following rubella immunization).
- Whooping cough vaccination should probably only be avoided where a child has a continuously changing pre-existing neurological handicap. It can be given to children with epilepsy, on a paediatrician's advice. The risk of brain damage is estimated at less than three cases per million vaccinations.
- Measles can cause pneumonia, heart disease and irritation of the brain (encephalitis). A recent epidemic of measles in the USA has resulted in 130 deaths.
- Five per cent of mumps sufferers also have a form of meningitis; inflammation of the testicles occurs in 30 per cent of boys, which can cause sterility. Other rarer risks from mumps are pancreatitis and inflammation of the heart.
- Whooping cough is distressing in itself and carries a high risk of bronchitis, pneumonia and convulsions.
- Prior to 1992, the MMR (see above) vaccine caused a temporary meningitis in about one in every eleven thousand vaccinations. That vaccine was withdrawn; the current one is held to carry a negligible risk, based on results from 150 million doses of the new vaccine given to date.

Recognition

Neither children nor adults like having needles administered, so a period of irritability and crying is only to be expected immediately after the injection. Crying or screaming for more than four hours is considered a significant reaction. Pain and swelling at the site of injection is common. Anything alarming, however, should be seen by your doctor.

Measles/mumps/rubella (MMR) can cause a fever beginning 7 to 10 days after vaccination and lasting for a few days. Swelling of the salivary glands by the angle of the jaw can happen three weeks after that vaccination.

Following whooping cough vaccination fever can occur and, rarely, screaming and convulsions or another allergic reaction. Whether there are any long-term reactions remains controversial. Although it is alleged that persistent fits and behavioural problems have followed whooping cough vaccination, the question is how many cases would have occurred by chance. This question is the subject of current legal action and the outcome cannot be prejudged.

ASK YOUR DOCTOR

- **What the balance of risks is for a child with a congenital neurological problem. Your doctor may wish to have a paediatric second opinion.**
- **About anything that specifically bothers you, if you feel unhappy about having your child vaccinated. Remember that your consent is needed to give vaccination, so a doctor cannot proceed without your agreement.**
- **About any reaction which you consider worrying. Sudden high fevers, convulsions, abnormal swelling around the vaccination site, long-term crying or discomfort, or, on the other hand, an unusual sleepiness or stillness can all be cause for concern.**

Remedy

Giving paracetamol syrup at or soon after immunization relieves the great majority of minor reactions. The very rare cases of convulsions or encephalitis are monitored in hospital. Encephalitis requires general nursing support while the child recovers.

Alternative Treatment

There are no scientifically respectable alternatives to immunization against the common infectious diseases. You may come across homoeopathic substitutes for immunization, the value of which is not proven. Until such time as there is a viable and infallible alternative, conventional vaccinations should be given to children.

Prevention

Immunization is all about prevention – the prevention of avoidable illness and its complications. Within living memory diphtheria, tetanus and polio were feared childhood infections, with a high risk of causing death or permanent disability. Measles vaccination was introduced in 1968 and mumps even later; many adults have had these illnesses and might consider them inevitable risks of childhood. In our modern low-risk world the deafness, birth defects or pain accompanying these illnesses are no longer acceptable, given the comparative safety of vaccines.

The problem which faces parents is that of giving consent to a procedure which carries a risk. Yet how many parents would willingly expose their child to diseases with known risks? Valid public concern has led to very close scrutiny of current vaccines, for which the overwhelming conclusion is that the risks of the vaccine are greatly outweighed by the risks of the diseases they prevent. It's important to remember that childhood diseases are every bit as capable of killing as they ever were.

There is current discussion on the advisability of vaccination against chicken-pox on the grounds of reducing the unpleasantness of the illness itself and the potential complications. The 250,000 cases of chicken-pox each year cause about eight child deaths, and many more cases of encephalitis and widespread infection.

Self-Help

Association of Parents of Vaccine Damaged Children
2 Church Street, Shipton on Stour, CV36 4AP
Tel: 01608 661 595

Campaign for Justice for all Vaccine Damaged Children
Erin's Cottage, Fussell's Buildings, Whiteway Road, Bristol BS5 7QY
Tel: 0117 955-7818

THE FEMALE REPRODUCTIVE SYSTEM

- Breast Cancer • Breast Pain • Cancer of the Uterus
- Cervical Cancer • Endometriosis • Infertility
- Menopause • Miscarriage • Ovarian Cancer
- Pre-Menstrual Syndrome (PMS) • Sexually
Transmitted Disease (STDs)

T HE REGULAR MONTHLY cycle of menstruation and the profound changes of pregnancy and the menopause make women far more closely attuned to their bodies than men. Much is understood about the delicately balanced hormone pathways which regulate these changes and the subtle interaction with emotion and with psychological factors.

Women have long promoted self-awareness, screening programmes for gynaecological disease and encouraged women to take some responsibility for their own health, all activities which men are belatedly taking up. It is relatively easy to investigate abnormalities in the reproductive tract and in the breasts, especially with the continual improvement in ultrasound scanning and the development of day case procedures for sampling the lining of the womb.

With a regular monthly cycle to act as a guide, women are well placed to spot deviations from what is normal for them and to have this checked.

BREAST CANCER

Possibly no other form of cancer is as feared as breast cancer; research into the causes has been enormous; 'breakthroughs' are announced almost weekly. A breast cancer screening service has been in place for several years. Modern medicine has much to offer anyone developing this disease, but the best way of improving your chances remains early recognition of abnormalities in the breast, as detailed below.

Risk

- 6 in every 100 women will develop breast cancer.
- It is the commonest form of cancer in women.
- Breast cancer accounts for about 20 per cent of all deaths from cancer in women in the UK; some 15,000 deaths per annum.
- Breast cancers are rare below the age of 25.
- It is still uncommon at thirty.
- The risk steadily increases with age; at 45 there are 140 cases per 100,000 women, rising to 240 cases per 100,000 women by age 85.

- The risks are slightly higher for women who: have never had children; have children late (twice the risk for a first child after thirty than for someone who has had children before twenty); have a close relative such as mother or sister who has had breast cancer (double the risk).
- The United Kingdom has one of the highest rates of breast cancer in the world, as do the USA and Canada. Yet it is relatively uncommon in Japan and Argentina. Why this should be so is unknown.
- Obesity doubles the risk in post-menopausal women.
- HRT for ten or more years increases risk by 50 per cent but this is outweighed by the beneficial effects on heart disease and osteoporosis.
- Men can develop the disease, though rarely.

Recognition

Be alert to breast lumps, pain, changes in the shape of the nipple, bleeding from the nipple. Report any of these to your doctor.

SIGNS AND SYMPTOMS

- Breast lumps

These are common and only about one in ten may be cancerous. Younger women, from teens to late twenties, will frequently feel a firm lump that seems to skate from under the fingers. These are known as breast mice, technically fibroadenomas (a firm lump made up of fibrous tissue), and are not forms of cancer. The warning signs of a serious lump are if it is hard, feels fixed to the skin, is painful and is associated with firm glands in the armpit on that side.

- Pain

It is suspicious to have an area of the breast which keeps feeling sore and uncomfortable, such as a prickling sensation under the skin. Of course most women experience some general tenderness of the breasts as a normal part of their regular monthly menstrual cycle. Learn to recognize what is normal for you so you can tell what is unusual.

- Change in shape of the nipple

If a nipple which previously stood out begins to retract into the breast, it is a sign of underlying breast cancer until proven otherwise. In older women one nipple may become cracked, itchy and sore, perhaps with a slight bloody ooze. This can be harmless, but may be a localized form of breast cancer called Paget's Disease of the Breast and must be checked.

- Bleeding from the nipple

There are several harmless reasons for this, including infection and inflammation but it should not be ignored as it may be the only sign of a small early cancer.

INVESTIGATIONS

- Mammography

In the UK all women from fifty to sixty-five years of age are offered mammography every three years. This test involves an **X-ray** (see page 301) of the breast aimed at detecting cancer even before any of the symptoms given above. There is little doubt that it does pick up early disease. What is less certain is whether this makes any difference to the woman's life expectancy. In the UK it is still too soon to tell. Some countries which have had enthusiastic screening programs for longer, such the USA and Sweden, are sure that it does reduce death rates. What is clear is that mammography allows treatment to start earlier, so reducing the severity of the treatment needed and giving more years of health.

● Biopsy

To make a definite diagnosis, at some point the breast has to be sampled. If possible this is done via a fine needle but it is frequently necessary to remove a lump or other suspicious area and analyze it. Once the exact nature of the cancer is known, appropriate treatment can be planned.

ASK YOUR DOCTOR
- **Is there a local specialist in breast disorders?**
- **When you should be reviewed, if symptoms persist.**
- **How quickly a second opinion can be arranged.**

Remedy

The mutilating surgery of fifty years ago is no longer routine in treatment. Where once the breast, the underlying chest muscles and all the glands in the armpit would frequently be removed, the trend has been to remove just the cancerous lump itself or, according to some specialists, not even that. Treatment will then usually be with **radiotherapy** (see page 301), **chemotherapy** (see page 298) or a combination of the two. There are different intensities of treatment available. At the one extreme there is high-dosage radiation and high-intensity chemotherapy. There are many distressing side-effects such as sickness, hair loss and radiation burns. Yet in pre-menopausal women this may offer the best chance of cure. In older women who have gone through the menopause, breast cancer often follows a more benign course and in such cases treatment may be simply to take long-term drugs; the most well known is called tamoxifen and works by counteracting the oestrogen or female hormone in the body.

Treatment should be an intensely individual affair and calls for close discussion between doctor, patient and family. There follows a long period of follow-up, checking for regrowth of the cancer or for signs of the cancer spreading elsewhere, such as to the bones causing bone pain, or to the liver causing jaundice.

Cure is difficult to define. Doctors talk not of cure but of survival, to one year after treatment, three years, five years, ten years. With the passage of each year cure is more likely.

Alternative Treatment

Alternative therapies have had wide media exposure but have yet to show results that stand up to scientific scrutiny. However, a therapy which offers support, encourages a positive mental attitude, determination and courage does much good and few doctors would argue against such an approach. Until unconventional treatments have been scientifically shown to make a difference, no woman should spurn a conventional medical assessment at some point in her disease.

Some therapies, like acupuncture and homoeopathy may encourage your body to become stronger, suffering less trauma from the illness and ensuring that recuperation is quick. In the event of radiotherapy or chemotherapy treatment, many alternative therapies can work to relieve stress, some of the worst side-effects, like nausea and burns, and, most importantly, stimulate the body to heal itself. Post-operatively, any of the relaxation therapies might help.

Prevention

- First and foremost, report symptoms early.
- If close members of your family have had breast cancer, it may be advisable for you to have regular breast checks or mammograms. Be sure to tell your doctor if this is the case.
- The contraceptive pill: there is controversy as to whether taking the pill as a teenager increases the risk of breast cancer later. Current evidence suggests a very small but possible increase in risk. This has to be weighed against the risks and long-term effects of a teenage pregnancy. Your doctor should be able to give more guidance on the latest evidence.
- There are ongoing trials to see if tamoxifen can be taken as a preventative treatment by women who are healthy. This may herald a time when breast cancer, like measles or lung cancer, becomes an avoidable disease.
- Two breast cancer genes have recently been identified, accounting for families where several members have had the disease and these genes may be a future target for screening.

Self-Help

Breast Cancer Care
15–19 Britten Street, London SW3 3TZ
Helpline: 0500 245 345

BREAST PAIN

This common symptom is experienced by most women at some time or other. Usually it is due simply to the effects of the changing levels of hormones during the monthly menstrual cycle. There will be a degree of discomfort which is normal for you; take notice of an increase or a localization of pain to one part of the breast. Painful lumps can also appear while breastfeeding, and represent milk building up behind, perhaps, a blocked duct. Breastfeeding can also produce sore nipples and pain when there is engorgement.

There may well be an emotional element in breast pain, especially a fear of breast cancer, and it is frequently a part of the **pre-menstrual syndrome** (see page 94). Though not all women can be made pain free, something can be done for most cases to give relief.

Risk

- 40 per cent of women experience breast pain at some point in their monthly cycle.
- Pain from breast infection is common during breastfeeding.
- Breast pain is common in the first few weeks after starting the contraceptive pill or hormone replacement therapy (HRT).
- Minor injury to the chest wall often bruises the breast but it may be a few days before pain begins, by which time the injury has been forgotten.

Recognition

SYMPTOMS

Generalized pain in the breast is self-evident. Note also whether it varies according to your monthly cycle, whether there is one specific site of pain, and, if so, whether there is a lump in that area.

SIGNS

Your doctor will look for:
- a breast lump (see **breast cancer**, page 71);
- puckering of the skin at the site of pain (see **breast cancer**, page 71);
- discharge or bleeding from the nipple;
- signs of infection especially if you are breastfeeding; a breast abscess causes severe pain in one breast;
- evidence of fluid retention such as swollen ankles.

INVESTIGATIONS

Further investigations may include **mammography** (see page 72).

ASK YOUR DOCTOR
- **If he or she is confident about the diagnosis.**
- **In what circumstances you should come back for a review.**
- **How your symptoms should be investigated, if you have a family history of breast disease.**

Remedy

- Breast pain which occurs in a regular monthly cycle is easier to treat than pain which occurs at any time in the month.
- If the cause seems to be a hormone preparation such as the Pill, it usually settles down in time. Occasionally a change of Pill is required.
- If it is related to your own monthly cycle there are several options. A simple diuretic 'water tablet' that makes you lose fluid may be sufficient, taken in the run-up to your period. There are other powerful hormones that help in extreme cases; for example, danazol and bromocriptine, but these do carry a risk of side-effects.
- Simple reassurance helps in many cases, especially where there is an underlying fear of breast cancer. American studies show that 75 per cent of women are helped by reassurance alone.
- Specific breast diseases will have their own remedy: an abscess is treated with antibiotics.

Alternative Treatment

Oil of evening primrose has been found to help some women. Many herbal remedies can work as a mild diuretic, particularly useful pre-menstrually. A trained homoeopath or acupuncturist would prescribe treatment according to your other symptoms. A reduction in dietary fat helps some women.

CANCER OF THE WOMB

The womb is a dynamic environment. Not only does it go through a regular monthly cycle of growth and breakdown, but it also undergoes the amazing changes of pregnancy. Its cells are influenced by hormones and these same hormones are intimately involved in causing cancer.

Risk

- There are 10 per 100,000 women at age 40 who contract the disease; 60 per 100,000 at age 50; 125 per 100,000 at age 70.
- About 75 per cent of cases occur at or after the menopause, especially between ages 50 and 60.
- There is a higher risk in women whose periods began early or which end in a later than usual menopause.
- There is a higher risk in women who have not had children.
- There is an increased risk in the overweight and in those with diabetes (possibly double).
- Certain hormones may increase the risk, especially hormone replacement therapy (HRT) (see page 86).
- Middle-class women are more prone to the disease than working-class women.
- Of all cases of abnormal bleeding at or about the time of menopause only 10 per cent will be due to cancer of the womb. Even in cases of bleeding after the menopause only 25 per cent will be due to cancer.

Recognition

SYMPTOMS

- Bleeding after the menopause

This is the prime symptom of which you should be aware. It may be bleeding after intercourse or a couple of spots of blood on your underclothes. There may just be a watery discharge tinged pink by blood. No matter how little blood you see it is essential to have it checked out.

- Irregular, heavy or prolonged menstrual bleeding

Although only 25 per cent of cases occur before the menopause, it may show itself as a change in your menstrual pattern. Unfortunately, similar changes occur frequently at that time anyway, most of which are down to perfectly benign variations in your hormone balance. Changes which are dramatic or persistent should be reported, to be on the safe side. One of the commonest causes for similar symptoms is fibroids. These are benign muscular growths in the wall of the womb which can grow to enormous size. Usually there is a characteristic feel on examination.

- Pain

Pain in the lower abdomen may be a feature of more advanced disease.

SIGNS

A doctor will feel for a hard enlargement of the womb with the womb feeling fixed and immobile. Blood may be visible, oozing through the cervix. In the case of a blood-tinged discharge, it may be that the walls of the post-menopausal vagina have become so thin that they bleed spontaneously. This is common, harmless and easily treated with a hormone cream.

INVESTIGATIONS

● Dilatation and curettage (D&C)

This was the standard method of diagnosis, by which a scraping of the lining of the womb is taken under anaesthetic. Analysis of the scrapings will detect cancerous cells. Many more D&Cs are undertaken than cases of cancer of the womb are found. It is a kind of screening test, as frequently no cause is found for the bleeding.

● Endometrial biopsy

In this procedure a sample is taken from the womb as an outpatient procedure and not requiring an anaesthetic (see **biopsy**, page 298).

● Ultrasound scanning

A good idea of whether there is a problem can be obtained by this technique, similar to the familiar method used to monitor a baby's growth during pregnancy. Painless and quick, it shows up the walls of the womb, picking out areas of unusual thickness which may harbour a cancer. It cannot give a diagnosis in itself, but it helps decide how urgently a woman should go on for further investigation (see **ultrasound**, page 301).

ASK YOUR DOCTOR
● **What is the latest thinking about the risks of taking hormone replacement therapy (HRT).**
● **To perform an internal check every year or so if you are on HRT.**

Remedy

A definite diagnosis of cancer of the womb will usually mean going on to a hysterectomy (removal of the womb) and bilateral oophorectomy (removal of both ovaries). The ovaries are removed because they produce female hormones which would encourage the growth of any deposits of the cancer elsewhere in the body. If the cancer has spread from the womb itself then more extensive surgery is done to try to remove as much tissue into which the cancer may have seeded itself.

It is usual to have **radiotherapy** (see page 301) a week or two after surgery; that is to say, a focused beam of radiation is aimed onto the pelvis to try to kill any remaining cancerous cells. In very advanced disease **chemotherapy** (see page 298) is used, in which a cocktail of drugs is given again with the aim of killing cells which may have spread elsewhere in the body,

The outlook for early disease is quite good, with something like an 85 per cent survival to five years. More advanced disease has a poorer outlook, but much can be done to relieve symptoms for at least a couple of years.

Alternative Treatment

General support and care through whatever school of alternative therapy appeals to you is sensible. There are no specific alternative treatments that can be recommended for treatment of the condition once established, although acupuncture, in particular, claims to be of some use. Post-operatively, many of the therapies can enhance recovery, strengthening the body and encouraging it to heal. Particular therapies of some use in this case may be acupuncture, homoeopathy, herbalism and nutritional therapy.

Prevention

Clearly the best way of catching this disease early is to take notice of and to report the kinds of unusual bleeding patterns detailed above. Doctors and gynaecologists are well used to investigating even minor irregularities of this kind, so you should not think that you are making a fuss about nothing. Statistics show that there will often be a benign cause for the bleeding, such as hormone disturbance, and very frequently no cause at all can be found even after careful investigation.

Women on hormone replacement therapy (HRT) should be especially alert to changes in their pattern of bleeding. Modern HRT treatments for women who still have their womb contain oestrogen, which is the hormone being replaced, and an additional hormone, called a progestogen, which is taken for a few days each month. The pills containing progestogen are a different colour from the pills for the rest of the month. The whole object of this additional hormone is to counteract the effect of pure oestrogen which would otherwise increase the risk of cancer of the womb.

Some women, realizing that those additional pills bring on monthly bleeding, may be tempted to omit them to avoid the inconvenience. This is highly dangerous as it will increase the risk of cancer. The latest HRT pills combine the hormones to make it impossible to miss out the progestogen.

Self-Help

BACUP (British Association of Cancer United Patients)
3 Bath Place, Rivington Road, London EC2A 3JR
Tel: 0800 181199

Women's Health Concern
83 Earls Court Road, London W8 6EF
Tel: 0171 938-3932

CERVICAL CANCER

The cervix is the neck of the womb, a fleshy structure that juts out into the top of the vagina. It is the channel through which the menstrual flow reaches the outside world and the conduit through which sperm swim en route to fertilize an egg. The cervix is similar to skin and is prone to many changes that ordinary skin shows. Polyps – fleshy wart-like growths – are common, as are erosions, which are sore areas that weep fluid causing a heavy or offensive vaginal discharge. But most worrying is the change to cancer.

Risk

- Cervical cancer accounts for some 2500 deaths per annum in the UK (1860 in 1992).
- It is commonest between the ages of 45 and 55.
- Cervical cancer is commoner in women beginning intercourse in their teens and with multiple partners.

- It is more common in lower social groups.
- Women who smoke have an increased risk.
- There is some evidence that use of the sheath (condom) for contraception is protective.
- There is increasing evidence that viruses are involved in causing the condition.

Recognition

The whole aim of the cervical smear screening program is to pick up pre-malignant changes, before a cancer has reached the stage of causing noticeable symptoms.

SYMPTOMS

- Bleeding between periods

The raw tissue of a cancerous cervix may ooze blood at any time of the month, often accompanied by a heavy vaginal discharge which may turn smelly or itchy. Perfectly innocent problems can also cause this symptom (for example, erosion of the cervix or harmless hormonal irregularities in the menstrual cycle). However, inter-menstrual bleeding at any age should not be ignored.

- Bleeding after intercourse

Another common symptom which often has an innocent cause such as an erosion or a polyp, but which again may be the earliest feature of cancer.

- Heavy/smelly vaginal discharge

A cancer of the cervix may become the focus of infection giving rise to these symptoms, though there are many other straightforward infections which may be to blame.

- Pain

It may come as a surprise to know that the cervix does not register pain. Internal pain is therefore a late feature of this condition, indicating that the cancer has spread from the cervix itself into surrounding structures which can feel pain, such as the womb or lymph nodes. Only through self-neglect would pain be the first symptom of the problem.

SIGNS

When the doctor examines the cervix it may look unhealthy, being raw, oozing blood on light touch, and feeling hard.

INVESTIGATIONS

A cervical smear involves taking a scraping of cells from the cervix for examination under a microscope. Skilled personnel can grade those cells into those which look normal, those which look suspicious and those which look frankly malignant.

A **colposcopy** (see page 298) is similar to taking a smear, but the cervix is examined under a high-powered microscope. This allows the doctor to select areas which look unusual and to take samples from those areas.

ASK YOUR DOCTOR

- **To examine you if you have any of the above symptoms.**
- **If you can have a smear every three years.**
- **Whether the local hospital offers colposcopy to women with mildly abnormal cervical smears (a so-called dyskaryotic smear). The latest research is suggesting that such a service should be available nationwide.**

Remedy

If you have taken advantage of the cervical screening service, any possible cancer should be detected at an early stage, meaning treatment can be quite minor.

PARTIAL REMOVAL OF CERVIX

This involves cutting out a section of the cervix, including any area shown to contain premalignant cells. The cutting may be done with a hot wire or a laser. The cervix heals rapidly. You still need regular review. The treatment can affect future pregnancies.

HYSTERECTOMY

This is used for more advanced disease, aiming to reduce the possibility of spread of the cancer into the womb and surrounding tissues.

RADIOTHERAPY

This is reserved for more advanced disease, or where it is shown at surgery that the cancer has spread elsewhere in the pelvis (see **radiotherapy**, page 301).

Treatment of early disease carries an excellent outlook, with a better than 80 per cent five-year survival. This drops dramatically with cases of advanced disease where survival at five years is 5 to 10 per cent.

Prevention

- Stop smoking, and avoid sexual relations with more than one partner; promiscuity and smoking increase the risk of the disease at an early age.
- The cervical smear screening programme offers the best chance of detecting this disease early. Yet the programme is surrounded by controversy. It is agreed that it detects early disease, but some experts argue that it has not resulted in a dramatic fall in deaths from cervical cancer in the UK. Other countries have produced better results, such as in Vancouver, Canada, one of the pioneers of the cervical smear screening programme, where the fall in death rates is impressive. Better evidence is expected within the next few years.
- It is known that those women most at risk of the disease (lower class with many sexual partners) are the hardest to persuade to come for screening. The government hopes that this will change in the UK where doctors are now financially encouraged to persuade women to have cervical smears.
- How frequently should you have a smear? Some women find it reassuring to have one every year. The cost of offering this to all women is very high. The government has adopted a five-yearly programme; many doctors feel this is too infrequent and would advise smears on a three-yearly basis. Unfortunately, not all hospitals agree to this and so in parts of the country women have to go privately if they wish to have smears every three years. Hopefully this will change. Of course women with any of the symptoms above would be offered a smear anyway, regardless of when they last had one.

Self-Help

Women's Nationwide Cancer Control Campaign
Suna House, 128–130 Curtain Road, London EC2A 3AR
Tel: 0171 729-2229

Most GPs have nurses who can provide advice and guidance.

ENDOMETRIOSIS

Endometriosis is a condition which has been recognized for years but which is just emerging into wider public awareness. It accounts for many cases of pelvic pain and infertility. Endometriosis occurs when the cells which normally make up the lining of the womb somehow are transported and grow elsewhere in the body, like seedlings. This happens most commonly in the pelvis, where the deposits can be seen scattered over the outside of the womb and on the ovaries. Less often the seedlings grow in the skin, lungs or navel. The cells may even seed themselves within the womb itself.

Since these cells are exactly like those in the womb they change through the menstrual cycle, even to the extent of bleeding regularly each month. You can imagine some of the odd symptoms that can result; coughing up blood for a few days each month or having a belly button that oozes blood each month.

Within the abdomen, as the blood cannot properly escape it acts as an irritant, causing thick layers of fibrous tissue to build up around the seedling. With time, these thick deposits bind down the womb or other internal structures, giving rise to the symptoms below.

The cause of this bizarre condition is unknown, though theories abound. The likeliest explanation is that at the time of menstruation, blood containing cells from the womb passes back up through the Fallopian tubes and spills into the pelvis, from where the cells then spread and seed themselves. This cannot account for all cases.

Risk

- Endometriosis is found in 14 to 21 per cent of women who have an exploratory operation for presumed gynaecological disease, often as an unexpected finding.
- About 14 per cent of infertile women prove to have endometriosis; some researchers report up to 33 per cent.
- 30 to 40 per cent of women with endometriosis are infertile.
- The condition is more common in those without children and in women of higher social class.
- The severity of symptoms bears no reliable relation to the extent of the physical findings.

Recognition

SYMPTOMS
- Painful, heavy periods
There are many causes for this, for example, infections, hormone imbalance, and the coil (IUDs); but of women with endometriosis some 50 per cent report progressively more heavy and painful periods.
- Infertility
Although 30 to 40 per cent of women with endometriosis are infertile, there are many other causes of infertility.
- Pain deep inside during intercourse (dyspareunia)
This is probably due to pressure on the ovaries due to the masses of fibrous tissue.
These are the classical features of endometriosis; if a woman presents with these symptoms the diagnosis should spring to mind, along with the possibility of chronic pelvic infection (see **sexually transmitted diseases**, STDs, page 96). Beyond these

classic symptoms there are many vague symptoms, such as lower abdominal pain, backache or a general lack of wellbeing. There may be no symptoms at all, the condition being discovered on investigation for infertility.

SIGNS

Large cysts and large amounts of fibrous tissue may give a characteristic feel on gynaecological examination. More often, however, the diagnosis is suspected from the patient's history rather than found on examination.

INVESTIGATIONS

● Laparoscopy

In this common procedure a thin tube is passed into the abdomen, allowing the gynaecologist to have a good look at the internal organs. This is the most reliable way of diagnosing endometriosis, as the characteristic cysts can be seen and samples taken for analysis. It also allows the specialist to check that the symptoms are not being caused by chronic pelvic infection, which gives rise to a very similar set of symptoms, but which is treated quite differently.

ASK YOUR DOCTOR

● **If you feel your symptoms fit; there is no harm in asking your doctor whether it is a possibility.**
● **Whether endometriosis has been considered as a cause of vague lower abdominal discomfort.**
● **Whether you should have a laparoscopy if you are having trouble becoming pregnant.**

Remedy

It has to be said that the treatment of endometriosis is not ideal. While it is possible to give some relief to minor symptoms, major symptoms of pain and infertility all too often end up in difficult choices for both the sufferer and her gynaecologist. Major surgery carries no guarantee of long-term cure; hysterectomy may be a final resort, but at the cost of sterility.

Not every case of endometriosis needs treating. It may have been found incidentally during surgery for some unrelated condition, or you may be past child-bearing age and can live with any symptoms. If it is causing symptoms then there are various options. Simplest is just to cut away the fibrous bands and to burn (cauterize) small deposits of endometriosis.

Next are hormone treatments ranging from the contraceptive pill to highly sophisticated hormones which interfere with the action of oestrogen (female hormone) on the deposits of endometriosis.

Lastly there is the option of major surgery to remove as much of the endometriosis as possible, together with the womb and ovaries. Of course this is an option to be used only when there is no desire for children or if there are severe symptoms which non-surgical options have not relieved.

Alternative Treatment

Some therapists believe that vitamins help in the treatment of endometriosis; for example, B vitamins and vitamin E. Calcium is said to help cramps. Acupuncture is another technique worth trying. There are also homoeopathic remedies, focusing on the painful periods, and treatment will be designed according to your constitution and symptom picture. Osteopathic treatment might encourage draining through the veins, which can help congestion of the uterus. There is long-term herbal treatment available, aimed at hormone levels and improving the function of the ovaries. Some women claim that aromatherapy has been useful.

Prevention

There is no known means of prevention of this condition. With increasing awareness it will be diagnosed earlier and this may prevent years of uncertainty about the cause of vague pelvic pains.

Self-Help

National Endometriosis Society
Suite 50, Westminster Palace Gardens, 1–7 Artillery Row, London, SWIP 1RL
Tel: 0171 222-2776

INFERTILITY

Infertility is defined as failure to fall pregnant after a year of regular sexual intercourse. It is an area which has seen an immense amount of research in the last twenty years, aimed at finding out more about the causes and in developing treatments. The successes of infertility treatments make front-page news, but responsible researchers in the field are more cautious about claiming breakthroughs. They know that the hopes of thousands of couples rest on their efforts and they are careful not to raise those hopes unrealistically. Nevertheless, the treatment of infertility has been one of the success stories of medicine in the late twentieth century. So much so that some suggest using the term subfertility instead of the term infertility, to reflect the modern possibility of improving the chances of conception.

Risk

- 90 per cent of couples will achieve a pregnancy after one year of trying.
- About 92.5 per cent of all couples will eventually achieve pregnancy.
- Of the 10 per cent of couples infertile at one year, about a quarter will eventually conceive, but the chances reduce with each year that passes.
- Smoking more than twenty cigarettes a day reduces the chances by 20 per cent.
- 30 to 40 per cent of cases are due to male infertility, not female.
- 30 per cent of cases involve the woman only.
- In about 15 per cent of cases no explanation can be found despite thorough investigation.
- Older women are less fertile than younger women.
- Any general disease, such as **diabetes** (see page 204), reduces the chances of pregnancy.

Recognition

Careful enquiry sometimes reveals a history of heavy, slightly late periods which could have been very early miscarriages, or infrequent intercourse which fails to give a true picture of the couple's fertility. It is also not unheard of for a woman to use the contraceptive pill or a coil without their partner's knowledge. Sensitive initial interviewing should uncover these potentially embarrassing factors which in turn may point to psychological uncertainty about achieving pregnancy on the part of one or other partner.

SIGNS AND INVESTIGATIONS
The doctor wants to check certain basic information:
- Are you having normal intercourse? Pregnancy cannot result from ejaculation into any other orifice than the vagina.
- Is the man producing good quantities of healthy sperm? Certainly only one is needed for pregnancy, but the wastage rate of sperm is huge and they have a daunting journey from vagina to egg.
- Is the woman releasing healthy eggs and can those eggs travel from the ovaries to the womb?
- Are there any diseases or problems in the womb preventing the egg from implanting and growing?

IN THE MAN:
- There will be an examination of testicles, a sperm count and checking for infections affecting the sperm.
- Excess consumption of alcohol reduces fertility and can cause impotence.
- It is thought that smoking affects sperm production.

IN THE WOMAN:
- A gynaecological examination might detect previous infection which is tethering down the womb and ovaries, or evidence of **endometriosis** (see page 81). Symptoms suggesting such problems include heavy painful periods, pain on intercourse and persistent vaginal discharge.
- Being underweight or dieting excessively can reduce fertility by suppressing periods.
- Blood tests check out hormone levels and coexisting disease, such as diabetes, which may play a part in reducing fertility.
- A Hystero-salpingogram involves a **laparoscopy** (see page 300) at which a harmless dye is introduced into the vagina. The gynaecologist checks whether the dye spills out from the Fallopian tubes. If no dye spills out there must be a blockage in the tube.

IN BOTH:
- Sperm is gathered from the vagina shortly after intercourse (a post-coital test). As well as checking whether adequate amounts of sperm are being delivered, this also shows whether the woman is producing antibodies to her partner's sperm, killing them off just like germs.

ASK YOUR DOCTOR

- **About any marital factors that may worry you.**
- **Whether treatment for infertility is available on the NHS in your area. Infertility treatment is increasingly being withdrawn from the NHS. Private treatment is carefully regulated and is generally of high quality, but can cost several thousand pounds.**
- **Who your doctor recommends for further treatment.**

Remedy

Treatment is directed at any identifiable cause.

IN THE MAN:

- An inadequate sperm count can be caused by abnormalities in the testicles, sometimes treatable by surgery (such as a varicocele). Otherwise the count can be raised by keeping the testicles cooler by wearing loose fitting underpants and avoiding hot baths. Some specialists, more controversially, give male hormones to boost the sperm count. Doxycline (an antibiotic) may enhance sperm count and motility.
- The male partner may have perfectly adequate sperm but there may be some reason such as impotence, why he cannot perform adequate intercourse. In these cases his sperm can be gathered and used to fertilize the woman This is AIH – artificial insemination by husband.
- If he is sterile, then AID can be offered to the woman, that is artificial insemination by donor. The donor is someone other than the husband and remains entirely anonymous.

IN THE WOMAN:

- It is now easy to stimulate the ovaries to produce eggs, using drugs such as clomiphene. Anatomical abnormalities in the womb or ovaries can often be treated surgically; e.g., opening up blocked tubes, or removing fibroids from the womb. Up to 40 per cent of women where this is the problem go on to conceive.
- Failing that, the woman's eggs can be harvested from the ovaries, fertilized outside the womb and then implanted directly into the womb. This is the so-called test-tube baby treatment properly called in-vitro fertilization (IVF). Even in the best centres there is only a 12.5 per cent chance of success (i.e. pregnancies carried to term) using this method.

Simple measures should not be ignored; increase intercourse at the time of the month when the egg is released; try different positions for intercourse to help sperm reach the womb. Couples going in for investigation and treatment of infertility must be prepared for a difficult time. The investigations can be unpleasant, sexual intercourse can all too easily be reduced to a mechanical act at the right time of the month. Only a small percentage of couples treated with in vitro fertilization succeed, even in the best centres, though the percentage is gradually improving.

The pace of investigation can seem infuriatingly slow; this is deliberate; whatever the treatment 25 per cent of couples infertile at one year will eventually conceive naturally so doctors will avoid operations until nature has been given a fair chance.

Alternative Treatment

Put an emphasis on a healthy diet, regular but not excessive exercise and avoidance of alcohol. A nutritional therapist would suggest supplementation with the mineral zinc, which appears to be low in many cases of male infertility, and some female. Slight deficiencies of vitamins or minerals is called a subclinical deficiency, and there is some evidence that these can affect the body enormously. Acupuncture can improve hormone balance in women, and claims to be able to improve the sperm count and quality of sperm in men. An aromatherapist might direct treatment at low oestrogen levels in the female, or at pelvic infection; in the male, sperm cell production might be increased. A homoeopath would address treatment to your constitution, that is one chosen to suit your individual nature.

Prevention

As with alternative therapy the emphasis is on a life of moderation. The major avoidable factors are:

- Cigarette smoking in either partner.
- Excessive intake of alcohol.
- Pelvic infection. Women are at risk of this if they have multiple sexual partners and if they ignore symptoms of infection such as heavy vaginal discharges, increasingly heavy and painful periods. Condoms may help reduce the risk.
- Wearing tight fitting underwear (men), which reduces sperm counts by increasing the temperature of the testicles.
- Dieting to excess; this destabilizes periods.
- Any general illness.

Dealing with the above factors is most successful if there is marginal infertility where a small improvement may make all the difference.

Self-Help

ISSUE – National Fertility Association
509 Aldridge Rd, Great Barr, Birmingham B44 8NA
Tel: 0121 344-4414

Women's Health Concern
83 Earls Court Road, London W8 6EF
Tel: 0171 938-3932

Fertility clinics advertise nationally; seek your doctor's opinion before committing yourself.

MENOPAUSE

The menopause is that time in a woman's life when her periods cease permanently. The ovaries stop producing eggs; the levels of oestrogen (female hormone) drop; the whole intricate system of monthly hormone regulation ceases. It is rarely a sudden event; it is more likely a gradual reduction in the regular monthly pattern. Women who have had a hysterectomy but who still have their ovaries will also experience menopausal symptoms when their ovaries eventually stop working.

The menopause attracts enormous interest, both for its physical and its psychological importance. It ushers out the time of fertility and ushers in what many women see as 'old age' in a way that has no parallel for men. Many, probably most, women cope with the menopause well, if a bit regretfully. For those who do not, there are a variety of effective treatments.

Risk

- 100 per cent of women will go through the menopause.
- On average it occurs around fifty but it can happen from the mid-thirties to the mid-fifties.
- The best guide to when it will occur is when your mother went through it.
- Removal of the ovaries causes an abrupt artificial menopause.
- Only a minority of women have serious trouble in the menopause.
- On average women who smoke go into the menopause two years earlier than non-smokers.

Recognition

SYMPTOMS

In the years just before the menopause, periods often become erratic; perhaps happening more or less frequently and either heavier or lighter than usual. This is due to a loss of fine control in the beautifully balanced hormone system that controls menstruation. Eventually the periods stop; by convention the menopause is taken to be when there have been no periods for a year.

As the levels of female hormone fall, so you start to have hot flushes and often night sweats. The skin becomes coarser; in particular the vaginal skin becomes thinner, which may give rise to soreness on intercourse. It is common to start having vague aches and pains in the joints.

The menopause has been blamed for each and every psychological symptom imaginable: depression, irritability, anxiety, decreased sexual drive, increased sexual drive, insomnia, tiredness, lack of concentration; the list goes on. It is quite uncertain which of these symptoms is directly due to the menopause. It is likely that the menopause forces a woman to confront the fact of her own ageing, with psychological symptoms flowing from how she comes to terms with that.

Some women welcome the menopause for relieving the nuisance of periods and for removing the risk of pregnancy.

SIGNS AND INVESTIGATIONS

Blood tests (see page 298) are useful if there is some doubt about the symptoms; perhaps the woman is unusually young; perhaps she has had a hysterectomy so that the absence of periods is no guide. The tests measure oestrogen levels or the levels of the other hormones – Follicle Stimulating Hormone (FSH), Luteinizing Hormone (LH) – involved in menstruation. An **overactive thyroid gland** (see page 211) can mimic some symptoms of the menopause; for example, hot sweats, irregular periods; a blood test will diagnose this.

ASK YOUR DOCTOR
- **To discuss the pros and cons of hormone replacement treatment (HRT, see below) in your case.**
- **To check out the significance of *any* vaginal bleeding after the menopause; this may be a symptom of cancer of the uterus (see page 76).**

Remedy

PSYCHOLOGICAL SUPPORT
Explanation and reassurance about the symptoms to be expected are very helpful. It goes without saying that support and tolerance by partners is invaluable but do not assume that every menopausal woman needs handling like a box of eggs. Nor should the menopause be made the scapegoat for every symptom. It is presumptuous to regard the menopausal woman as no more than a chaotic jumble of hormones; such an attitude, apart from being demeaning in itself, can delay the recognition of serious psychological or physical illness that is as likely to occur at the menopause as at any other time.

HORMONE REPLACEMENT THERAPY
Commonly known as HRT, this gives back to the woman the oestrogen her body is no longer making. This can be done by a daily tablet; by wearing a patch which releases oestrogen through the skin or by injection every few months. This is fine for women who have had a hysterectomy.

Women who still have their womb need to take an additional hormone, progestogen, for a few days each month. This protects the womb against the increased risk of cancer of the uterus which would result from taking oestrogen alone.

HRT has many benefits, including:

- a general sense of well-being;
- reduction or cessation of the hot flushes and sweats;
- protection against post-menopausal thinning of bone (*osteoporosis*, see page 174), so reducing the chances of fractures in old age;
- reduction of vaginal dryness, relieving soreness and making intercourse more comfortable.
- probably protection against heart disease;
- relief of many of the aches and pains women experience at the menopause.

There are some drawbacks to HRT:
- it increases the risk of breast cancer, though quite how much is uncertain;
- it increases the risk of cancer of the uterus, unless taken with a progestogen (see above);
- it may increase blood pressure and the risk of blood clots (thrombosis) in the legs;
- some women start to have periods again; this can be unacceptable.

The current climate of opinion is that for most women the benefits of taking HRT for a few years outweigh the risks. Certainly taking it for a year or two can bring huge relief of symptoms. The controversy is over how long it should be taken. At least five to ten years is needed to give protection against osteoporosis into old age. Yet taking it for years on end increases the risks of cancer of the breast and womb. There is no certain answer at present although the balance is tending to favour HRT more and more; trials are continuing and meanwhile it can only be left to individual discussion in the light of personal circumstances and the latest evidence.

OESTROGEN CREAM
This can be very useful in relieving vaginal dryness if that is the main symptom.

NON-HORMONAL TREATMENTS
Hot flushes can be helped by drugs such as clonidine or a beta-blocker. It is a good idea to have a diet rich in calcium and vitamin D to protect against osteoporosis, whether or not on HRT.

Alternative Treatment

Check whether tablets contain calcium or vitamin D. These will be helpful. Other than vitamin D, there is no evidence that vitamins in general help the symptoms of the menopause, although vitamins B and E are often recommended. See a nutritional therapist for individual treatment. Some people benefit from acupuncture. Aromatherapy claims to redress hormonal imbalances causing symptoms; homoeopathic treatment would address the unpleasant symptoms of the menopause; some herbal remedies, tailored to your symptoms and prescribed by a registered herbalist, may help with symptoms and with their cause (namely hormonal imbalances). Exercise (walking at least two miles per day) will reduce the risk of post-menopausal osteoporosis.

Self-Help

The Amarant Trust
11–13 Charter House Building, London EC1N 7AN
Tel: 0171 490-1644

MISCARRIAGE

Miscarriage occurs when a pregnancy fails to progress beyond a few weeks or months. It is a very common event; probably more common than is realized as sometimes it may show itself simply as a heavier than usual period which was just a few days late. Most people have in mind the loss of a pregnancy which has reached eight to ten weeks, though miscarriages happen up to the twentieth week of pregnancy and beyond. However early or late, miscarriage can be a great sadness. Increasingly it is recognized that parents can feel a sense of bereavement after a miscarriage and that they should have the chance of coming to terms with this.

Risk

- Between 15 and 25 per cent of all pregnancies end in miscarriage.
- Most miscarriage happens during the first twelve weeks of pregnancy.
- In up to 50 per cent of miscarriages there is some serious abnormality in the fetus.
- A woman who has had a successful pregnancy but who then has a miscarriage, has a 70 per cent chance of her next pregnancy proceeding normally. That falls to 50 per cent if she has not had a previous successful pregnancy.

- There is only a 1 in 200 to 300 chance of having three miscarriages in a row.
- Women who have previously had a termination of pregnancy run a risk of being left with a lax cervix and therefore a somewhat increased chance of miscarriage in mid-pregnancy.

Recognition

There is an assumption made that you know you are pregnant because of a pregnancy test and the typical symptoms of pregnancy: missed periods; tender breasts; nausea; a desire to pass urine frequently; and fatigue.

Symptoms

Vaginal bleeding is the earliest symptom; it may or may not be accompanied by pain low down in the abdomen. If painless, it is called a threatened miscarriage, because things may yet settle down. If the blood contains jelly-like material it is more likely that a complete miscarriage will occur. If the bleeding becomes heavy you need immediate medical attention.

Pain is typically central lower abdominal pain. Pain which is tending to one or other side suggests the possibility of an ectopic pregnancy (see below.)

Signs and Investigations

The doctor feels whether the neck of the womb (the cervix) is open, by trying to insert the tip of a finger. If it is still closed there is a chance that the threatened miscarriage will settle down. If open, complete miscarriage is much more likely.

The doctor also examines for tenderness in the Fallopian tubes on either side of the womb, especially if there is one-sided abdominal pain. Another test is to see if you have pain when the cervix is moved. These tests both check the possibility of an ectopic pregnancy in which the fertilized egg has lodged not in the womb but inside the Fallopian tube. This is a very serious condition, because there is a risk of the tube being burst open by the growing egg, causing heavy internal bleeding.

Ultrasound (see page 301) is a quick, painless procedure which allows a search for the fertilized egg or the fetus. If implantation has occurred in the Fallopian tubes, it is an ectopic pregnancy needing an urgent operation. If there is no heartbeat or if the fetus cannot be located then miscarriage has occurred.

Ultrasound is so reliable that it is replacing internal examination especially if there is a chance of an ectopic pregnancy, where internal examination can cause an ectopic pregnancy to rupture.

ASK YOUR DOCTOR
- **About the possibility of pregnancy in any case of lower abdominal pain.**
- **About ectopic pregnancy; the combination of feeling faint, one-sided lower abdominal pain and vaginal bleeding adds up to ectopic pregnancy until proven otherwise.**

Remedy

IMMEDIATE TREATMENT

Doctors will always advise rest, though in truth there is little evidence that this really makes much difference to the outcome. Once it is clear that miscarriage is inevitable the woman will usually be offered a D&C (dilatation and curettage) in order to sweep the womb clean of debris. This prevents infection. It is good advice to then wait for one normal period before trying to conceive again.

RECURRENT MISCARRIAGE

A woman who has had three miscarriages in early pregnancy should be investigated. A woman who has had even one miscarriage in later pregnancy, especially after twenty weeks, should also be investigated. Sometimes the womb is malformed or has bands running across it. These can be dealt with by surgery.

Commonly the neck of the womb (cervix) is lax and simply cannot hold the developing pregnancy. If so, early in the next pregnancy the cervix is stitched shut until late pregnancy when the stitch is removed. Specialists will also check whether the levels of hormones involved in pregnancy are adequate; low levels can be treated with drugs.

Alternative Treatment

If there is any question of an ectopic pregnancy, it must be considered a medical emergency and orthodox medical treatment sought immediately. Miscarriage cannot be halted by alternative medicine; where the therapies come into their own is post-miscarriage. Following a miscarriage many alternative therapies offer sound advice on diet and exercise to put your body into best form for your next pregnancy. There are homoeopathic remedies offered for recurrent miscarriage. Some therapies may be helpful for women who have a history of spontaneous abortion, in particular, homoeopathy, herbalism and nutritional therapy. Remember not to take anything while trying to conceive without checking first with your orthodox medical practitioner.

Prevention

The fetus is a foreign object which the mother's body ought to reject, in the same way that someone rejects a transplanted kidney unless they take powerful drugs to suppress the immune system. So it is a great mystery how any pregnancy manages to survive the mother's immune mechanisms at all. Thus there is great interest in whether antibodies or other immune mechanisms are involved in recurrent miscarriage.

Various ongoing trials are testing ways of dampening down the immune system in cases of recurrent miscarriage. Drugs being tested include steroids, heparin (an anticoagulant) and aspirin, that humble substance which is emerging as the wonder drug of the late twentieth century. (Do not, however, take aspirin while pregnant without the permission of your doctor. It can cause abnormalities in the fetus.)

It is neither likely nor desirable that all miscarriages will be preventable as so many miscarriages involve a malformed fetus with no chance of survival. Research is suggesting that about 50 per cent of miscarriages may be preventable.

Self-Help

The Miscarriage Association
c/o Clayton Hospital
Northgate, Wakefield, West Yorkshire WF1 3JS
Tel: 01924 200 799, 01926 843 223

Cervical Stitch Network
c/o The Miscarriage Association (see above)

OVARIAN CANCER

Although it is a low-profile disease, ovarian cancer (cancer of the ovaries) is the fourth commonest cancer in women, after breast, lung and bowel. Growths of the ovary are very frequent, ranging from simple cysts to outright cancer. Whether benign or malignant, ovarian growths tend not to give any symptoms until they are well advanced, which means that treatment is less effective than it would be for growths which show themselves early, such as **breast cancer** (see page 71).

In about 15 per cent of cases the growth is of a bizarre nature – termed a dermoid cyst – in which hair, teeth, skin or other tissues are found; these are not always malignant.

Risk

- There are nearly 6000 cases a year.
- There are 4500 deaths per annum in the UK.
- Ovarian cancer is found at all ages, including during childhood.
- There is a 1.5 per cent overall lifetime risk of the disease.
- Risk increases with age, especially between fifty and seventy years of age.
- It is commoner in women with few children.
- Ovarian cancer is more common in higher social classes.
- Risk is increased in women who began periods early or who have a late menopause.
- Having a close relative affected increases the risk three to ten times.
- Taking the contraceptive pill reduces the risk by up to 40 per cent.

Recognition

SYMPTOMS

These tumours can grow to a large size without causing any symptoms at all; however, the following symptoms may occur. It is important to realize that none of these symptoms, whether alone or together, is proof of a cancerous growth, let alone of an ovarian growth; there are many other explanations for each of them. However, they should prompt you to see a doctor.

- Swelling of the abdomen
Generally in the lower abdomen and usually midline, though it can be on one side only.
- Vague recurrent abdominal pain or indigestion
This can be difficult to pin down to anything specific as there may be nothing at all to

feel on examination. Indigestion happens if the growth is large enough to be putting pressure on the stomach (this is a very rare cause of indigestion).
- Sudden pain in the abdomen

Occurs if the tumour bursts or if the growth twists on itself, cutting off its blood supply. As the cancer grows it outstrips its blood supply and this too can lead to pain, though less abruptly.
- Swelling of the legs

This results from the pressure of a large growth on the blood supply to the legs.
- Disturbances of menstruation

Certain less common forms of ovarian cancer can alter the menstrual pattern, causing bleeding after the menopause or other lesser upsets.

SIGNS
It may be possible to feel a mass in the abdomen or on gynaecological examination. There is a typical feel to a malignant ovarian tumour which may alert the doctor.

INVESTIGATIONS
An **ultrasound scan** (see page 301) is good for showing swellings on the ovary, though this investigation cannot itself tell whether the swelling is benign or malignant. A **laparoscopy** (see page 300) is a diagnostic procedure which lets the gynaecologist look inside the abdomen and inspect the internal organs.

Open surgery might happen as part of the investigation of sudden abdominal pain.

ASK YOUR DOCTOR
- **Whether pregnancy is a possibility.**
- **To give you a gynaecological check every year or two, especially if you are on the contraceptive pill.**
- **To examine your abdomen in the event of any persistent indigestion or swelling of your legs.**

Remedy

Overall, some two-thirds of these tumours are inoperable by the time they are diagnosed. This means that treatment is aimed at relieving symptoms rather than curing. However, depending on the precise type of cancer, cure rates vary enormously, from 95 per cent to just 10 per cent, five-year survival.

Surgery removes the ovaries and as much spread of the tumour as possible; usually the womb has to be removed as well. **Radiotherapy** (see page 301) may be tried after surgery to try to kill off cancerous cells remaining within the pelvic organs.

Chemotherapy (see page 298) is usually recommended in order to control spread or recurrence of the disease.

Alternative Treatment

Cancer therapies which emphasise a positive frame of mind can only help. There are homoeopathic remedies for benign ovarian cysts, if the diagnosis is certain. Post-operative therapies like acupuncture, reflexology, homoeopathy, aromatherapy and herbalism may enhance recuperation, strengthening the body and encouraging it to heal.

Prevention

With ovarian cancer causing 4500 deaths a year, a screening test is desperately required. Some rare ovarian tumours produce chemical 'markers' which can be monitored by blood samples. Most forms of ovarian cancer release a blood marker known as Ca 125; measuring this is a useful check on whether a treated tumour is recurring. As yet there is no evidence that screening for this marker in the general population reliably detects previously undiagnosed ovarian cancer earlier but there are ongoing trials to see whether screening using combinations of blood markers might be worthwhile. However, it is worth screening women who have a family history of cancer of the ovary.

Regular **ultrasound** (see page 301) checks might in theory pick up early changes; however, a **biopsy** (see page 298) would be needed to confirm any abnormality shown; there is no firm evidence that the benefits would outweigh the drawbacks of so many women having unnecessary surgery, but trials are being undertaken.

Women taking the contraceptive pill enjoy a 40 per cent lower risk of cancer of the ovary; it has been suggested that women in their forties should take the Pill in order to reduce their risks of ovarian cancer. This is something to discuss with your gynaecologist, as other risks associated with the Pill may outweigh any benefit.

At all ages the possibility of ovarian cancer should be considered in any case of vague lower abdominal pain or swelling.

Self-Help

Women's Health Concern
83 Earls Court Road, London W8 6EF
Tel: 0171 938-3932

PRE-MENSTRUAL SYNDROME (PMS)

This term is more accurate than the commonly used term 'pre-menstrual tension' as it recognises that women may suffer from a much wider range of problems other than tension. It is hard to know why the subject should be so controversial. It is a matter of common knowledge that pre-menstrual changes exist and the real debate should be on the best methods of treatment. Instead the subject has acquired feminist overtones which at times seem to have more to do with encouraging women to actually suffer from PMS as a token of their womanhood rather than to agree that, for most women, it is just a damn nuisance which generates more frustration than femininity. Over 150 different symptoms have been attributed to PMS, so not surprisingly there is no one treatment that will help everyone.

Risk

- It is very hard to assess, but perhaps 10 per cent of women suffer severely enough to make it a real problem in their lives
- For another 20 to 30 per cent of women it is a moderately severe problem.
- It is more common from 30 to 35 years of age.

Recognition

SYMPTOMS

● Cyclical change

PMS builds up from seven to ten days before the period is due, disappearing within a day or two of the start of the period. It is essential to show this pattern, otherwise the diagnosis is less certain and the possibility of a psychological problem is more likely.

● Fluid retention

Fluid retention, as a result of changing levels of hormones is a central feature, showing itself as weight gain, a bloated feeling, constipation and breast engorgement.

● Low blood sugar

This may account for headaches, tiredness, a desire for sweet things, an increased appetite.

● Psychological features

These commonly include irritability, depression, headaches, difficulty concentrating and tiredness. More extreme psychological features extend to suicidal feelings and uncontrollable swings of mood, including aggressive outbursts.

SIGNS

There are no generally agreed signs. A doctor will want to check that the symptoms do follow a cyclical pattern, enquiring also about sleep disturbances, mood during the rest of the month and your general feelings about relationships. This is to check the possibility of a depressive illness or other psychological state showing itself as PMS.

There is no generally agreed **blood test** (see page 298), though some authorities say that it is useful to measure hormone levels.

ASK YOUR DOCTOR
● **Whether it is essential to take any tablets they recommend, if you feel reassurance has been sufficient.**
● **Whether there is a local specialist in PMS to whom you can go if you feel desperate.**

Remedy and Prevention

● Reassurance

This alone can be very helpful; it can give permission for you to feel unwell for part of each month and it validates that feeling to the rest of your family.

● Diuretics (water tablets)

As many physical features of PMS are due to fluid retention this is a logical form of treatment. It is especially useful for tender breasts and for a bloated feeling. Diuretics have potentially serious side-effects, so that doctors will advise you to take them for just a few days when you feel most bloated. As an alternative, try restricting your fluid and salt intake at those times.

● Vitamin B6 (Pyridoxine)

Several trials have shown this to be helpful. There is no need to buy an expensive form; the simple vitamin in a dose of 50 mg once or twice a day is sufficient, beginning when your symptoms begin; in fact, higher doses can cause side-effects. Vitamin B6 is found naturally in a wide range of foods, including fish, bananas, pork, kidney and peanuts.

● Oral contraceptive pill
This is a useful treatment if you also wish for some form of contraception. As with other hormone treatments, not all women benefit.

● Tranquillizers
Sufferers from really severe PMS may benefit from a tranquillizer. The modern ones are safe when used responsibly and the risk of addiction is much overstated, so long as they are used for just a few days each month.

● Danazol and bromocriptine
These drugs work on the hormone system and may be helpful especially for breast pain. However they both cause side-effects and so are reserved for severe cases of PMS. Common side-effects are nausea, constipation and dizziness. Nevertheless, these drugs are very effective and women with disabling PMS may be willing to accept some level of side-effects.

Alternative Treatment

Many other naturopathic remedies will be found to be some combination of mild sedative or mild diuretic. Acupuncture, relaxation techniques and homoeopathic treatments all have their advocates. A nutritional therapist might suggest vitamin and mineral therapy, and oil of evening primrose has proved successful in dealing with symptoms. They might also suggest cutting down on tea, coffee and alcohol, which encourage mood swings, and eating small, regular meals to encourage a steady level of blood sugar. This can also prevent cravings. Symptoms can also be alleviated by aromatherapy and herbalism.

Self-Help

National Association for Pre-Menstrual Syndrome
PO Box 72, Sevenoaks, Kent TN13 1XQ

The Pre-Menstrual Society
PO Box 102, London SE1 7ES

SEXUALLY TRANSMITTED DISEASES (STDS)

Venereal disease was the old-fashioned term for these, but it came to be associated just with gonorrhoea and syphilis. The modern term is used because it recognizes the much wider array of diseases that can be spread by sexual contact. These range from the annoying but harmless thrush to **AIDS** (page 13). Most sexually transmitted diseases produce symptoms that should alert a woman to have a check-up. Some, especially gonorrhoea, can cause nothing by way of symptoms until well advanced.

For this reason in the UK there is a sophisticated system to find and offer treatment to sexual contacts of men or women who have a sexually transmitted disease. The system works anonymously; not even your own doctor is informed without your specific permission. This is designed to preserve the trust of those using the service, so you should have no reservation about going to a genito-urinary (GUM) clinic if you are worried.

We have included thrush in this section because it can be sexually transmitted. However, most cases of thrush occur spontaneously, because the naturally warm and moist conditions of the female genital tract are ideal for the growth of the fungus that causes thrush. Therefore, neither you or your partner should assume that a case of thrush has necessarily been sexually transmitted.

Risk

- There are nearly 600,000 cases a year in the UK seen in GUM clinics.
- Many more cases of thrush and vaginitis are dealt with by family doctors or self-treated.
- The more sexual partners, the higher the risk.
- There is an increased risk in many countries in Asia and Africa.
- Condoms protect against sexually transmitted diseases.
- Apart from causing illness in women, there is a later risk of infertility or of recurrent miscarriage.

Recognition

SYMPTOMS
There are too many sexually transmitted diseases to detail each one. The symptoms below can only be pointers to the possibilities. Often specialized tests are needed to make a definite diagnosis.

VAGINAL DISCHARGE
All women have a normal level of vaginal discharge, which should be clear, non-smelly and non-itchy. Be alert to a discharge which becomes very heavy, offensive in smell and appearance or is itchy.

- A white, itchy discharge is typical of thrush (candida), a fungal infection.
- A frothy yellowish discharge suggests trichomonas.
- A heavy discharge with a fishy odour accompanies bacterial vaginosis.
- A very heavy, very offensive discharge may be due to a tampon which has been forgotten.
- Disease of the cervix, e.g., cervical erosion, causes a heavy, clear discharge.

ULCERS, WARTS AROUND THE GENITALIA
- Painful ulcers in groups are typical of genital herpes.
- A single painless ulcer can be the first sign of syphilis.
- Syphilis causes typical warts which spread in a sheet-like form around the genitalia or the anus.
- Genital warts are commonly caused by viral infections passed venereally.
- Not all ulcers are venereal in origin; the hairy genital area is a common site for boils and infections at the root of the hairs.

PAIN ON PASSING URINE
- This is usually down to a straightforward urinary infection or irritation of the outlet from the bladder (the urethra). However if accompanied by a discharge from the urethra or other symptoms it may be a feature of disease, in particular gonorrhoea or chlamydia.

OTHER GYNAECOLOGICAL SYMPTOMS

- An acute infection of the ovaries and Fallopian tubes gives rise to severe lower abdominal pain plus a heavy discharge. Chronic pelvic infection is suggested by a combination of pain on intercourse, heavy painful periods and, in time, infertility. Chronic infection of the tubes and ovaries can follow gonorrhoea and chlamydia. Unfortunately the first symptom may well be **infertility** (see page 83). This reinforces the importance of contact tracing of sexual partners.

GENERAL SYMPTOMS

- Syphilis can cause widespread skin rashes, swollen glands in armpits and groin and, in its later stages, dementia, difficulty walking. **AIDS** (see page 13) eventually causes general decline in health, with chest infections and weight loss especially noticeable.

SIGNS AND INVESTIGATIONS

- A diagnosis can often be hazarded on the basis of the appearance of a discharge, its smell and the associated symptoms. Swabs taken from the vagina, the anus and the opening from the bladder are analyzed. Blood tests check on the possibility of syphilis and AIDS. Chronic pelvic infection may be suspected but only really proven by surgery to look inside the abdomen.

ASK YOUR DOCTOR

- **To take account of your pattern of sexual behaviour; it may be crucial in deciding how urgently to investigate and treat your symptoms.**
- **About any persistent vaginal discharge.**
- **About the implications of venereal disease in your partner.**

Remedy

- Many women recognize thrush, treatable with over-the-counter anti-fungal creams or pessaries. For really persistent cases there are highly effective anti-thrush antibiotics taken by mouth.
- Chlamydia, trichomonas and bacterial vaginosis all respond well to antibiotics.
- Antibiotic treatment of gonorrhoea and syphilis is also effective if diagnosed early. It requires specialised care and follow up. The late stages of these diseases are difficult to treat.
- Genital herpes responds to an anti-viral cream such as acyclovir, but may again be difficult to cure completely.
- Genital warts should be removed for analysis.

Alternative Treatment

There is logic in treating recurrent thrush using live yoghurt douches. Similarly there are douches using aromatherapy or herbal preparations which may be soothing, anti-fungal or anti-bacterial. Some work by changing the acidity of the vagina to one that the fungus cannot survive in. There is no place for alternative treatment in the other conditions mentioned, as effective conventional treatment exists and there are serious long-term consequences from inadequate treatment. Alternative therapies can, however, work on the immune system alongside conventional medical care, and build up the body in order to make it strong enough to resist further attacks of a condition.

Prevention

- Thrush is unavoidable for most women at some time; for example, after a course of antibiotics. As mentioned earlier, most cases of thrush do not arise as a result of sexual transmission. Nevertheless this route of transfer must be considered if thrush is persistent. In cases of severe or recurrent thrush, have your urine tested for sugar, as occasionally it is due to unsuspected **diabetes** (page 204).
- Avoid a sexually promiscuous lifestyle; otherwise, encourage your partner to wear a condom.
- Do not neglect unusual vaginal symptoms, nor vague lower abdominal pains.
- Have regular smear tests.
- Do not be afraid of going to a clinic for sexually transmitted diseases if you suspect an infection. Nor should you turn down screening as a result of one of your sexual partners attending a clinic.

You may feel your lifestyle is no one's business but your own. This is not true if you may be passing on syphilis, gonorrhoea or AIDS, which carry the threat of chronic disease, infertility or death.

Self-Help

Pelvic Inflammatory Disease Network
52 Featherstone Street, London EC1Y 8RT
Tel: 0171 251-6580

Herpes Association
41 North Road, London N7 9DP
Tel: 0171 609-9061

THE MALE
REPRODUCTIVE SYSTEM

- Cancer of the Testicle • Impotence
- Prostate Cancer • Sexually Transmitted Diseases
(STDs) • Torsion (twisting) of the Testicle

M EN'S RELUCTANCE TO talk about health matters has changed in recent years. Heart disease led the way, bringing with it a new readiness to consider diet, exercise and lifestyle. Now there is that same readiness to admit to other major health problems, of which the most important is cancer of the prostate. This enthusiasm has not quite reached the stage of setting up screening programmes; if the American experience is a guide then screening will be here within a few years.

The other topics included here are, apart from impotence, less common but are avoidable causes of future problems so that men should be aware of the symptoms of these illnesses.

CANCER OF THE TESTICLE

This is not a common tumour but it is increasing in frequency for reasons unknown. Caught early it is curable, making early detection a priority.

Risk

- In the UK there are about 1250 cases a year and 123 deaths.
- The incidence varies from 0.8 per 100,000 per annum in Japanese men, 2 to 3 per 100,000 per annum in USA, to 6 to 7 per 100,000 in Scandinavians.
- It is twice as common in men of higher social class.
- The commonest malignancy is in men in the late 20s and early 30s (50 per cent of all cases).
- There is a 1 in 20 risk in testicles which have not descended from the abdomen.
- There is about 2 per cent risk if there is any history of undescended testicles, even if treated.
- If cancer is found in one testicle there is a 5 per cent chance of finding it in the other one.

Recognition

SYMPTOMS
The earliest symptom is a lump in the testicle. Often the testicle feels heavy; only occasionally is there any pain.

SIGNS

Skilled examination can differentiate from other lumps in the testicle. Some are simply normal structures which become enlarged; for example, the epididymis at the back of the testicle. There are **blood tests** (see page 298) of hormones produced by the tumour which help in diagnosing the type and extent of a growth.

ASK YOUR DOCTOR
- **For an examination as soon as you feel a lump in your testicle.**
- **What to do if you have an undescended testicle.**

Remedy

A **biopsy** (see page 298) is needed to show the type of tumour, as different types have different treatment. **Radiotherapy** (see page 301) alone cures some types. Other types have to be removed together with the testicle, followed by some combination of radiotherapy and **chemotherapy** (see page 298).

Cure rates for early growths are very high – up to 100 per cent. If the tumour has spread widely, the five-year survival is still 90 per cent and recent years continue to see a steady improvement in rates of cure. Follow-up needs to be for many years; blood tests are useful to check on recurrence.

Prevention

All men, but especially those in their twenties and thirties, should check their testicles regularly, reporting any unusual lump or sensation. Baby boys are screened for undescended testicles which should always be brought down by surgery.

In theory, high-risk men (for instance, those who had undescended testicles), might benefit from a biopsy of the testicles from time to time but the value of this in practice is undecided.

Self-Help

Save Our Sons
Tides Reach, 1 Kite Hill, Wootton Bridge, Isle of Wight PO33 4LA
Tel: 01983 882876

IMPOTENCE

Impotence means the inability to achieve an erection firm enough to have normal intercourse. It is not an absolute abnormality; all men experience it at times due to some combination of tiredness, alcohol or stress. It becomes a problem when it regularly interferes with sexual life.

For many years psychological causes were believed to account for most cases of impotence. Recent research, stimulated perhaps by an ageing population more open about sex in later life, is showing that physical factors are much more common than once thought. With this knowledge have come improved methods of treatment.

Risk

- Sexual activity diminishes with age; even so most men up to seventy are still interested in sex.
- After seventy, perhaps 20 per cent of men remain interested in sex.
- Unknown numbers of men suffer from the problem; physical reasons are more likely in the elderly, and psychological reasons in the young.
- It is more common in men with **diabetes** (see page 204) or with poor blood flow to the lower body.
- Many drugs can cause impotence; commonest are beta-blockers and diuretics used for **high blood pressure** (see page 150) and certain antidepressants.

Recognition

SYMPTOMS

This may seem obvious but it is important to distinguish true impotence from premature ejaculation, failure of orgasm or disease of the penis preventing full erection. It is useful to know whether the man ever has a satisfactory erection; for example, on waking in the morning. If he does not, it makes a physical cause more likely.

A psychological factor is more likely if a man experiences impotence with one partner or in certain circumstances.

SIGNS

The doctor really has to go by the man's description of his problem. However, a physical check may give clues to the cause. Small testicles and absent body hair suggest a hormone problem. Peyronie's disease results in a hard band around the penis which prevents normal erection and causes the penis to curve. A tight foreskin can make a full erection painful. There may be bad circulation to the legs or signs of neurological disease in the legs such as **multiple sclerosis** (see page 255). Perhaps there are features of **alcohol abuse** (see page 268). Impotence can be a symptom of **depression** (see page 278) or other severe psychological illness. The urine should always be tested for sugar; diabetes is a common cause of impotence.

Simply changing a drug, for example, one used to treat high blood pressure, may solve the problem.

ASK YOUR DOCTOR
- **If any drugs you are taking might be to blame.**
- **If your consumption of alcohol could be a cause.**
- **If you also have pain in your legs when walking or if you notice numbness around your bottom; these suggest respectively blood flow or neurological causes for impotence.**

Remedy

PSYCHOLOGICAL

Anxiety or **depression** (see pages 275 and 278) can be treated, remembering that the very drugs used for this can make the problem worse to begin with. There is a very common vicious circle of anxiety about past impotence resulting in impotence the next time. To treat this there is a programme of psycho-sexual counselling that puts the emphasis on sexual foreplay but which bans intercourse till later in the programme. This same method is used in treating premature ejaculation.

PHYSICAL TREATMENTS
Self-injection has become a widespread effective treatment for those who can learn to do it. The drug papaverine is injected into the shaft of the penis; this will produce a satisfactory erection in most cases. The main risk is of the erection lasting for several hours. There is also a possibility that repeated use will cause fibrous changes in the penis.

Very recently the gas nitrous oxide was discovered to be involved in erections, suggesting the possibility of completely novel drugs that could be used in treatment.

MECHANICAL DEVICES
Patent suction devices placed over the penis will cause it to swell enough to have intercourse. A pump or a semi-rigid tube fitted inside the penis is quite successful especially in younger men

SURGERY
Poor blood flow to the lower body or Peyronie's disease can be treated by surgery.

Impressive results from surgery to improve blood flow to the penis are reported, mainly from the USA; such operations may become more widely used but are likely to remain an option only in the private sector in England.

OTHERS
Injections or tablets of male hormone are worth a try if only to break a vicious circle of anxiety. Their long-term use cannot be recommended because of side effects.

Alternative Treatment

Ideas about treatment for impotence are often fad-related. There is a school of thought which insists that Ginseng is useful; many men swear by it. A nutritional therapist might uncover a zinc deficiency, which would account for low testosterone levels. Acupuncture and reflexology might be useful to stimulate the circulation, reduce tension and address any physical causes. All of the relaxation therapies could help; aromatherapy, T'ai chi, massage and hypnotherapy are suggestions.

Prevention

- Stop smoking; it is a common cause of poor blood flow to the lower body.
- Avoid excessive alcohol consumption.
- Be alert for symptoms of **diabetes** (page 204).
- If affected by impotence, and you are bound to be at sometime or other, try to make light of it and defer intercourse to another time when you are relaxed, so as to avoid that vicious circle of fear of failure.

Self-Help

In most areas there are psycho-sexual counsellors to whom you can self-refer; for instance, The Brook Advisory Centres.

Impotence Information Centre, PO Box 1130, London W3 OBB

PROSTATE CANCER

The prostate gland lies between the root of the penis and the anus. It encircles the urethra, the tube which carries urine from the bladder through the penis. The function of the prostate gland is uncertain and in practice it is nothing but a nuisance.

It is a mystery why prostate cancer, which is so common, should have been so little publicized until recently. This is changing as there is an increasing openness about all aspects of men's health.

Risk

- There are 14,000 new cases a year.
- Deaths from prostate cancer are the second most common cause of death from cancer in men in the UK, after lung cancer; this is over 9,000 a year.
- It accounts for about 7 per cent of all cancers in men in the UK.
- There is wide international variation in occurrence; it is much commoner in the USA, rare in Japan and the Far East.
- Only 2 per cent of cases occur below age 55; 16 per cent under age 65; but it is common by the age of 80.
- Small areas of cancer are a frequent finding in men who have had what appears to be a perfectly benign gland removed.
- Cancer causing no symptoms can be found in about one-third of men in their 70s and two-thirds of men by their 80s.

Recognition

SYMPTOMS

The symptoms may be from the prostate gland itself or from spread of a cancer. The prostate gland is like a cuff circling the urethra. As the gland enlarges it squeezes the urethra causing partial obstruction. The result is a poorer flow of urine and difficulty in starting to pass urine. Often a man finds he needs to pass small but frequent amounts of urine day and night. These symptoms are identical to the symptoms caused by simple benign overgrowth of the prostate gland.

Symptoms from spread of prostate cancer are usually due to spread of the disease into the bones of the pelvis. So there may be pain in the hip or lower back.

SIGNS

By passing a finger into the anus a doctor can feel the prostate gland; it should feel smooth and rounded. Cancer of the prostate feels hard and irregular.

INVESTIGATIONS

A **biopsy** (see page 298) can be take from suspicious areas using a fine needle. There are two chemicals that can be measured with a **blood test** (see page 298); raised levels make cancer very likely. These are acid phosphatase and prostate specific antigen (PSA).

Further information is gathered by doing an **ultrasound** (see page 301) examination of the gland; this shows up suspicious areas. Scans of various kinds (**CT scan, MRI scan,** see pages 298 and 300) will show whether the cancer has spread into bone.

ASK YOUR DOCTOR
- **About alterations in your flow of urine.**
- **About any blood in the urine.**
- **About pain in any bone which is persistent and especially if it keeps you awake at night.**

Remedy

If cancer is found unexpectedly in a gland removed for some other reason, current opinion is to just watch and wait. This is because only a small percentage of such growths progress to serious disease.

The treatment for cancer which is causing symptoms is **radiotherapy** (see page 301) or surgical removal of all the prostate gland. Both options offer 80 to 90 per cent five-year survival; 60 to 80 per cent ten-year survival. The main drawback of surgery was a high risk of urinary incontinence or of impotence but newer forms of surgery are overcoming these problems.

If the cancer has spread outside the prostate gland then treatment is with radiotherapy. Often hormone treatments are used as well, to reduce the amount of male hormone in the body. The oldest method was removal of both testicles. Many men find this unacceptable and with newer drugs this can be avoided. However it is not known how effective these are in the long run. Once spread has happened five-year survival is 50 to 70 per cent; ten-year survival is 30 to 50 per cent. Where there is spread into bones, survival falls to about 20 per cent at five years.

Alternative Treatment

Herbal and vitamin therapies are suggested for this condition, if you do not wish conventional drugs. It is very important first to have a conventional medical assessment of the risks of cancer of the prostate. There are also homoeopathic remedies, which will be prescribed according to your symptoms. Acupuncture is commonly used.

Prevention

A strong body of opinion is building up favouring screening for cancer of the prostate using two simple methods. One is for men over a certain age, perhaps fifty-five, to have a yearly rectal examination. The other is for regular blood tests of the PSA (Prostate specific antigen). In the USA already men are being offered surgery for disease detected in these ways but which is causing them no symptoms; it is unknown whether this aggressive approach will improve survival.

What is clear is the striking difference in survival between cases of localized cancer and cases where it has spread into the bone. This does reinforce the need for early detection but how to weigh this against the side-effects of surgery or radiotherapy is an unanswered question.

Increasing numbers of specialists are recommending that men over fifty have the screening tests as a first step to gathering the data that will eventually answer this question. Without doubt this will be one of the great health screening debates of the next decade.

Self-Help

BACUP (British Association of Cancer United Patients)
3 Bath Place, Rivington Street, London EC2A 3JR
Tel: 0800 181199

SEXUALLY TRANSMITTED DISEASES (STDS)

These used to be known as venereal diseases, but that phrase became associated with just gonorrhoea or syphilis. A much wider range of sexually transmitted diseases is now recognized. The special case of **AIDS** is dealt with elsewhere (page 13).

In general, for men sexually transmitted diseases are unpleasant but not a long term threat to health. Also the symptoms are usually obvious. This is quite the opposite of the situation for women where symptoms may be few and the risk of permanent damage high. This puts a special responsibility on men to have treatment for sexually transmitted disease. To avoid treatment simply because of embarrassment may result in infertility for future sexual partners.

Most towns have a genito-urinary clinic for rapid diagnosis and treatment. An important part of the work of the clinic is to trace sexual contacts in order to pick up unsuspected disease. This is done in strictest confidence.

Risk

- The more sexually promiscuous the higher the risk.
- Gonorrhoea and syphilis are relatively uncommon in the UK but very common in Asia and Africa.
- Homosexual sexual activity increases the risk.
- Condoms reduce the risk.

Recognition

SYMPTOMS
Discharge from the penis
  This may be yellow and itchy or just clear. It may be noticed as staining on underwear. Thrush, a fungal infection, gives an itchy white rash on the penis.

BURNING ON PASSING URINE
This often goes together with a discharge. It may be a feature of gonorrhoea or chlamydia. It can be simply due to urinary tract infection, though this is far less common in men than women.

ULCERS, WARTS AROUND THE GENITALIA
- Painful ulcers in groups are typical of genital herpes.
- A single painless ulcer can be the first sign of syphilis.
- Syphilis causes typical warts which spread in a sheet like form around the genitalia or the anus.
- Genital warts are commonly caused by viral infections passed venereally.
- Not all ulcers are venereal in origin; the hairy genital area is a common site for boils and infections at the root of the hairs.

GENERAL SYMPTOMS

Syphilis can cause widespread skin rashes, swollen glands in armpits and groins and, in its later stages, dementia, difficulty walking. AIDS eventually causes general decline in health, with chest infections and weight loss especially noticeable.

SIGNS

Though appearances may be typical of a particular illness, blood tests and swabs are needed to make a precise diagnosis.

ASK YOUR DOCTOR

- **About your symptoms or if you have reason to suspect an STD. Ensure that you disclose details of your pattern of sexual behaviour; it may be crucial in deciding how urgently to investigate and treat your symptoms.**
- **About any discharge from the penis.**
- **About the consequences for you of venereal disease in your partner.**

Remedy

- Thrush gives a typical itchy rash, treated with over-the-counter anti-fungal cream. For really resistant cases there are highly effective anti-thrush antibiotics taken by mouth.
- Chlamydia and trichomonas cause minimal symptoms in men and therefore are often found by tracing sexual contacts. They respond well to antibiotics.
- Antibiotic treatment of gonorrhoea and syphilis is also effective if diagnosed early. It requires specialized care and follow-up. The late stages of these diseases are difficult to treat.
- Genital herpes responds to an anti-viral cream such as acyclovir, but may again be difficult to cure completely.
- Genital warts should be removed for analysis.

Alternative Treatment

It is essential that STDs are diagnosed and treated by conventional medical practitioners in the first instance. Some carry the risk of death and infertility, so it does not seem prudent to experiment with alternatives. Alongside conventional medicine, there are a number of complementary therapies which can help to encourage healing and the immune system of the sufferer, in order to fight off the disease. Some reputable therapies which claim to offer useful treatment are: aromatherapy; homoeopathy; nutritional therapy; herbalism; and, to some extent, acupuncture.

Prevention

- In cases of severe or recurrent thrush, have your urine tested for sugar, as occasionally it is due to unsuspected **diabetes** (page 204).
- Avoid a sexually promiscuous lifestyle; otherwise wear a condom, especially if you follow homosexual practices.
- Do not be afraid of going to a clinic for sexually transmitted disease if you

suspect an infection. Nor should you turn down screening as a result of one of your sexual partners attending a clinic.

- You may feel your lifestyle is no one's business but your own. This is not true if you may be passing on syphilis, gonorrhoea or AIDS, which carry the threat of chronic disease, infertility or death.

TORSION (TWISTING) OF THE TESTICLE

Each testicle hangs on a spermatic cord, a tube which carries sperm away from the testicles. Torsion happens when that cord becomes twisted, giving rise to severe pain. Unless the torsion is released within eight to twelve hours there is a high chance of permanent damage to the testicle, threatening future fertility.

Risk

- It is commonest in adolescent boys.
- It can occur at any age.
- A testicle which is undescended is more likely to twist.

Recognition

SYMPTOMS
Sudden severe pain in the testicle. Within a few minutes it begins to swell; frequently there is nausea and vomiting. In babies and infants torsion may occur without so much pain but the child will still clearly be in discomfort, with a hard, reddened scrotum.

SIGNS
The testicle is extremely tender; often it hangs higher than the other testicle. It is the testicle itself which is tender; tenderness at the back of the testicle suggests an infection.

Orchitis, which is inflammation of the testicle, happens occasionally in adult men and can be indistinguishable from torsion, except that there is an accompanying fever. It is not a safe diagnosis to make in children or adolescent boys.

ASK YOUR DOCTOR
- **To examine a case of testicular pain as soon as possible.**

Remedy

With young boys, surgery to inspect the testicle is nearly always advisable. The testicle is untwisted and stitched to prevent another torsion. The other testicle should also be surgically fixed in place. With adults an infection is more likely and is treated with antibiotics.

Prevention

Never ignore pain in the testicles. In boys it is torsion until proven otherwise.

THE DIGESTIVE SYSTEM

- Crohn's Disease
- Cancer of the Colon and Rectum • Cancer of the Oesophagus (Gullet) • Cancer of the Pancreas
- Cancer of the Stomach • Diarrhoea • Gallstones
- Irritable Bowel Syndrome • Pancreatitis
- Peptic Ulcers • Ulcerative Colitis

T HE DIGESTIVE SYSTEM is a factory for turning what we eat into substances that the body can use. Everything we take through our mouths, from pop-tarts to haggis, must be worked on by the digestive juices until all that culinary artistry is reduced to simple sugars, fats, protein, vitamins and minerals.

The body produces specialized chemicals called enzymes which achieve this task at a rapid rate; the first of these is contained in saliva, which begins the breakdown of carbohydrates while food is still being chewed. Later food is exposed to more enzymes, powerful stomach acids, detergent-type substances, and bacteria which further break down food. Meanwhile, the walls of the intestines contain systems which actively select and absorb nutrition from the watery slurry passing through. Finally, water and a few extra minerals are absorbed in the large intestine before the residue is passed out, a mixture of unwanted material, unabsorbable fibrous matter and bacteria from the large intestine (these in fact make up the bulk of faecal material).

The control of this whole effort is achieved by a combination of nerve pathways and hormones which is far from being completely understood. The cells lining the intestines have a rapid turnover, which is one reason why cancers of the digestive tract are so common. People come to recognize their 'bowel habit' and a persistent change in the usual pattern should alert you to the possibility of disease.

CROHN'S DISEASE

This disease causes inflammation of the digestive tract, anywhere from the mouth to the anus. In mild forms it causes abdominal discomfort and diarrhoea, which are irritating but not serious. In more advanced disease it can cause severe pain, profuse diarrhoea, bowel obstruction, abscesses around the anus, poor growth in children and a constant feeling of being unwell. It is a lifelong illness with no known cure, but with effective treatment for flare-ups.

Since first recognized in the 1930s it has become four times more common, though recently it may be diminishing in frequency again. The increase may have been through better recognition of the disease, rather than a true increase in its frequency. The cause remains unknown. It seems logical to think that diet plays a part or some immunological cause; neither of these has been proven. A persistent theory is that it is due to an infection, but again no firm evidence yet supports this.

Risk

- There are 5 new cases per 100,000 population per annum.
- There are 30,000 sufferers in the UK at any one time.
- It is more common among Jews.
- Crohn's disease is more common among close relatives of sufferers.
- It is more common in the Western world.
- The condition is four times commoner in smokers.
- It is slightly more common in women on the contraceptive pill.
- Peak onset is between 20 and 40 years, but it occurs in children and the elderly.
- Many years of relatively normal life are possible.
- The overall mortality is about twice the average.

Recognition

SYMPTOMS

In the typical case there is recurrent abdominal pain and **diarrhoea** (see page 119). Sometimes there is bleeding from the back passage and the individual may feel generally unwell and lose weight. These symptoms usually fluctuate over some months though it is possible for the disease to begin suddenly. The non-specific nature of the symptoms plus the fact that sufferers may feel perfectly well in between flare-ups means that it is often some while before the diagnosis is made.

SIGNS

Tenderness is common in the lower right side of the abdomen. Mouth ulcers and painful cracks around the anus are other frequent findings. Otherwise there is rarely much to find so investigations are needed to clinch the diagnosis.

INVESTIGATIONS

X-rays (see page 301) of the intestines show up the typical changes of Crohn's disease, which are narrowing of the walls of the intestines. **Colonoscopy** (see page 298) is a technique allowing inspection of the wall of the bowel; **biopsies** (see page 298) taken from the wall will show the microscopic changes of inflammation typical of the disease.

Blood tests (see page 298) detect **anaemia** (see page 186), which is common, and also give an idea of how active the disease is.

ASK YOUR DOCTOR

- **To investigate recurrent abdominal pain.**
- **About rectal bleeding.**

Remedy

For mild cases it is just a matter of controlling diarrhoea and correcting any anaemia. The abdominal pains improve on a high protein, low bulk diet. Even so it can be a problem to deliver sufficient nutrition to maintain weight or to keep children growing.

Bad flare-ups of pain, diarrhoea or infection need vigorous treatment with steroids and other anti-inflammatory drugs such as azathioprine. Often the sufferer has to be admitted to hospital for fluids by drip. At some time nearly all sufferers from the disease will need surgical treatment to cut out an obstructed part of bowel. Where there is persistent ill-health and weight loss there may be no alternative but to remove a large part of the diseased bowel.

Alternative Treatment

Many sufferers find that particular foods make things worse. With guidance these can be identified. It is also sensible to take vitamin supplements. A nutritional therapist might suggest a special diet, but this must only be undertaken with the consent of your medical practitioner. There are several homoeopathic and herbal preparations for the condition, and an acupuncturist might be able to redress an imbalance which causes flare-ups. There are a number of therapies which will address specific symptoms like pain and diarrhoea.

Prevention

As the cause of the disease is unknown, there are as yet no strategies for prevention.

Self-Help

National Association for Colitis and Crohn's Disease
98a London Road, St Albans, Herts AL1 1NX
Tel: 01727 844296

CANCER OF THE COLON AND RECTUM

These are the second most common cancers in the UK, after lung cancer. Everyone should be aware of the early symptoms because the outlook varies enormously, depending on how early the disease is caught. Not only that, but early disease can be treated with relatively modest surgery, whereas advanced disease may need far more extensive therapy.

Risk

- One in every 50 people will suffer from these cancers.
- There are over 30,000 new cases and about 20,000 deaths per annum.
- They are most common from the age of sixty onwards.
- It is rare in Africa and Asia but common in the West.
- The risk is three times higher in first degree relatives of those who have had these cancers.
- There is a high risk in sufferers from **ulcerative colitis** (page 132) or familial polyposis (see **prevention**, below).

Recognition

Symptoms

These can occur as individual symptoms or in combination. None on their own is diagnostic of cancer but the more symptoms the higher the chances of cancer.

● Rectal bleeding

Ignore this at your peril. Although there are several innocent causes, it is the serious ones that have to be excluded. So even the slightest streak of blood should be checked. In those below forty years there may well be another reasonable explanation, such as a haemorrhoid which has clearly bled recently or a tear around the back passage. As you become older, so the index of suspicion must rise. By the ages of fifty or sixty even though your doctor may see haemorrhoids or a tear it is not safe to leave it at that.

Passing motions which are black is another symptom of rectal bleeding; the black is due to a chemical change in blood oozing into the bowel. Confusion can result if you are taking iron tablets, which also turn motions black. In these cases a sample should be sent for analysis.

● Change of bowel habit

Everyone is different in how frequently they open their bowels. It may vary from twice a day to once a week. Similarly there will be a typical type of motion that you pass – firm, loose or pellet-like. This is more subject to day-to-day change, depending on variations in diet. By change in bowel habit is meant a change in what is normal for you; perhaps constipation, perhaps diarrhoea, perhaps motions which have to be forced out in a way unusual for you.

● Abdominal pain

This may be a symptom of more advanced disease, where there is some obstruction of the bowel by the tumour or spread of the tumour outside the bowel. In complete obstruction there is severe abdominal pain, swelling of the abdomen and vomiting.

● Weight loss, loss of appetite

These are non-specific features of many cancers; probably they are caused by chemicals released by cancer cells. They are a feature of more advanced disease.

Signs

It may be possible to feel a lump in the abdomen; similarly it may be possible to feel an abnormality through rectal examination. Otherwise investigations are needed to locate the tumour.

Investigations

Common investigations are: **sigmoidoscopy** (see page 301), where a rigid tube is passed into the rectum: **colonoscopy** (see page 298), where a flexible tube is guided around the colon, and a **barium enema** (see page 297) to show up the lining of the bowel.

Some tumours present as bowel obstruction, the tumour being found during surgery to relieve the obstruction.

ASK YOUR DOCTOR
- **About rectal bleeding, no matter how innocent or obvious the cause may seem to you.**
- **About weight loss in the absence of dieting.**
- **If you are found to be anaemic** (see page 186), despite having a good diet ask if you need further investigation for possible bleeding into the bowel.

Remedy

Except in the very frail the treatment is always surgery. This has two aims: one is to remove the cancer; the other is to check whether it has spread. Modern surgical techniques mean that most cases can be dealt with without the need for a colostomy – a bag into which waste material is collected.

In the case of early growths the results of surgery are excellent; 95 to 100 per cent of patients are still alive after five years. More advanced growths are treated with **chemotherapy** (see page 298) as well as surgery. In these cases there is a 30 to 75 per cent five-year survival depending on how far the tumour has invaded.

Cancers which have already spread outside the bowel at the time of surgery have a much poorer five-year survival; about 10 to 20 per cent.

Alternative Treatment

Therapies which put a stress on sharing worry and providing support have much to offer, but this should always be combined with having a conventional surgical opinion. Post-operatively, many therapies can offer treatment which encourages healing. Some, like acupuncture, can deal with the pain. Any cancer sufferer that cannot be treated by conventional medicine might find some relief from symptoms, and indeed the cancer itself, through alternative medicine. Because of the strong mind-body relationship, there is evidence that some therapies work precisely because they are thought to do so by the sufferer. It is, however, a field full of charlatans and you should beware of anyone making miraculous claims. Homoeopathy, herbalism and acupressure may help. Healing and hypnotherapy are also used.

Prevention

There is much enthusiasm for a screening programme to reduce the frequency of bowel cancer. There is such a big difference in the chances of survival between early and late disease that this is seen as an important public health measure.
- Diet

The fact that the cancer is common in the West yet rare elsewhere suggests that diet is involved in some way. Current theory is that we in the West should eat a diet higher in fibre, in the hope that this will protect against cancer of the colon as well as the extremely common diverticular disease.
- Screening for blood in the motions

There are modern tests which are very sensitive to blood in the motions and are relatively cheap and quick. They will detect blood even though to the naked eye all is well and the individual feels fine. The problem is that the tests are over-sensitive. They will show positive even if your gums have bled after brushing your teeth. This is called a false positive; that is, the test is positive but not because of the disease it is supposed to detect.

Many people would be investigated unnecessarily if this test alone were used for screening. For this reason the test has not yet been recommended in the UK, although elsewhere it has shown to be worthwhile in the detection of early disease. Research is currently being undertaken to find a test as simple to perform but which is more specific in detecting bleeding from the lower bowel.

● Sigmoidoscopy

In theory everyone over a certain age (for instance, 55) could have a sigmoidoscopic inspection of their rectum. Some people estimate that this could prevent between 3000 and 5000 deaths from bowel cancer each year. Quite apart from doubts about how many would accept this uncomfortable procedure, there are just not the resources to do it. It is justified in three specific groups (see below).

● At-risk groups

There are three well-known groups at high risk of cancer of the bowel who merit regular reviews and sigmoidoscopy or colonoscopy. First degree relatives of sufferers from the disease have a three times increased chance of also having this form of cancer. There are even higher risks in sufferers from familial polyposis, a disease where there are many polyps scattered throughout the bowel. Finally people with **ulcerative colitis** (page 132) active for more than ten years have up to a forty times increased risk of bowel cancer.

The costs and benefits of these screening programmes will be urgent issues in the next ten years. Meanwhile it cannot be over-emphasized that you should take seriously the symptoms given earlier.

Self-Help

BACUP (British Association of Cancer United Patients)
3 Bath Place, Rivington Street, London EC2A 3JR
Tel: 0800 181199

CANCER OF THE OESOPHAGUS (GULLET)

The gullet is a somewhat sophisticated mechanism. Its walls are muscular; they contract in waves, pushing food down and preventing it coming back up again; if you wish you can swallow a glass of water while standing on your head. Most disorders of the gullet are to do with acid problems giving rise to heartburn. Cancer of the oesophagus may cause similar early symptoms.

Risk

● Cancer of the gullet accounts for 2 to 3 per cent of deaths in the UK.
● There are 3000 to 5000 new cases per annum.
● It is much more common in certain countries like China and South Africa, due to effects of chewing tobacco and other harmful substances.
● Heavy consumption of alcohol and of tobacco increases the risk.
● It is commonest in the 60 to 70 age range.
● There is a small increased risk in conditions causing chronic acid reflux into the oesophagus; for example, hiatus hernia.

Recognition

SYMPTOMS

Difficulty swallowing is the commonest symptom; it begins as a feeling that solid food is not going down easily. The food seems to stick behind the breastbone. Often you can point precisely to where this happens. Later there is difficulty in swallowing fluids; in really advanced cases even saliva fails to go down. This stage can be reached in a matter of weeks.

Pain behind the breastbone is unusual and generally means more advanced disease. Weight loss is a consequence of inability to swallow and the slow starvation that results.

Similar symptoms can be caused by severe acid disease, although in that case there are additional features such as acid coming into the mouth, belching and relief from antacids.

SIGNS

There are no specific signs. Diagnosis relies on **X-rays** (see page 301) of the gullet or taking a look down with an **endoscope** (see page 299), when any narrowing can be identified and **biopsies** (see page 298) taken from suspicious-looking areas in the walls of the gullet.

ASK YOUR DOCTOR

- **About any degree of difficulty swallowing, even if associated with acid problems**

Remedy

In the vast majority of cases the disease is well established by the time it produces symptoms. **Chemotherapy** (see page 298) plus **radiotherapy** (see page 301) offer the best hope but are suitable only for certain types of oesophageal cancer; even then the five-year survival is only around 25 per cent. Poor as this is, it is much better than the outlook for the rest of the tumours where five-year survival is less than 10 per cent.

The difficulty in swallowing can be relieved by inserting a tube into the oesophagus or by cutting away part of the tumour with a laser. Sadly these measures give only temporary relief because the tumour inevitably continues to eat its way into the tissues surrounding the oesophagus. Treatment then consists in keeping the sufferer as comfortable as possible.

This is a highly upsetting disease for everyone involved in caring for the patient. With most other cancers the sufferer can at least gain some pleasure from food and drink but in this condition they are condemned to a relentless starvation which is all the more pitiful to watch for being impossible to help.

Prevention

Keep to a moderate intake of alcohol and stop smoking all together. This advice is recommended for general health and not only because they are avoidable risk factors for cancer of the oesophagus. In those countries where the cause is thought to be chewing harmful substances like tobacco, prevention is obvious.

Modern treatment for acid diseases is highly effective (see **peptic ulcer**, page 129) and over the next few decades should reduce the small associated risk of developing cancer of the oesophagus. Be alert to any unusual change in your digestion especially any hint of difficulty in swallowing.

Self-Help

BACUP (British Association of Cancer United Patients)
   3 Bath Place, Rivington Street, London EC2A 3JR
   Tel: 0800 181199
   Oesophageal Patients Association
   16 Whitefields Cresent
   Solihull, West Midlands B91 3NU
   Tel: 0121 704-9860

CANCER OF THE PANCREAS

The pancreas is a large organ (called a gland) which lies at the back of the abdomen. It produces hormones important in digestion including insulin. Because of its position, abnormalities in the gland are not easily detected, while pain from the gland tends to be of a vague nature not readily pinned down.

It may come as a surprise to learn that cancer of the pancreas, though little discussed, is the fourth most common cause of death from cancer in the UK. It rarely produces any symptoms in its early stages and so tends not to be diagnosed until it is already well advanced.

Risk

- There are between 7000 and 8000 cases a year.
- Men are at higher risk than women.
- The incidence is increasing, why is unknown.
- Smoking probably increases the risk.
- **Diabetes** (see page 204) may increase the risk.
- The role of alcohol is uncertain.
- It is commonest from 60 years of age.

Recognition

SYMPTOMS
There are no early symptoms of the condition; the sufferer may just feel unwell with nothing to localize the disease. Weight loss is common. There may be abdominal pain, typically felt deep inside and seeming to gnaw into the back. Jaundice, if it occurs, is painfree, as opposed to the jaundice associated with painful **gallstones** (see page 122).

SIGNS
Frequently there is little to find. Only occasionally can a swelling be felt in the abdomen.

INVESTIGATIONS
Modern body scans using **ultrasound** (see page 301) or **X-ray** (see page 301) have greatly simplified the diagnosis of cancer of the pancreas, though not improved how soon it is diagnosed.

ASK YOUR DOCTOR
- About recurrent abdominal pains.
- About back pain appearing for the first time and which interferes with sleep.

Remedy

There are few diseases met with unremitting gloom but cancer of the pancreas is one of them. Five-year survival is just 2 per cent, with many sufferers dying within six months of diagnosis. In a very few cases it may be worth going for rather heroic surgery to remove the pancreas, an operation hazardous in itself and with many after-effects.

On the other hand jaundice, which is a major problem with this cancer, can be relieved by surgery in many cases. Otherwise treatment consists of adequate pain relief and general support.

Alternative Treatment

Techniques such as aromatherapy can be greatly soothing during the illness, and a number of therapies can help to relieve some of the pain. Acupuncture and reflexology would address the body systems appropriate (the endocrine system and the digestive system), and generally improve the overall health of the sufferer, with the intention of encouraging healing and a stronger immune system. Many sufferers suggest that different therapies work for them; indeed, it is probably worth experimenting for one that is suitable for you. Bear in mind, however, that there is no cure and it is wise to be wary of anyone who suggests there is. There is a strong mind–body relationship and if you think a therapy is working, it likely is.

Prevention

There is no method of prevention yet known. Smoking is the one avoidable risk factor. Scares about the effects of drinking coffee have proved to be without foundation.

CANCER OF THE STOMACH

There is a high level of awareness of this cancer; quite rightly, people recognize it as a possibility in the case of upper abdominal pain. Doctors also have a high index of suspicion of the disease, in the knowledge that the earlier it is detected the better the outlook.

Risk

- It is the third most common cause of death from cancer, with about 15 cases per 100,000 population per annum.
- There are 8000 cases a year in the UK.
- Men are affected twice as often as women.
- The incidence varies greatly from country to country; it is, for instance, very common in Japan.
- There is a 20 per cent increased risk in people with group A blood.

- The lower the social class the higher the risk.
- It is commoner in smokers and in the elderly.
- Overall it is becoming less common in the west; why is unknown.
- There is a 1 per cent risk in people with **pernicious anaemia** (see page 199).
- The exact role of diet is uncertain.

Recognition

SYMPTOMS

There is no one symptom of the condition. The general rule is to be suspicious if anyone over the age of forty has the following symptoms, alone or in combination.
- Upper abdominal pain

That is, pain felt just below the breastbone. The pain may be gnawing in nature or it may be a burning pain, exactly like the pain of indigestion. Food and antacids will relieve the pain, as they do in indigestion, serving only to confuse the possible diagnosis.
- Weight loss, loss of appetite

Many cancers cause these symptoms, probably due to chemicals released by the cancer.
- Vomiting, difficulty in swallowing

This may result when tumours cause a partial obstruction (but see also **cancer of the gullet** page 114).
- General effects

Constant bleeding from a stomach cancer can cause anaemia. If cancer spreads into the abdomen there may be abdominal swelling. If the liver is involved there may be jaundice.

SIGNS

It may be possible to feel a firm mass in the upper abdomen or an enlarged liver.

INVESTIGATIONS

The most reliable test is a **gastroscopy** (see page 300), where a tube is passed into the stomach allowing direct vision of the walls of the stomach and allowing samples to be taken from any suspicious looking area. A **barium meal** (see page 297) is commonly performed; if of high quality these can detect up to 90 per cent of tumours, but the results cannot distinguish a tumour from an ulcer in the wall of the stomach. Other tests will show whether the tumour has spread.

ASK YOUR DOCTOR
- **If you have indigestion or pains which are new and you are over forty years of age.**
- **How confident the doctor is of the results, if you have just had a barium meal.**

Remedy

In most cases the cancer is already advanced by the time of diagnosis. In one-third of cancers it is worth removing the tumour together with part of the stomach. It is only at operation that the decision can be made because only then is it possible to see whether the cancer has spread to surrounding tissues or to the liver. This form of surgery offers a 25 to 30 per cent five-year survival.

Sometimes the whole stomach has to be removed; this is a dangerous procedure, with a 10 per cent risk of death in itself. Even if the cancer cannot be removed it is usually possible to perform surgery to relieve obstruction and difficulty in swallowing.

If treated early the outlook is good: 90 per cent survive up to five years. Unfortunately this is the exception and overall there is no more than a 10 per cent chance of five-year survival, with many surviving just a few months from the time of diagnosis. The results of chemotherapy are disappointing.

Alternative Treatment

Any medical condition which cannot be treated successfully by conventional medicine attracts much experimentation in the world of alternative health. There are a number of therapies which are useful, but it is important to beware of charlatans, who proliferate in this field. Having said that, there is a strong mind-body relationship and there is no doubt that if you believe the treatment you are undergoing is working, it is likely to work for just that reason. An acupuncturist might treat symptoms and aim to prevent the cancer from spreading, as well as building up the constitution of the sufferer. There are herbal and homoeopathic remedies for symptoms, and post-operatively, many of the therapies will be useful to encourage the body to heal.

Prevention

The key to prevention is early detection. This is more difficult than it sounds. Indigestion is so common at all ages that not everyone can be investigated instantly. Nor is it feasible to perform gastroscopy on the population as a screening procedure. In Japan, where cancer of the stomach is much more common, screening is on offer and it is true that many 'precancers' are picked up and operated on. But in the UK where the cancer is less common the pick-up rate is too low to justify the cost.

For now the following advice holds:
- stop smoking;
- anyone over forty should have a medical opinion about indigestion of recent onset or persistent abdominal pain;
- doctors need to keep the diagnosis in mind.

Self-Help

BACUP (British Association of Cancer United Patients)
   3 Bath Place, Rivington Street, London EC2A 3JR
   Tel: 0800 181199

DIARRHOEA

Though usually more of a nuisance than a serious threat to health, diarrhoea is included because it is so common and because it may herald more serious illness. Most cases are just gastro-enteritis, otherwise known as a 'tummy bug'. Many countries have popular local names for gastro-enteritis. Regardless of the cause, diarrhoea can be dangerous in infants and in the elderly, where there is risk of rapid dehydration. In Third World countries simple gastro-enteritis is a major cause of death in childhood, through dehydration. Diarrhoea is often accompanied by vomiting. This increases the risks of serious fluid loss.

Risk

- This condition is too common to estimate.
- Episodes lasting for a day or two are rarely of any significance.
- Travellers are at special risk.
- It is extremely common in children through viruses and through changes in diet.

Recognition

Symptoms

- True diarrhoea is the frequent passage of loose or watery motions. That is different from the passage of small quantities of normally formed motions, more likely to be a symptom of an **irritable bowel syndrome** (page 124).
- Toddler's diarrhoea is a common normal finding; the child's motions are persistently a little looser than usual and contain recognizable remains of food, especially vegetables such as corn, peas or carrots. The child thrives and grows normally. No treatment is needed.
- Breastfed babies pass small amounts of loose motions; this looks like diarrhoea but is entirely normal.
- Diarrhoea can co-exist with constipation, a combination common in the elderly. What happens is that solid waste builds up to constipation but liquid motions find their way past the constipated blockage, as if overflowing. The treatment for this is, of course, to relieve the constipation rather than to treat the diarrhoea, which would only make constipation worse.

Signs

When assessing a case of diarrhoea a doctor will be thinking of the following questions:

- Has it caused serious loss of fluid (constant vomiting, thirst, drowsiness, reduced output of urine)?
- Is it likely to recover without treatment; for example, is it just a few episodes of diarrhoea and stomach cramps after eating food that was slightly off?
- Could it be a symptom of more serious illness, because of features such as persistence, blood in the motions, high fever, weight loss, a return from abroad, or abdominal pain?

Investigations

In most cases these are unhelpful; by the time the results arrive the diarrhoea has ended. Where there may be a serious underlying cause, possible investigations range from analysis of motions (to detect infection and blood) to **barium X-rays** (see page 297) of the bowel (if cancer is suspected) or samples of the lining of the bowel (querying a disease such as **Crohn's disease** or **ulcerative colitis** see pages 109 and 132). **Blood tests** (see page 298) can point to unusual diseases which cause diarrhoea as part of a more general picture of malabsorption.

ASK YOUR DOCTOR
- About diarrhoea lasting more than 24 hours in infants.
- About any episode of diarrhoea containing blood or mucus.
- About diarrhoea which happens at night.
- About persistent diarrhoea, especially if you also have abdominal pains or weight loss.
- Whether any drugs you are on might be causing diarrhoea; for example, antibiotics.

Remedy

Any but the mildest episodes need fluid replacement; a useful formula is one teaspoon of sugar and a pinch of salt to every pint of water. Simple as it may seem, this formula greatly improves the uptake of fluid through the walls of the intestine in comparison to drinking water alone. In poor countries where diarrhoea is common this simple public health treatment is life-saving.

On its own this will not stop the diarrhoea, only replace the fluid loss; there are several drugs which do stop diarrhoea, such as kaolin (for children), and codeine and loperamide for adults. Some doctors frown on giving these, because diarrhoea is often the body's means of ridding itself of an invader. If vomiting is a problem anti-nausea drugs can be given by injection or by suppository. In extreme cases – for instance, in children – it may be necessary to replace fluid by drip.

Where infection is proven or suspected, as it might be in recent travellers from abroad, the appropriate antibiotic is used.

It used to be taught that you should stop eating while you had diarrhoea; this is no longer thought necessary; adults and children can have a light diet, comprised perhaps of eggs, rice, bread, etc. It is, however, a good idea to avoid milk, fizzy drinks, sugar and fruit juice (which can have a diarrhoeal effect). Underlying causes are treated as required.

Alternative Treatment

No alternative therapist would take steps to stop the diarrhoea. Diarrhoea is caused by something and it is this which would be addressed. There are a number of therapies which would supply treatments to replace lost fluids. There are others which would ease the discomfort. All, however, would be aimed at treating the cause of the condition. Acupuncture, homoeopathy, herbalism, nutritional therapy, reflexology and acupuncture all may have something to offer.

Diarrhoea in children and in the elderly can be a medical emergency and it is essential that conventional medical treatment is obtained first and foremost.

Prevention

- Basic common-sense measures in dealing with food will reduce the risk of infective gastro-enteritis.

- Breastfeeding provides a certain degree of immunity to the baby, because the milk is clean in itself as well as containing antibodies protective against a range of illnesses.
- Maintain hygiene in any area where food is prepared; that means washing hands frequently, keeping uncooked food away from cooked food, not using the same utensils on cooked and uncooked food, covering food to protect from contamination. Look at your ingredients and smell them, discarding anything that could be off.
- Choose food from shops with a rapid turnover, where food is less likely to go off. Take-away food is one of the pleasures of life but again chose an outlet with a rapid turnover and with known high levels of hygiene. Check sell-by dates.
- When abroad wash fruit, avoid salad unless certain how well it is washed and drink bottled water. Beware of ice; it may be made from contaminated tap water. Use bottled water to clean your teeth. Buy food from roadside vendors with care; look for some evidence of hygiene, rapid turnover and food the raw ingredients for which are recognizably edible.
- Heat food to recommended temperatures and test to see it is cooked through; this is very important if reheating food. Avoid recipes using uncooked eggs, especially for pregnant women, infants and the elderly.
- Be sure your fridge is cold enough by using a fridge thermometer. Follow guidelines for keeping food in the freezer. Do not refreeze food which has thawed and freeze fresh food quickly.

Self-Help

Many organizations and food retailers publish useful guides to food handling. For travellers there is a Department of Health booklet.

GALLSTONES

The gall-bladder is a hollow sac a couple of inches long which nestles under the liver, below the ribs on the right. It connects up with the part of the small intestine called the duodenum through the biliary duct. The gall-bladder produces bile, a complex fluid which helps digestion. It is a kind of detergent which aids the absorption of the fatty elements of the diet. Bile also contains yellow-green pigments formed from the breakdown of old red blood cells.

The gall-bladder churns out a litre of highly concentrated bile every day; not surprisingly deposits build up over time inside the gall-bladder. These deposits can progress to actual gallstones. These are rather greasy pebble-like objects up to a centimetre or two in size. There may be dozens in the gall-bladder.

Surgery to remove the gall-bladder (cholecystectomy) is one of the most common operations performed in the West.

Risk

Generations of doctors were taught that the high-risk group for gallstones was fair, fat, female and forty. Now that it is known just how common gall-stones are, this aphorism should perhaps be amended.

- Gallstones are extremely common; 10 to 20 per cent of the population have them.

- They are twice as common in women.
- Most remain silent, causing no symptoms of illness.
- They are commoner in the West and seem to be increasing in frequency.
- Gallstones are more common with age.
- Risk is increased by the contraceptive pill and a high fat diet.

Recognition

SYMPTOMS

Typically, things begin with a few niggles of discomfort under the right ribs. This is due to the gallstones blocking the exit from the gall-bladder or lodging somewhere in the pipework (biliary duct). With more complete blockage pain increases to 'biliary colic'. That is a very severe persistent pain under the ribs, spreading across the upper abdomen, accompanied by sweating, nausea and vomiting. Some people find that the pain also affects the tip of the right shoulder.

A mild degree of jaundice is common during an attack; the skin and the whites of the eyes become yellow. Often there is fever due to infection in the blocked-off part of the gall-bladder.

Recurrent pains of this sort suggest a condition of chronic inflammation of the gall-bladder.

SIGNS

At the time of an attack there is tenderness under the right ribs and jaundice may be seen. **Peptic ulcer** disease (see page 129), severe indigestion (see page 129) and even a **heart attack** (see page 144) may give a similar picture, which may be difficult to tell apart without tests.

INVESTIGATIONS

An **ultrasound scan** (see page 301) of the gall-bladder is excellent as a quick reliable painless test. **Blood tests** (see page 298) show whether there is any liver damage or **pancreatic disease** (see page 127). If it is thought that there is a gallstone lodged in the pipework, then sophisticated **X-rays** (see page 301) can localize that stone. This procedure glories in the name endoscopic retrograde cholangio-pancreatography, mercifully shortened to **ERCP** (see page 299) and performed via an endoscope, which is a flexible tube passed down the gullet. Sometimes the stone can be dislodged through the endoscope.

ASK YOUR DOCTOR
- **About even mild niggly upper-right-sided abdominal pain; this may be the earliest warning of gallstones.**
- **About any episode of jaundice, no matter how slight.**

Remedy

SURGERY

If you have been unfortunate enough to have biliary colic or infection in the gall-bladder from stones then surgical removal is sensible. It is a far less clear-cut decision if you have suffered from rather vague upper abdominal niggles, and on investigation been found to have gallstones. As they are so common it may be simply coincidence and have nothing at all to do with your symptoms, which may be caused by indigestion or **irritable bowel syndrome** (below). In these circumstances wise doctors will advise a wait-and-see strategy, using other medication to see if they can relieve your symptoms.

The trend is to remove gall-bladders via so-called keyhole surgery. The advantages of this technique are that recovery takes just days and there is only a small scar. Drawbacks are that it is a technically more difficult procedure than the classical operation so you need a highly skilled operator; there also seems to be a slightly higher risk of unforeseen complications.

DRUGS

There are some drugs which will dissolve gallstones over a period of time — up to two years. The early excitement has died away as it has become clear that only a minority of stones are suitable and that it really only buys time until surgery. Still there is a role for this form of treatment in those who neither wish nor are strong enough for surgery.

Alternative Treatment

A low-fat diet may reduce the frequency of attacks of colic. Evidence suggests that a cholesterol-lowering diet may actually increase the chances of developing gallstones (see also **prevention**, below). Acupuncture and homoeopathy may be suitable for treating gall-bladder problems.

Prevention

Gallstones are becoming more frequent in affluent countries so presumably something in our lifestyle is predisposing to them. What exactly is unclear. **Obesity** is one strong association, the treatment of which is under our control (see page 208). Women on the contraceptive pill have a higher risk of developing gallstones, but in practical terms are unlikely to see that as a hazard when weighed against the benefit of controlling their fertility.

Other than these clues there seems nothing else to prevent them. In fact, it is an irony that diets to reduce cholesterol, increasingly popular, increase the risk of gallstones so if anything gallstones are likely to become even more common.

IRRITABLE BOWEL SYNDROME

Also known as irritable colon, spastic colon, and functional bowel disorder, irritable bowel syndrome (IBS) is not a positive diagnosis but rather the name given to what is left when other serious bowel disorders have been ruled out. No one dies from the condition; the greatest hazards are over-vigorous drug treatment or unnecessary surgery. Many cases will improve over six to twelve months.

There is no agreement as to what causes irritable bowel syndrome; the likeliest explanation is that it is something to do with the control of the muscular wall of the bowel, but more than that is unknown. There is undoubtedly a large psychological element as many sufferers are clinically depressed.

Risk

- At least 40 per cent of the population suffer frequent mild abdominal pain and about 20 per cent of the population is considered to suffer from IBS.
- Only a minority (25 to 40 per cent) report that pain to their doctors.
- Sufferers from recurrent abdominal pain make up the majority of people sent to see bowel specialists; irritable bowel syndrome is by far the commonest diagnosed bowel disorder in that group.
- It is most commonly reported by women between 20 and 40 years of age, but surveys suggest that the syndrome is suffered by equal numbers of men and women.
- Symptoms of bowel upset often date back to childhood.

Recognition

There is a core of symptoms recognized by doctors; there may be an array of other nebulous symptoms reported in individual cases.

SYMPTOMS

There is recurrent abdominal pain, perhaps every single day, often described as a 'squeezing' colicky pain. There is a feeling of abdominal distension or bloating. The bowels tend to swing between constipation and diarrhoea, with neither lasting more than a day or two; or they may be normal.

The motions are often pellet-like. Opening the bowels relieves abdominal pain. The abdomen feels distended. The symptoms are made worse by stress or by the menstrual cycle. These symptoms go on for months and years, yet general health is good; there is no weight loss.

SIGNS

There is nothing abnormal on examination; perhaps a little abdominal tenderness but of a non-specific nature. What the doctor is looking for is what is not there: weight loss, ill-health, masses in the abdomen, blood in the motions. There may be signs of stress or depression, which it is important to spot.

INVESTIGATIONS

Certain basic investigations are sensible, no matter how certain the diagnosis appears. These would include **blood tests** (see page 298) and analysis of the motions and urine. Sometimes a **barium enema** (see page 297) is called for or examination of the rectum through a sigmoidoscope. Someone over forty presenting for the first time with these symptoms needs more thorough tests than the young girl who has had symptoms for years.

ASK YOUR DOCTOR

- About any rectal bleeding, mucus or weight loss.
- About a persistent change in bowel habit, whether it is constipation or diarrhoea.
- Do not be afraid to mention if you are worried about some underlying disease or cancer; this worry may be feeding on itself to give rise to the very symptoms that are worrying you. Always admit stress and depression and mention any unusual feature of your diet.

Remedy

REASSURANCE

Simply knowing that there is nothing serious underlying the symptoms is a great relief in itself. Though the symptoms may not go the worry associated with them does. Doctors do not all want to medicalize irritable bowel syndrome.

DIETARY CHANGE

A high fibre diet is a good thing for most sufferers, preferably by adding fruit and vegetables to the diet. Otherwise, there are concentrated fibre drinks to do the same. Occasionally laxatives are needed.

DRUGS

Anti-spasmodic drugs relax the muscles of the bowel, causing less vigorous squeezing actions and therefore less by way of colic. The effect is rather unpredictable, some people reporting great relief, others none at all. Similar effects are obtained by taking peppermint oil, available in a convenient capsule form. If diarrhoea is a feature there are standard drugs that can be used.

Where stress or depression seems important it is worth a trial of a low dose of an anti-depressant.

FOOD ALLERGY AND INTOLERANCE

Many people with the condition believe that certain foods make it worse. Foods commonly blamed are chocolate, bananas, oranges and onions. The way to test this possibility is to keep a careful diary of symptoms over a couple of weeks, then exclude the food you suspect and keep a further note for at least two more weeks. The final step is to reintroduce the food and see what happens. It is important to make no other changes in diet or lifestyle which might otherwise account for any improvement.

Whether food additives might be to blame for vague bowel symptoms is highly controversial; it is possible to test for this by avoiding foods containing additives but in practice this calls for a degree of obsession few can tolerate. If you really suspect this it is best to see a professional dietician for a skilled assessment.

Alternative Treatment

Stress is believed to have an important role in the condition; alternative treatments to relieve stress may well help; for example, aromatherapy, hypnotherapy, massage, yoga or T'ai chi. There are many homoeopathic and herbal remedies which will be prescribed according to your specific symptoms and the triggers for flare-ups. A nutritional therapist will address dietary changes. An acupuncturist will address any fundamental problems causing the condition, and can help to ease discomfort and stress.

Prevention

No breakthroughs have been found to prevent the condition. Most doctors find that by stressing the benign nature of irritable bowel and by suggesting attention to diet and stress, that most sufferers manage to control it and that many grow out of it.

Self-Help

IBS Network
Centre for Human Nutrition, Northern General Hospital, Sheffield, S5 7AU
Tel: 01142 611531

PANCREATITIS

There is a surprising lack of general awareness of this serious, relatively common condition which is a possible diagnosis in anyone with severe upper abdominal pain. The pancreas is a gland at the back of the abdomen which produces hormones and juices needed in digestion. The best known is insulin. In pancreatitis, the gland becomes inflamed, releasing those juices into the abdomen where they go about their function which is to digest tissues. In this case the tissues are the body's own substances – the pancreas itself, the intestines, liver, etc. The result is excruciating pain and a very ill patient.

There is a less dramatic form, chronic pancreatitis, causing recurrent milder upper abdominal pain which may persist for weeks at a time. In that condition eventually the pancreas becomes 'burnt out' with resulting **diabetes** (see page 204) and failure to absorb food properly.

Risk

- There are 13,000 to 14,000 cases causing about 1000 deaths a year.
- **Gallstones** (see page 122) cause 50 per cent of cases of acute pancreatitis.
- Alcohol abuse causes 20 per cent of cases of acute pancreatitis and 80 per cent of cases of chronic pancreatitis. The cause of the rest is often uncertain.
- It is more common in women than men.

Recognition

SYMPTOMS

In acute pancreatitis there is upper abdominal pain which rapidly worsens and becomes excruciating. Vomiting and nausea are common.

In chronic pancreatitis pain comes and goes over months or years, often felt also in the back. The symptoms of diabetes may develop; for example, thirst, excess output of urine and weight loss (page 204).

SIGNS

The patient with acute pancreatitis is clearly ill – in pain, with a low blood pressure and with upper abdominal tenderness. It can be hard to tell it apart from other causes of severe upper abdominal pain such as a bleeding **peptic ulcer** (page 129) or pain from a **gallstone** (page 122). In cases of chronic pancreatitis there may be little to find except for features of **alcoholism** (see page 268).

INVESTIGATIONS

As part of the disease enzymes normally confined to the pancreas spill out into the bloodstream where they can be detected by **blood tests** (see page 298). **CT** or **MRI scans** (see pages 298 and 300) will show whether the gland is inflamed and help differentiate from other causes of upper abdominal pain. Sometimes surgery is needed to clinch the diagnosis.

ASK YOUR DOCTOR
- **About the effects of alcohol. The safe limit for men is 21 units a week, for women 14 units a week (see page 268).**
- **To check recurrent upper abdominal pain; do not assume it is simply indigestion.**

Remedy

Acute pancreatitis is a highly dangerous illness; severe attacks carry a 50 per cent chance of death. Even mild attacks have a 1 per cent risk of death. All cases should be in hospital, where the patient is put on a drip and given pain relief. There are many possible complications from pancreatitis which scans can detect early, especially cysts of the pancreas and abscesses. These are dealt with by surgical drainage. Recovery takes weeks to months.

Chronic pancreatitis is treated with pain relief and replacement of the enzymes no longer produced by the pancreas, like insulin and other enzymes available in capsule form. Sometimes it is possible to remove diseased parts of the gland. If the sufferer stops drinking there is an 80 per cent ten-year survival, but otherwise just 40 per cent ten-year survival.

Alternative Treatment

Use all means of support to give up alcohol. There are therapies which will help to ease the pain of, and control chronic pancreatitis. Acute pancreatitis is a medical emergency and should be treated as such. Acupuncture, homoeopathy, reflexology and medical herbalism might be the most useful therapies to treat the symptoms of pancreatitis and all will take steps to ascertain and then treat its cause.

Prevention

- Where acute pancreatitis has been caused by gallstones they should be removed.
- Have a review of any drugs you are taking as a few can cause pancreatitis, most commonly certain diuretics (water tablets).
- There is a rare form of raised blood fats (raised tri-glycerides) which causes the condition. This is detected via a blood test.
- Stop drinking; this applies to either form of pancreatitis but especially to chronic pancreatitis,.where continued drinking is a self-imposed sentence of death.

Self-Help

Alcoholics Anonymous
PO Box 1, Stonebrow House, Stonebrow, York YO1 2NJ
Tel: 01904 644026
61 Great Dover Street, London SE1 47F
Tel: 0171 352-3001

PEPTIC ULCER AND ACID PROBLEMS

Each day, the stomach produces three litres of highly concentrated hydrochloric acid, required for the digestive process. A thick layer of mucus protects the lining of the stomach from the corrosive action of the acid, but the tubes entering and leaving the stomach – the gullet and the duodenum – are less well protected. Good as the protective mechanism is, it is not totally effective so that acid-related problems are extremely common. They vary from soreness of the lining of the stomach (gastritis) to actual ulceration of the stomach or of the duodenum or the gullet. At worst these ulcers can wear through the walls of the stomach or duodenum, causing a perforation. This is a medical emergency.

Over the last twenty years the diagnosis of these conditions has become more precise while treatment has been transformed by a range of drugs which reduce acid production. 'Peptic ulcer' is a general term which includes ulcers of either the stomach or the duodenum.

Risk

- There is a 15 per cent lifetime risk of having a duodenal ulcer.
- Men have up to four times the risk.
- There is a 5 to 7 per cent risk of having a stomach ulcer.
- Duodenal ulcers are four times commoner than stomach ulcers in the young; both sorts are more common with age.
- Indigestion is so common as to be virtually normal at some time or other.
- Smoking increases the risks of both indigestion and ulcers.
- Aspirin or drugs related to aspirin (widely used for arthritis) frequently cause indigestion or ulceration.
- There is a small genetic tendency for close members of the same family to suffer from peptic ulcers.
- Ulcers can be caused by the stress of major trauma or surgery and it is presumed that the stress of everyday life causes excess acid production, too.
- In the older age group stomach cancer can cause symptoms indistinguishable from a gastric ulcer (see below).

Recognition

The relationship between symptoms and cause is a loose one; it used to be taught that certain patterns of symptoms pointed more to a duodenal ulcer than a stomach ulcer. While this is probably true it is really only of academic interest now; the treatment is the same and diagnosis via endoscopy is precise.

SYMPTOMS

The most reliable feature is pain felt just under the breastbone. The pain is of a burning nature which food may either relieve or make worse. Pain at night is common. Often there is heartburn and a feeling of hunger. More vague symptoms include bloating, wind and nausea. Vomiting is a feature of neglected disease. Symptoms can be highly variable, coming and going from week to week.

Occasionally bleeding is the first symptom. There may be obvious blood in the vomit or the vomit may contain so-called coffee grounds, an excellent description of the gritty fine brown vomit seen when blood has been partly digested before being vomited.

Passing black motions is another important symptom of serious internal bleeding.

> *If a peptic ulcer perforates, it causes sudden severe upper abdominal pain followed by collapse. Urgent medical help is essential.*

Signs

There is rarely anything other than some tenderness under the breastbone. The doctor is on the lookout for weight loss or evidence of bleeding, these suggesting more serious disease.

Investigations

Not everyone needs investigation. It is entirely reasonable to treat someone under the age of forty without investigation, so long as they have none of the worrying features given above. Otherwise, the best investigation is **endoscopy** (see page 299), in which a flexible tube is passed into the stomach and duodenum, under mild sedation. This allows a good look at the lining of the stomach, ulcers can be seen and **biopsies** (see page 298) taken. Increasingly a test is made for helicobacter (see below).

A **barium meal** (see page 297) is good for spotting stomach ulcers, but invariably endoscopy is required in order to take a biopsy to exclude stomach cancer.

ASK YOUR DOCTOR

- **About indigestion which seems to gnaw into your back; this may be a peptic ulcer threatening to perforate.**
- **About any indigestion with associated loss of weight.**
- **If you vomit blood or pass black motions.**

Remedy

Twenty years ago the choice was simple: continual antacids or surgery on the stomach. The more sadistic doctors also prescribed endless boiled fish in milk. All this has changed thanks to two developments. The first has been the discovery of drugs which block acid production. The second is the realization that a 'bug' called helicobacter somehow links with acid disease and that eradicating the bug cures the disease. There is a generation of surgeons who have found that a large chunk of their workload has been lost at one swoop.

Antacids

Simple antacids give rapid relief and are a useful first step in treatment. They do not actually cure any excess acid or ulcers but work by chemically neutralizing the acid.

Acid-reducing drugs

Few treatments deserve the term revolutionary but these drugs do. Their development is an epic of pure science. Starting from a theory that histamine controls how acid is secreted in the stomach, researchers tailored molecules to block histamine – so called H2 receptor antagonists. The result was cimetidine, one of the most effective and commercially successful drugs ever. Soon son of cimetidine appeared, ranitidine, and this has gone on to world acclaim. Both these drugs are remarkably free of side-effects and are effective in treating peptic ulcers and acidity. If necessary, they are safe to take for months or years to keep acid under control.

Very recently a new class of drugs has appeared, proton-pump inhibitors. These are even more effective than the H2 blockers and may well replace them in time. Thanks to these drugs surgery is rarely necessary.

The Helicobacter Story
Helicobacter pylori is a bacterium long thought to be a coincidental finding in peptic ulcer. Just a few years ago an Australian researcher had the thought that far from being a coincidence, it may cause the disease. This has proved to be the case, though its importance is not yet fully understood. Current research is looking at the best way of eradicating this bacterium, thereby curing both gastric and duodenal ulcers for years at a time.

SURGERY

Rare cases resistant to all the considerable fire power of modern drugs may yet come to surgery. The operation cuts the nerves which control the secretion of acid or removes the acid-secreting part of the stomach. In skilled hands these are effective operations but do carry annoying side-effects and so are reserved for selected cases only.

If an ulcer perforates, blood and gastric juices pour into the abdomen. This is a medical emergency for which urgent surgical repair is essential.

Alternative Treatment

Stress is often a cause of peptic ulcer and any therapies which encourage relaxation are useful. A nutritional therapist will provide a diet tailored to your symptoms. There are herbal antacid preparations, and homoeopathic remedies which will be prescribed according to your constitution and symptom picture. Acupuncture and acupressure claim some success in treating this condition. An old wive's tale suggests eating fresh pineapple following every meal (tinned won't do, but only a small slice is necessary). A substance in the pineapple is a natural antacid and relieves the discomfort of an ulcer, and of indigestion and heartburn.

Prevention

- Stop smoking. Quite how nicotine is involved in peptic ulcers is obscure: what is sure is that giving up smoking aids healing and reduces the chances of recurrence. It is probable that excess intake of alcohol worsens acid problems and should be moderated.
- Change of diet is not necessary; however, it is sensible to eat regular meals and to try to have those in an unhurried way.

- Many drugs irritate the stomach, of which by far the commonest are aspirin and others in the class of NSAIDS (non-steroidal anti inflammatory drugs). Examples are ibuprofen, indomethacin, naproxen. Several are available over the counter for treatment of arthritis, sports injuries and back trouble. They are useful drugs but carry a serious risk of stomach irritation when used frequently. Older people and those who drink or smoke run a higher risk. You should discuss with your doctor whether you need to keep taking these drugs; report any acid problems you notice. If your doctor considers they are essential it is possible to prescribe with them a drug which helps protect the lining of the stomach from their irritant effect.
- It cannot be stressed too much that the symptoms of **stomach cancer** (page 117) can be indistinguishable from those of a peptic ulcer. The older the individual the more this possibility must be thought about.

ULCERATIVE COLITIS

This disease of the bowel has some similarities to **Crohn's disease** (page 109) but tends to be more dramatic in onset. It is a generalized inflammation of the colon, (the large intestine and rectum) giving rise to pain, **diarrhoea** (see page 119) and rectal bleeding. Like Crohn's disease the cause is unknown, with infection or immune problems being currently suspected. For most people it is a lifelong illness, where periods of inactivity mingle with flare-ups of varying degrees of severity. There is an increased risk of cancer of the bowel, needing regular specialist follow-up. On the other hand there is a form of the disease, proctitis, confined to the rectum where the long-term outlook is excellent.

Risk

- There are 5 to 10 new cases per 100,000 of population per year.
- There are about 60,000 sufferers in the UK.
- It is more common in Jews.
- Ulcerative colitis is commoner in the Western world.
- It is commoner in relatives of sufferers.
- It begins mainly between the ages of 20 and 40.
- Women are affected more often than men.
- It is half as common in smokers (this is about the only benefit of smoking ever detected!).
- In cases of proctitis, only 10 per cent go on to full-blown ulcerative colitis.

Recognition

Even in the first attack there is usually little doubt that there is a serious disease going on.

SYMPTOMS
The main feature is profuse bloody **diarrhoea** (see page 119), often mixed with mucus and often accompanied by abdominal pain especially when opening the bowels. There may be a general feeling of illness plus high temperatures and dehydration to the point of collapse.

In about 10 per cent of cases the individual has just one attack, another 10 per cent of sufferers have persistent symptoms and the rest fall somewhere in between.

Proctitis shows itself as blood streaking on the motions and pain on opening the bowels.

SIGNS

The individual is clearly unwell, with left-sided abdominal tenderness.

INVESTIGATIONS

The diagnosis is made by taking a **biopsy** (see page 298) from the rectum, which looks raw and oozes blood. **Blood tests** (see page 298) give a good indication of how active the disease is, as do **X-rays** (see page 301) of the colon.

There are infections which can give a similar picture, as can poor blood flow to the bowel. **Cancer of the colon** (see page 111) does not usually cause such a dramatic picture but has to be kept in mind in older patients.

ASK YOUR DOCTOR

- **About any rectal bleeding, no matter how slight.**
- **About regular checks on the possibility of cancer of the bowel, if you have ulcerative colitis.**
- **To be sure to test your motions for infection, following a first attack, as amoebic dysentery mimics ulcerative colitis but is curable.**

Remedy

Mild attacks are treated with steroids and anti-diarrhoeal agents. Severe attacks must be handled in hospital as there is a major risk of dehydration and of the bowel bursting; this carries a high mortality.

The drug sulphasalazine and other equivalents reduce the frequency and severity of flareups; most sufferers need to take it continuously. As ulcerative colitis affects the colon, surgical removal of the colon may be sensible in patients whose disease is continuously active, especially after more than ten years of activity, when there is a sharp rise in the risk of cancer of the bowel.

By contrast, proctitis responds to steroid foam introduced into the rectum.

There is no evidence that allergies cause the condition. However, sufferers do find that certain foods make symptoms worse and it is sensible to follow those instincts.

Alternative Treatment

Stress may trigger a flare up, so alternative therapies to reduce stress may help. These include yoga, T'ai chi, hypnotherapy, massage, aromatherapy, among others. Conventional medical treatment must be sought in a flare-up, which must be considered a medical emergency. However, in order to prevent further flare-ups, acupuncture, homoeopathy and herbalism, undertaken by registered practitioners, might be helpful. A nutritional therapist might address aspects of diet which exacerbate the condition.

Prevention

Although the disease itself cannot be prevented it may be possible to reduce the frequency and severity of flare-ups by avoiding stress. Some people find that antibiotics set off attacks and so these should be used sparingly.

A major but preventable long-term risk is of cancer of the bowel. Those at greatest risk are sufferers whose whole bowel is affected by ulcerative colitis and where the disease has been active for more than ten years. Here the risk of cancer may up to forty times that of the general population. Ideally these individuals should have regular inspections of their colon (**colonoscopy**, see page 298) to detect early tumours. There is interest in the use of nicotine patches to reduce the risk of flare-ups.

Self-Help

National Association for Colitis and Crohn's Disease
98a London Road, St Albans, Herts AL1 1NX
Tel: 01727 844296

HEART, BLOOD VESSELS AND CIRCULATION

- Aneurysms • Cardiomyopathy
- Deep Vein Thrombosis • Endocarditis
- Heart Attacks • Heart Failure
- High Blood Pressure (Hypertension)
- High Cholesterol • Ischaemic Heart Disease
- Poor Circulation

DURING THE COURSE of the twentieth century, diseases of the heart and circulation have become the single biggest cause of death in most of the developed world and the cause of much chronic ill-health. All the evidence suggests that something about the Western way of life increases the chances of arteries becoming furred up with atheroma, a mixture of blood clot and cholesterol leading to poor blood flow and eventually heart disease or blockage of blood flow to a limb.

Although there is general agreement thus far, controversy surrounds the specific reasons for this change. The candidates are high blood pressure, raised cholesterol, stress, smoking, lack of exercise and obesity. Smoking apart, the evidence linking these factors to heart disease is of variable strength. Smoking stands on its own as an unquestionable risk factor.

The problem with proving the weight of those other risk factors is the time scale needed to show the effects of changes in diet, exercise patterns, etc. These studies are being done, but out of necessity they extend over decades. Within this section we have tried to give a fair account of the current weight of evidence. In summary, it carries no great surprises: reduce your intake of animal fats (saturated), increase exercise, maintain a recommended weight, have high blood pressure treated, drink in moderation and stop smoking.

ANEURYSMS

An aneurysm is the term describing a ballooning out of the wall of an artery. Arteries have muscular walls to cope with the high pressure of blood within them. At certain sites in the body, the walls of arteries are especially liable to weaken. Eventually the artery widens until there is a large bulbous swelling of part of the wall. Blood within that section no longer flows smoothly but swirls around. This increases the chances of a blood clot forming in that section. The blood clot has the effect of further weakening the artery. The wall can become so weak that it bursts. If the artery is one of the major ones, the result is instant death. If the swelling is detected before that stage there is a good chance of successful surgical repair.

The commonest artery affected is the aorta, the large main artery which carries blood away from the heart. In the abdomen this is about an inch wide; if an aneurysm is present, this can increase to as much as three to four inches. Small aneurysms are also found within the brain, where they are a cause of strokes, especially in younger people (see **subarachnoid haemorrhage**, page 266).

Aneurysms are so common that surgeons are increasingly arguing for a system to screen for them in older age groups.

Risk

- Aneurysms are rare until late middle age.
- Asymptomatic aneurysms are found in 5 per cent of 65-year-olds; and in 10 per cent of 80-year-old men.
- People at higher risk of atherosclerosis are also more prone to aneurysms (see **ischaemic heart disease**, page 157)
- Those with **high blood pressure** (see page 150) have a two to three times increased risk of having an aneurysm.
- A 3 per cent death rate in elective surgery compares to a 50 per cent death rate in emergency surgery, which excludes those who die before receiving medical help.

Recognition

In many cases there are no symptoms until the aneurysm bursts, causing sudden abdominal pain and, usually, inevitable death.

Symptoms
You may notice a pulsation in your abdomen, more prominent when lying flat. This can be normal in very thin people but it is suspicious if it is new for you. The book in bed test is useful; if a book balanced on your tummy bounces up and down, there is cause for concern. Backache can be a feature of a large abdominal aortic aneurysm, which is pressing against the back of the abdomen. This is an unusual cause of backache, but must be considered in an older person developing backache for the first time. Chest pain can happen if the aneurysmal artery extends up into the chest.

Signs
If the aneurysm is a large one, it can be felt by pressing down on the abdomen. There may be signs that tiny blood clots have escaped from within the aneurysm; these are seen as little purple specks on the toes. There may be signs of poor blood flow into the legs.

Investigations
Abdominal **ultrasound** (see page 301) shows up aneurysms well, allows them to be precisely measured and is an easy way of checking whether they are expanding. A chest **x-ray** (see page 301) may show features suggestive of an aneurysm of the aorta within the chest. Occasionally an abdominal aortic aneurysm shows up on an abdominal x-ray taken for some other reason.

There are a few rare conditions which can cause aneurysms which may need to be considered. Syphilis used to be a significant reason for aneurysms, but is now uncommon.

ASK YOUR DOCTOR
- **About any gnawing form of backache.**
- **If one of your toes suddenly goes white, blue or painful; this may be due to a blood clot cutting off the blood flow.**
- **If you notice a pulsation within your belly.**

Remedy

The treatment depends on the stage of the aneurysm.

If an aneurysm has been found before it causes any symptoms, and as long as it measures no more than 5 cm across, the surgeon will keep it under regular review using ultrasound scans. Once the aneurysm grows above that size surgery is recommended. This involves cutting out the diseased section of artery and replacing it with a graft. It is a major operation, but the success rate in the best centres is 97 per cent.

If the aneurysm is leaking (causing backache or bleeding), then emergency surgery is the only option, again replacing the diseased section with a graft. The mortality in such cases is 50 per cent of those who survive long enough to reach hospital. A ruptured abdominal aortic aneurysm is a common cause of sudden death. If the individual does not die immediately and if a specialized surgical team can operate rapidly, the death rate is still 50 per cent.

Alternative Treatment

There is no substitute for surgical repair of an established aneurysm. Post-operatively, and preventatively, alternative therapies can be useful for improving your overall level of health and well-being. See **heart disease**, page 157.

Prevention

There is great interest in screening for asymptomatic abdominal aortic aneurysms. This is based on the fact that 5 per cent of men aged sixty-five and 10 per cent of men in their eighties have an aneurysm. With detection being simple and safe and with surgery being very successful, screening seems an excellent idea. As always it comes down to cost and organization; it is likely that it will become part of a recognized screening process before too long.

Self-Help

Coronary Prevention Group
102 Gloucester Place, London W1H 3DA
Tel: 0171 935-2889

CARDIOMYOPATHY

Cardiomyopathy is a general term for a number of different diseases that affect the actual muscle of the heart, as opposed to its blood flow or valves. Sometimes there is an identifiable cause, such as alcohol, or the effects of a virus. In most cases no cause can be found. The disease weakens the heart muscle; in one form this gives rise to heart failure.

In another form, it is a cause of sudden death in young adults, thought to be due to a sudden abnormality of the rhythm of the heart.

Risk

- There are an estimated 20,000 to 24,000 people affected in the UK.
- Some forms of the condition run in families.
- Once identified treatment is essential to prevent deterioration or sudden death.
- There is a 2 to 3 per cent annual risk of sudden death.

Recognition

SYMPTOMS

There may be the symptoms of **heart failure** (see page 147); these include breathlessness, swelling of the legs, tiredness. It is a possible cause of **angina** (see page 158), which is pain from the heart on exertion.

One particularly important symptom is feeling faint or even falling unconscious on exertion. All these symptoms are a reflection of the heart's inability to keep pumping an adequate supply of blood to the rest of the body.

SIGNS

There are not likely to be any signs unless there is heart failure. A cardiologist may be able to detect slight but significant changes in the way the heart sounds through a stethoscope.

INVESTIGATIONS

Ultrasound (page 301) imaging of the heart has made the diagnosis of cardiomyopathy far easier by showing on screen the abnormally thickened or stiff heart muscle. As a screening test, chest X-rays and the **ECG** (recording of the heart, see page 299) sometimes pick up suggestive features. The few rare treatable diseases which can cause cardiomyopathy are found by **blood tests** (see page 298). In really puzzling cases a **biopsy** (see page 298) of the heart muscle is taken via a catheter guided into the heart from the large femoral artery in the groin.

ASK YOUR DOCTOR

- **If cardiomyopathy was the cause of death in a member of your family who has died young; if so, other members of the family should be screened for the condition.**
- **If, despite no change in your fitness or exercise level, you start to feel faint on exertion.**

Remedy

If there is a treatable cause (excess alcohol intake, high blood pressure), that is dealt with. Next, drugs are given to relieve any heart failure; these are the familiar diuretics (water tablets) which force the body to lose fluid, thereby reducing strain on the heart. Drugs are given to stabilize the heart in a normal rhythm and these have to be taken for the foreseeable future.

Despite these measures some individuals remain in heart failure or at considerable risk of sudden death. These sufferers are candidates for a heart transplant, a procedure which has long stopped being experimental and which is now successful in most cases. The five-year survival of people having a heart transplant is 70 per cent. This may sound unimpressive, but not if you consider that these are individuals who would otherwise have been certain of steady deterioration or sudden death.

Alternative Treatment

Alternative therapies should not be undertaken to treat this condition, unless they are taken alongside conventional medicine and with the approval of your doctor. Some therapies are designed to enhance health and well-being, and these are complementary to the aims of orthodox medicine. Homoeopathic remedies can be taken by anyone, under the supervision of a registered homoeopath. Gentle exercises like T'ai chi or yoga are useful and may help to relax the sufferer. Acupuncture and acupressure may be used with conventional medicine.

Prevention

Alcohol is the one common preventable agent. Otherwise take note of any cases of early sudden death from heart disease within your immediate family. Not only should this lead to tests for raised **cholesterol** (see page 153) but also to consider screening other young members of the close family for cardiomyopathy. If a previously fit young adult starts to experience faintness on exercise, this should not be shrugged off as it can be the earliest symptom of a cardiomyopathy.

Self-Help

Association for Children with Heart Disorders
26 Elizabeth Drive, Helmshore, Rossendale, Lancs BB4 4JB
Tel: 01706 213632

HOCM Association
40, The Metro Centre, Tolpits Lane, Watford WD1 8SB
Tel: 01923 249977

DEEP VEIN THROMBOSIS AND PULMONARY EMBOLISM

Thrombosis means clotting of blood. This can occur anywhere in the circulation, but is far more common in the more sluggish blood flow in the veins than in the rapid circulation within the arteries. Deep vein thrombosis (abbreviated to DVT) is unpleasant in itself, but its main importance is the risk it poses of a pulmonary embolus. That happens when a portion of the blood clot breaks away, flies off towards the heart, where it is pumped off into the lungs. The blood clot lodges in the lungs, with the result that the blood supply to an area of lung is obstructed. This is termed a pulmonary embolus. An embolus is the obstruction; the term embolism refers to the condition of having an embolus.

What happens next depends on how big the clot is; a small one can pass entirely unnoticed; larger ones cause pain and breathlessness. The largest clots completely obstruct blood flow to the lungs, this being a significant cause of sudden death after operations. This is why the prevention of DVT has been of major importance in reducing the risks of surgery.

Risk

- There are 20,000 known deaths from pulmonary embolus per annum and probably many more unrecognized ones.
- DVT occurs in 50 per cent of people after a **stroke** (see page 262), and there are about 100,000 strokes per annum.
- DVT occurs in one-third of people after a **heart attack** (see page 144), and there are up to about 150,000 heart attacks per annum.
- It is likely that many more DVTs happen but go unrecognized.
- There is increased risk in the immobile, the obese, and those in heart failure.
- DVT occurs in about 1 of every 1000 users of the contraceptive pill per annum.
- Cancer sufferers are at higher risk of DVT, for unknown reasons.
- There is a slightly increased risk in pregnancy.

Recognition

Many DVTs go unrecognized until they cause a symptom such as a pulmonary embolus.

SYMPTOMS
Most commonly you notice a sudden pain in the calf, followed by swelling of that leg. This suggests a blood clot in the deep veins of the calf. If there is painful swelling above the knee it points to a thrombosis extending up into the great veins of the leg or of the pelvis.

A pulmonary embolus produces a sudden knife-like pain in the chest, which is worse when breathing in. It may be accompanied by breathlessness and the coughing of fresh blood. Really large pulmonary emboli cause sudden faintness with chest discomfort, to the point of unconsciousness.

Do not confuse a DVT with the far less important thrombophlebitis, which is also a blood clot, but in a superficial vein. It can be felt as a tender cord just below the surface of the skin. If in doubt, ask your doctor to check.

SIGNS
The lower leg is swollen and the calf feels tense and painful. Swelling may extend up the leg, in which case there is usually a lot of pain. In the lungs it may be possible to hear a rubbing noise where the embolus has lodged.

INVESTIGATIONS
These are always necessary, firstly to confirm the diagnosis and secondly to see how far the thrombosis extends. An **ultrasound scan** (see page 301) is quick at diagnosing a large DVT; otherwise a **venogram** (see page 301) is performed which involves injecting a dye into the veins of the leg.

To detect a pulmonary embolus a **lung scan** (see page 300) is the most sensitive test, although an **ECG** (see page 299) can help, plus knowledge of the obvious signs and symptoms.

ASK YOUR DOCTOR
- **To advise on prevention of DVT before you go into hospital for surgery.**
- **About alternative contraception; if you have ever had a DVT you must not take the contraceptive pill.**

Remedy

If you suspect a DVT you need urgent assessment, while for a pulmonary embolus you should have emergency treatment. The immediate aim is to anti-coagulate the blood, by reducing its tendency to clot. This is done by injections of heparin for a few days, after which you will be switched to warfarin by mouth. How long you stay on warfarin depends on the reasons for the DVT; six to twelve weeks is usual.

Additional treatment for a major pulmonary embolus is with a drug that dissolves the blood clot; such a one is streptokinase; this is occasionally also used for large DVTs in the pelvic veins. Rarely and only at high risk, it may be possible to surgically remove a large blood clot from the lung.

Following a DVT the chances are that the leg will always be prone to swelling, because the deep network of veins has been destroyed. There will always be an increased risk of another DVT.

Alternative Treatment

Many therapies will advise you to switch to fish oils and to take vitamin E and garlic, and this is probably worthwhile as a general measure to reduce circulation problems. An established DVT or pulmonary embolus should only be treated by conventional methods. Post-operatively, there are a number of therapies which can encourage the body to heal.

Prevention

The main opportunity for prevention is at the time of major surgery; especially repair of a fractured hip and abdominal surgery. These individuals should have heparin or warfarin until they are mobile, unless they have one of the few conditions where this is inadvisable (for example, a bleeding stomach ulcer). During and after surgery individuals can wear special compression stockings. There is also risk following an immobilizing illness such as a heart attack, when anticoagulants may be advisable.

The earlier you become mobile the better – most DVTs occur within three days of immobility; that is why there is such an emphasis on walking even after major surgery.

If you are faced with having major surgery, including hip replacement, it is entirely reasonable to ask what measures are taken by that hospital to prevent DVT; if they do not propose to use heparin ask why not; there may be some good medical reason in your individual case but otherwise push for a satisfactory explanation.

ENDOCARDITIS

Endocarditis is an infection of the lining or valves of the heart. Although it can occur as a rapidly progressive disease, more usually it smoulders away for weeks and months producing rather non-specific symptoms until well advanced.

Infection can attack the healthy heart but the main risk is where there is any abnormality in the heart. With modern investigation of minor heart conditions, these are increasingly recognized and therefore increasing numbers of people are being advised to have antibiotic treatment to avoid endocarditis (see **Prevention**, below).

Bacteria can enter the bloodstream any number of ways; for example, during operations or even when brushing the teeth. The body has superb systems for mopping up these germs but it only takes a few to make it through the net to cause endocarditis. The disease is far more common in the developing world.

Risk

- Estimates range from 1500 to 3000 cases a year, causing 450 deaths.
- The risk increases if there are even minor changes in the smoothness of heart valves.
- Anything increasing the risk of infection in the bloodstream increases the chances of endocarditis; for example, intravenous drug users and those on dialysis for kidney disease.
- The elderly are at higher risk.

Recognition

SYMPTOMS
The symptoms are those of a chronic infection, that is a general feeling of malaise, weight loss, drenching sweats at night and fevers. In untreated cases there is more damage to heart valves, ending up with heart failure, strokes and kidney damage. If untreated, the disease is almost always fatal. Even treated there still is a 30 per cent mortality.

SIGNS
The best sign is suspicion of the condition in someone known to have a heart abnormality and who becomes vaguely unwell over a few weeks. Hence there may be a murmur over the heart, or the individual may have an artificial valve and have recently had some operative procedure which could have introduced infection into the bloodstream.

More specific signs are the effects caused when clumps of bacteria detach themselves from the main infection and lodge in small blood vessels elsewhere (emboli). In the nail beds there may be a few dark lines left from tiny bleeds under the nail. Perhaps there are some painful spots on the limbs due to other haemorrhages. If this happens in the brain it can cause a **stroke** (see page 262).

Over several weeks the nails themselves become highly curved in a special way called clubbing. The person looks anaemic and it may be possible to feel a spleen. Subtle signs all of these, but they are highly suggestive to the observant physician.

INVESTIGATIONS
The ease of diagnosis has improved since the availability of **echo–cardiograph scans** (see page 299) of the heart. These can show up the actual clumps of bacteria clinging to the valves and lining. It can also tell whether valves have been so damaged that they must be surgically replaced. The other crucial investigation is **blood culture** (see page 298),

trying to grow organisms from the bloodstream. Blood cultures may need to be repeated many times before obtaining a positive result. Other blood tests help follow progress of the condition.

ASK YOUR DOCTOR

- If you suffer from night sweats; the causes range from benign (the menopause, see page 86) to very serious (leukaemia and endocarditis, pages 194 and 141).
- If your fingernails become clubbed. There are many causes for this, with chronic infections and chronic lung disease (including lung cancer) being possibilities.
- If you have heart valve problems and become generally unwell.
- Whether you should have preventative antibiotics before any form of surgery, including dental work.

Remedy

The object is to identify the organism and then to hit it with long, strong concentrations of the antibiotics to which it is sensitive. To start with this has to be via a drip in hospital, switching to therapy by mouth after two to three weeks, for several weeks more. Surgery may be necessary to replace hopelessly damaged valves or those where the infection just cannot be eradicated any other way. Complications from the infection have to be dealt with as they arise; for example, heart failure, strokes, kidney damage.

Alternative Treatment

Not recommended for this dangerous illness. Some therapies may be used recuperatively, but if you are advised to have preventative antibiotics for whatever reason, do not be tempted to substitute natural remedies.

Prevention

As echo-cardiographs are more widely used, increasing numbers of people are being found to have minor abnormalities of their heart valves. Thus increasing numbers of people are advised to take antibiotics before any surgical procedure. This includes dental polishing and scaling – although there is a theoretical risk of infection from vigorous brushing of teeth it is impractical to stay on antibiotics continuously for this eventuality. A single high dose of antibiotic is normally all that is recommended.

Obvious sources of infection should be dealt with; including chronically inflamed teeth and recurrent boils. As has been said earlier, the best prevention for this condition remains a high index of suspicion in at-risk individuals.

Self-Help

British Heart Foundation
14 Fitzharding Street, London W1H 4DH
Tel: 0171 935-0185

HEART ATTACKS

Also known as a coronary thrombosis or a myocardial infarction, frequently abbreviated to MI, heart attacks occur when the blood supply to part of the heart is interrupted. This is nearly always associated with narrowing of the coronary arteries with atheroma, the sludge of cholesterol and fat which coagulates and blocks the arteries (see **cholesterol**, page 153). It is thought that a blood clot forms on the atheroma, blocking the artery with a mixture of atheroma and clot.

The result is to cut off the blood supply to the heart muscle downstream. The muscle might have more than one blood supply; if so it may survive. If its only supply is lost, then the chances are that some portion of the heart muscle will die – this is the true meaning of the term infarction.

Why should such an event be so serious? One reason is that the heart's output is geared to the usual demands of the individual; that is why people in training have bigger hearts than those out of training. So to lose a large part of the heart muscle suddenly leaves the heart unable to cope with the body's demands for blood supply. The result is **heart failure** (see page 147).

The second reason is to do with the control of the heart's speed and output. This is partly controlled by electrical impulses that flow around the heart in a wonderful system of 'cabling', the effect of which is to ensure that the whole contraption pumps away in a coordinated, efficient way. When part of the muscle is damaged it causes all sorts of abnormal electrical interference which distorts that normal electrical activity. The result can be a simple irregular heart rhythm or it may be the dreaded ventricular fibrillation, a chaotic quivering of the heart which achieves nothing and, untreated, is the prelude to death.

Heart attacks were unheard of before the twentieth century. Early, somewhat puzzled reports of heart attacks in the first decades of the century are curious reading to modern eyes, which are only too familiar with the condition. The frequency of heart attacks is falling. The reason for this is unknown.

Risk

- Heart attacks are the single most common cause of death in the UK and much of the Western world.
- There are an estimated 150,000 per annum.
- Men are at higher risk than women.
- Smokers, the overweight, those with high blood pressure and with raised cholesterol are all at greater risk.
- The more risk factors the greater the overall risk; that is, someone who smokes and has high blood pressure is at much greater risk than someone who smokes but has normal blood pressure.
- 50 per cent of those who are going to die from an MI do so within the first two to three hours; 75 per cent within the first 24 hours. Overall, 40 per cent of people who have an MI die within a month.
- For survivors, there is about a 20 per cent risk of death in the year after the MI, and 5 to 10 per cent each year after that. That means there is a 75 per cent, five-year survival, 50 per cent ten-year survival.

Recognition

SYMPTOMS

The fundamental symptom is chest pain. It comes on at rest (unlike **angina**, see page 157), persists and can be very intense. In severe cases there is sweating, breathlessness, nausea and vomiting. In mild cases the pain may be relatively modest, unusual only for its persistence.

In a few cases (an estimated 20 per cent) the heart attack is 'silent', in that it causes no pain. It is recognized only through the complications it may cause, such as sudden breathlessness.

SIGNS

The sufferer may look ashen and pale, sweating and breathless. There are fine crackles in the lungs, indicating the ominous build-up of fluid from a failing heart. There may be unusual heart rhythms. If it has been a 'silent' heart attack, all there is to go by is a sudden unexplained deterioration in someone's general condition, with breathlessness, an abnormal heart rhythm or, in the elderly, confusion.

INVESTIGATIONS

The fundamental investigation is an **ECG** (see page 299), to display the electrical activity of the heart. Abnormal wave forms appear from the damaged heart muscle and the ECG also reveals unusual rhythms. Characteristic enzymes spill out of the damaged muscle and show up on **blood tests** (see page 298) but these take a day or so to become abnormal. In dubious cases it is possible to make a **radioactive scan** (see page 301) of the heart, but this is rarely done.

In the first hour or so the ECG may be normal. The wise physician does not treat the ECG but treats the patient. If the symptoms and signs all point to a heart attack, the patient is treated for that, regardless of the ECG appearance.

ASK YOUR DOCTOR
- **About chest pains which are persistent.**
- **About a chest pain which is unusual for you, even if you already suffer from angina.**

Remedy

The last few years have seen a revolution in the treatment of heart attacks. Until recently treatment concentrated on dealing with pain, heart failure and abnormal heart rhythms. Those are still crucially important but now the most immediate emphasis is on limiting the area damaged by the infarction, using the drugs below.

ASPIRIN

This familiar drug reduces the tendency of the blood to clot; it therefore reduces the size of the thrombosis in the heart and the blockage resulting from it. Aspirin therapy is continued for some while after a heart attack, some specialists recommend forever.

FIBRINOLYTIC TREATMENT

The blood clot doing the damage is made up of a protein called fibrin. Fibrinolytic drugs dissolve that fibrin as long as they are given soon enough. For maximum effect fibrinolytic therapy must be started within six hours of the heart attack, though there is still some benefit from having them within twenty-four hours. The drugs are given in an intravenous drip. Their use has reduced early mortality from heart attacks by a staggering 30 per cent, the biggest single improvement in treatment seen this century.

Supportive treatment

It remains as important as ever for heart failure to be dealt with, for pain to be relieved and to detect those heart rhythms which can suddenly threaten death. In most cases this is best achieved in hospital in a coronary care unit. A few centres perform emergency surgery to bypass the blocked arteries which have caused the heart attack.

Rehabilitation

Rehabilitation aims to return the individual to a normal life within two to three months via a programme of supervised activities. The psychological after-effects of having a heart attack can be overwhelming for some individuals, who need sympathetic reassurance about their prospects.

Alternative Treatment

Once the individual is on the road to recovery, alternative therapies emphasizing a good diet, gentle activity, and mental relaxation have much to offer. This should be taken in the context of general advice on lifestyle as below. Many therapies are excellent in the rehabilitation stage of the illness; see a registered homoeopath, herbalist or acupuncturist for advice that is tailored to you, your condition and your constitution.

Prevention

The risks factors for heart attacks are the same as those for **ischaemic heart disease** (see page 157). In summary stop smoking, treat **high blood pressure** (see page 150), reduce weight (see **obesity**, page 208) and deal with raised blood fats (see also **high cholesterol**, page 153).

The biggest single avoidable risk factor is smoking; no survivor from a heart attack should smoke again unless their attitude to taking risks sees early death as part of life's rich tapestry. If you have had a heart attack you may be advised about medical treatment to prevent another one. Aspirin has been mentioned. Some specialists advice anti-coagulants to thin the blood for perhaps a year after a heart attack. Drugs called beta-blockers reduce complications if taken for about a year after the attack; they work by reducing the chances of an abnormal heart rhythm.

The rise and fall of the heart attack is a twentieth-century story. Figures from the USA show that the frequency of heart attacks there has been falling since the 1960s, long before there was such an emphasis on healthy living and treatment of high blood pressure or cholesterol. It may turn out that the medical profession is wrong about the reasons for heart attacks, but for now the advice on prevention is based on current theory and recommendations.

Finally a reminder about having rapid treatment; the necessary drugs have to be given within six hours, if possible. Doctors in country areas may carry these drugs, but in town areas it may be better to call an ambulance in order to reach hospital as soon as possible.

Self-Help

British Heart Fandation
14 Fitzhardinge Street, London, W1H 4DH
Tel: 0171 935 0185
Family Heart Association
Wesley House, 7 High Street, Kidlington, Oxford OX5 2DH
Tel: 01865 370292

HEART FAILURE

Heart failure is the inability of the heart to keep up with the body's requirements for blood flow. It can cover all degrees of severity, from a bit of breathlessness on exertion to an individual swollen up with retained fluid and breathless on the slightest exertion. Although a common disorder, heart failure has been seen very much as an inevitable consequence of ageing. Advances in treatment now mean that more can be done.

Risk

- Heart failure affects an estimated 1 per cent of the over sixty-fives.
- It is most often caused by **ischaemic heart disease** (see page 157) or as a consequence of a **heart attack** (see page 144).
- It is an end result of severe uncontrolled high blood pressure.
- It can result from disease of the valves of the heart.
- Heart failure is occasionally a consequence of other disease; e.g., **over-active thyroid gland** (see page 211), **anaemia** (see page 186) and **cardiomyopathy** (see page 137).
- Despite modern advances 50 per cent of sufferers from severe heart failure survive no more than two years.

Recognition

SYMPTOMS
- Breathlessness

This is the commonest early symptom. In severe cases this may occur even at rest, but more commonly only on exertion. Breathlessness can occur if lying flat. In these cases the sufferer learns to prop themselves up at night, using more and more pillows until eventually sleeping virtually upright. The reason for the breathlessness is the pooling of fluid in the lungs when lying flat.

- Fatigue

The body is being under-provided with oxygen, while waste products tend to accumulate. The net result is tiredness.

- Accumulation of fluid

Fluid in the lungs causes breathlessness. Very commonly fluid accumulates around the ankles, then the legs and, untreated, within the abdomen itself. This is different from the benign, mild degree of ankle swelling seen in so many elderly people which does not deteriorate in the same way.

Signs

These really confirm in more precise ways the above features. Crackles in the lungs reflect the build-up of fluid, changes in heart sounds reflect the heart under pressure and there may be murmurs from diseased heart valves. Signs of fluid may be found in the abdomen even though the individual had no suspicion of fluid.

There might be features of disease contributing to the heart failure such as **high blood pressure** (see page 150), the racing pulse and staring eyes of **thyrotoxicosis** (see page 212) or the pallor of **severe anaemia** (see page 186).

Investigations

A chest **X-ray** (see page 301) will show shadows from fluid on the lungs; an **ECG** (see page 299) may show an enlarged struggling heart or perhaps signs of a silent **heart attack** (see page 144), or a rhythm that is making the heart less efficient. **Blood tests** (see page 298) detect effects on the kidneys or anaemia. If there are abnormal heart sounds or murmurs, then an **echocardiogram** (see page 299) will reveal which valves are damaged.

Angiography (see page 297) is a way of demonstrating blood flow around the heart; this is not a routine investigation but reserved for cases where the sufferer may benefit from **coronary artery bypass grafting** (see page 160).

ASK YOUR DOCTOR

- **About unusual breathlessness or odd heart rates; do not ignore these as expected consequences of ageing.**
- **About ankle swelling that seems to be progressing.**
- **If you are unable to lie flat in bed through breathlessness.**

Remedy

In a minority of cases investigations detect a specific cause for heart failure with its own specific treatment; for example, anaemia or abnormal heart valves which can be replaced. The majority of cases are down to ischaemic heart disease. Sometimes it will be possible to replace the blood supply by coronary artery grafting.

Diuretics (water tablets)

These are the mainstay of treatment whatever the underlying cause. Diuretic drugs force the body to excrete more urine than normal (hence the name water tablets) so reducing the volume of fluid that the heart has to pump. In sudden heart failure diuretics given intravenously in large doses are life-saving. Many sufferers remain on a low dosage.

ACE inhibitors

These are the big recent success story in the treatment of heart failure. They are drugs with a complex series of actions on the kidney and on blood vessels, the net result of which is to improve the heart's performance. They need to be given with diuretics in most cases and need careful monitoring at the start of treatment. Thereafter they are well tolerated. Probably all sufferers from heart failure should have at least a trial on these drugs.

DIGOXIN

There was a time (up till the late nineteenth century) when digoxin was the most potent drug in the doctor's armoury; some would say the only one of any use at all apart from aspirin. Then familiarity bred contempt. In the last decade digoxin has been welcomed back as a treatment for heart failure, especially in the elderly.

OTHER DRUGS

New drugs for heart failure are always appearing and are used in severe cases resistant to the above therapy.

SURGERY

Diseased heart valves can be replaced with a high degree of safety even in the elderly. For others coronary artery bypass grafting may be recommended, assuming that the rest of the heart is healthy. As a final option there is heart transplantation, reserved for those with specific disease such as **cardiomyopathy** (page 137).

Alternative Treatment

Herbal treatments for water retention might be useful in this condition, and acupuncture and acupressure claim to be able to redress imbalances in the body which exacerbate the condition. Nutritional therapy is helpful to ensure a balanced diet, low in saturated fats which would place extra strain on the heart and circulatory system. Heart failure is a dangerous condition and all alternative treatment should be undertaken alongside orthodox medical treatment. Gentle exercise, like yoga or T'ai chi can help to relieve stress, and encourage relaxation.

Prevention

The prevention of ischaemic heart disease offers the best hope of avoiding heart failure in later life. These strategies include avoiding smoking, treating high blood pressure, maintaining an ideal weight and keeping cholesterol under control.

There was a time when heart valve abnormalities caused much heart failure. These were linked with rheumatic fever, a disease now so uncommon in the UK that there is no section on it in this book, though it is still an important cause of heart disease from a global perspective. **Endocarditis** (see page 141) is about the one fairly common condition in the UK which may still damage heart valves.

Take notice of irregularities in your pulse and heartbeat. Often these are quite benign and need no treatment; there are those which, untreated, may precipitate heart failure and other complications. Treatments include digoxin and pacemakers.

Above all do not put every symptom down to age. The elderly do tire easily and breathlessness is common; but if these symptoms arise suddenly or deteriorate suddenly have a medical check as there may well be a treatable cause.

Self-Help

Coronary Prevention Group
  Plantation House, Suite 5/4 D&M, 31–35 Fenchurch Street, London EC3M 3NN
  Tel: 0171 626-4844

HIGH BLOOD PRESSURE (HYPERTENSION)

Blood pressure is what drives blood through the circulation. The two figures doctors measure are the upper (systolic) and lower (diastolic) limits of blood pressure as measured in millimetres of mercury. The World Health Organization has recommended levels of blood pressure at different ages, above which there is an increased risk of heart disease, heart failure, strokes and kidney disease. This is the condition of hypertension.

There is no one correct level of blood pressure. Although most doctors will agree on what is normal and what is clearly abnormal there is much less agreement about the middle ranges of blood pressure and what to do about them.

Risk

- Blood pressure increases with age.
- Depending on the definition used, up to 15 per cent of the population is classified as hypertensive; of those perhaps half are on treatment.
- Even mild hypertension is increasingly being regarded as abnormal; by this definition an even higher percentage of the population is at risk.
- A systolic blood pressure of 190 versus 130 carries approximately twice the normal risk of a stroke, heart attack or heart failure.
- In 90 per cent of cases no cause is found for hypertension.
- Those under thirty-five are more likely to have some unusual underlying cause.
- Those with kidney disease are at increased risk of hypertension.
- Certain drugs can cause hypertension, notably steroids and the contraceptive pill.
- Anyone with rapidly increasing blood pressure (malignant hypertension) has a 90 per cent chance of death within two years; such cases are uncommon.

Recognition

SYMPTOMS

Mild to moderate hypertension does not cause any convincing symptoms. Though people often ask if a headache can result from hypertension this is only likely if blood pressure is extremely high, when there would also be blurring of vision or heart failure (breathlessness, chest pains, swelling of ankles) and a significant risk of strokes.

SIGNS

The doctor determines if the blood pressure is causing some damage; perhaps there is mild heart failure, with breathlessness and ankle swelling. Perhaps you have angina (chest pain on exertion). Maybe you have had a stroke or a heart attack in the past. Tests may show that your heart is enlarged, that your kidney function is reduced or that tiny blood vessels are bleeding in the retina of the eyes. These are all significant findings, which make all the difference to whether your doctor decides to keep an eye on you or recommends treatment.

INVESTIGATIONS

When taking blood pressure readings, the physician measures two values. If the figure was 120/80: the first reading is the systolic blood pressure, that is the peak blood pressure reached when the heart contracts. The second value, here 80, is the diastolic pressure, the level to which blood pressure drops while the heart is in between beats. In adults 120/80 to 139/89 is normal; 140/90 to 155/95 is borderline hypertension. Figures above that, for instance, 160/100, are true hypertension.

In an older age group, perhaps above sixty-five, a reading of up to about 160/100 would be accepted as reasonable; above that and treatment might be advised.

An **ECG** (see page 299), tests of **kidney function** (see page 300), blood cholesterol and lipids, a chest **X-ray** (see page 301). These are the basic tests. In the young or if odd features turn up, you have more sophisticated tests looking for underlying conditions that can cause high blood pressure. These are rare.

ASK YOUR DOCTOR
- **To check your blood pressure every two to three years.**
- **For checks every three to six months, if you are on treatment.**
- **To discuss side-effects of medication; there is a great choice of treatment so it should be possible to find medication that controls your blood pressure without causing unacceptable side-effects.**

Remedy

Sometimes there is no doubt about the need for treatment. Such would be the case in someone with so-called malignant hypertension, where the blood pressure rises steadily over a short period of time. Without treatment 90 pcr cent of such individuals will be dead within two years from a heart attack, heart failure or a stroke.

Then there is hypertension of a mild to moderate degree but where there are already signs of damage, such as an enlarged heart. Here too the decision to treat is not difficult. The biggest grey area is that of mild and borderline hypertension, as defined earlier. Here doctors are guided by the results from huge trials of treatment, some of which have been going on for decades. These trials say that treating even borderline hypertension reduces the risks of stroke by 2.5 per cent for every 1 mm mercury reduction in blood pressure. There is a reduction too in the risks of heart failure and kidney damage.

Strangely, there is no reduction in the chances of having a heart attack. Worryingly, there is no reduction in deaths except in the elderly, who paradoxically, are the ones doctors may feel more reluctant to treat.

MEDICATION
There is a vast array of drugs for treating hypertension. Most trials have been on the effects of using either beta-blockers, or a drug called bendrofluazide. It is assumed that the same benefits extend to using the new drugs available; e.g., calcium blockers or ACE inhibitors, but the firm evidence will be years in coming.

NON-DRUG TREATMENT
- Salt

Reducing the salt in the diet may be just enough to drop borderline hypertension into a normal range.
- Diet and smoking

You will be advised to reach an ideal weight. Stopping smoking goes without saying. Excess alcohol consumption causes hypertension and should be reduced. However, a modest alcohol intake is protective against heart disease (men up to 21 units a week, women up to 14).

● Cholesterol and blood fats

This is a complicated area; in a nutshell, if you have high blood pressure and smoke and drink, high blood cholesterol is one more risk factor you can do without and so you should attempt to lower it (see **cholesterol**, page 153, for a fuller account).

Alternative Treatment

Vegetarians appear to have a lower risk of both hypertension and of heart disease in general. It is not known why this should be but it is a consistent finding in several surveys. Many therapies suggest a sensible diet, which should make a difference to hypertension.

Techniques to reduce stress have been shown to reduce mild hypertension; suitable therapies might be yoga, meditation, dance or music therapies, visualization or hydrotherapy. There seems little harm in trying homoeopathic or herbal remedies to reduce borderline hypertension, but be sure to have regular blood pressure checks. Treatment should always be tailored to you and to your symptom picture.

Prevention

The reason for treating blood pressure is to prevent its consequences of strokes, heart attacks, or kidney damage. Only in the elderly can it be said that reducing blood pressure reduces the risk of death and even then many hundreds have to be treated to save one life. When drugs for treating hypertension had unpleasant side-effects it could well be argued that their benefits were outweighed by their side-effects.

Modern anti-hypertensive drugs are better tolerated and have fewer side-effects, though they are not completely free of effects such as gout, **diabetes** (see page 204) or **impotence** (see page 101). The argument for using them rests on the assumption that the lower the blood pressure the lower the risks of complications to the heart, brain and kidneys. With well-tolerated drugs it becomes increasingly difficult not to treat mild hypertension, although the enthusiasm for treating hypertension still runs well in advance of the hard evidence for doing so. This is even more so if doctors were to treat borderline hypertension, found in 15 per cent of the population.

We come back to the concept of overall risk. The non-smoking individual, who exercises regularly, who takes moderate alcohol and who has reasonable levels of cholesterol might well feel that he or she can ignore mild hypertension, whereas someone overweight, who is a smoker and heavy drinker should take a different view despite having exactly the same level of blood pressure.

Ante-Natal Influences
Fascinating evidence is gradually accumulating that the foundations for hypertension are programmed into the baby while still in the womb. Babies who are lighter than average at birth and who may therefore have had slightly inadequate nutrition during pregnancy seem to have a higher risk of developing high blood pressure and diabetes as adults. This is a finding with enormous public health implications. For example it has long been known that babies born to mothers who smoke in pregnancy are lighter by 8 oz to one pound. Does this mean that they are also programmed to heart trouble years later? Doctors just do not yet know for certain; prudent people will ask, why take a chance of disadvantaging your children?

Self-Help

British Heart Foundation
14 Fitzhardinge Street, London W1H 4DH
Tel: 0171 935-0185

HIGH CHOLESTEROL

There is now general agreement that high blood fats and high cholesterol increase the risks of heart disease. Cholesterol, which is not a fat, is an essential element in the working of the body. A high level of blood cholesterol is called hyper-cholesterolaemia. Fats are specific chemical structures also called lipids. To have raised blood fats is to have 'hyperlipidaemia'; a diet to reduce blood fats is a 'lipid lowering' diet. You may come across certain fats called triglycerides; this refers to technical features in their chemical structure.

Cholesterol is a natural component of animal foods being found mostly in animal fat and in eggs. Food of vegetable origin contains only tiny amounts of cholesterol, not readily absorbed. The average Western diet contains 600 to 800 mg a day of cholesterol. One single egg contains about 250 mg of cholesterol, but only the minority of the cholesterol the body needs comes from what you eat. The rest is made, mainly in the liver, amounting to about 1000 mg a day.

The main use of cholesterol is in the formation of bile by the liver, which is then stored in the gall bladder. Bile is a detergent; it turns fat into a water-soluble form more easily absorbed by the body – think of the deposits of grease that remain in a washing-up bowl if you do not use a detergent washing-up liquid. Thus bile helps to absorb essential fats in the diet, including fat-soluble vitamins such as vitamin D (for bones) and vitamin E. Cholesterol is also used to synthesize certain hormones; for example, the female hormone oestrogen, and is a component of the membranes of cells.

Fat is defined by its chemical structure. Saturated fats are solid at room temperature and unsaturated fats are liquid. Fats which are very unsaturated are polyunsaturated. Polyunsaturated fats are thought to be less likely to cause heart disease.

Despite their bad name, fats are an excellent source of energy and they are vital building bricks in the metabolism of the body. Both cholesterol and fat are essential; liquid fats are better than solid fats. Things go wrong in the formation of atheroma; this is a greasy sludgy deposit made up of cholesterol and fat which can accumulate in the arteries, especially those to the heart. It is atheroma which greatly increases the chances of a **heart attack** (see page 144) or disease due to poor blood flow through the arteries (see page 161).

The whole great debate on cholesterol and lipids is to do with: the links between diet and atheroma; the reliability of the link between atheroma and heart and circulatory disease; and whether the benefits of diet/drugs to reduce cholesterol and lipids outweigh their side-effects. The debate is of enormous significance, because heart disease is the greatest threat to health in the Western world, accounting for between 40 to 50 per cent of all deaths. If diet or drugs can make even 10 per cent difference in death rate, that implies hundreds of thousands of lives saved each year.

Numbers for Cholesterol Watchers

Cholesterol is measured in units called millimoles per litre. A figure of 4 is considered extremely low in the West (though is normal in some parts of the world; e.g., China). Forty per cent of British adults have cholesterol above 6.5. The present UK public health target is to reduce cholesterol to below 5.2. Lipids measurements are complex; there is no single number which is meaningful without reference to the type of lipids measured.

Risk

- The higher the blood cholesterol the higher the risk of heart disease.
- It is estimated that every 1 per cent reduction in cholesterol reduces the risk of heart attack by 2.5 per cent.
- Men with cholesterol of 4 risk one death from heart disease per 2000 men per annum.
- Anyone with a blood cholesterol of 5 has twice the risk of someone with a cholesterol of 4; i.e., one death from heart disease per thousand men per annum.
- Compared to a cholesterol of 4 a cholesterol of 7 carries five times the risk of fatal heart disease, but that still translates into only about 2.5 deaths per 1000 men per annum.
- In 1 out of every 500 of the population raised cholesterol is genetically determined.
- Another genetic form of raised lipids affects 1 in 200 of the population.
- Common reasons for increases in cholesterol are obesity and diabetes and alcohol excess, but many other diseases can contribute.
- The significance of raised cholesterol is vastly magnified by additional risk factors for heart disease; for example, smoking and high blood pressure.

Recognition

Symptoms

Raised cholesterol gives no symptoms. Raised lipids may rarely cause abdominal pains, being an unusual reason for **pancreatitis** (page 127). Where atheroma is already affecting the heart and blood vessels you may notice **angina** (see page 157) or **poor circulation** (see page 161).

- Angina

This is pain arising from the heart on exertion. You feel a squeezing sensation in the chest after going up hills, climbing stairs, at moments of excitement or physical exertion. The pain goes within a few minutes of resting.

- Poor circulation

The basic symptoms are cold toes and a cramp-like pain in the calves on exertion.

SIGNS

Modest increases in cholesterol or blood fats cause no signs. Higher levels may produce some of the following signs.

- Arcus senilis

This is a white ring around the iris (the coloured part of the eye). As the name implies it is a normal finding in the elderly but is suspicious in a younger person, where it is frequently associated with raised cholesterol.

- Xanthelasma

This condition is comprised of little yellow raised patches found below the lower eyelids. These are deposits of cholesterol in the skin.

- Cholesterol nodules

These may be found over tendons in the hands, elbows or Achilles tendon. They are a feature of the rare but serious genetic types of hyperlipidaemia.

INVESTIGATIONS

A random **blood test** (see page 298) of cholesterol and lipids is a useful screening test. Where an abnormality is detected more sophisticated tests are done on blood taken after fasting, analyzing in detail the types of fat. Depending on the pattern, treatment (or no treatment) may be advisable. For the investigation of angina and of poor circulation see the references given above.

ASK YOUR DOCTOR

- **To check your blood cholesterol/fats if any close relative develops heart disease at an early age.**
- **About xanthelasma, they are common and important.**
- **If you are on treatment for high blood pressure or diabetes, to see if your cholesterol has ever been checked.**
- **If you develop angina or poor circulation.**

Remedy

The cholesterol issue is one of great debate. Here are the arguments:

PROS

- There is a clear and accepted relationship between the average levels of cholesterol in a country and the levels of heart disease in that country.
- Within individual countries, the higher the individual's cholesterol the higher is his or her risk of heart disease.
- In the USA cholesterol levels have been falling over three decades and with them the incidence of heart disease.
- Several scientific studies have shown that reducing cholesterol can reduce the risk of non-fatal heart disease and other disorders of circulation.
- Sufferers from familial disorders of cholesterol or lipids have high risks of cardiovascular problems which are greatly reduced by treatment.

CONS

- Although drug treatments to reduce cholesterol are effective and reduce heart deaths, they do not reduce overall death rates because deaths from causes other than heart disease increase.
- It remains unproved that reducing cholesterol reduces the deaths from heart disease except in people who already have heart disease.
- It is difficult to reduce cholesterol significantly by diet alone.

Diet

In the UK the aims are clearly recommended: reduce fat intake to no more than 30 per cent of total calorie intake; reduce your intake of saturated fat and increase that of polyunsaturated and mono-unsaturated fats; reduce cholesterol in the diet to below 300 mg day. Overall, you should be aiming for the recommended weight for your height and build. In practice it all means cutting down on eggs, animal fats and dairy products.

Unfortunately there is little evidence that such diets work in reducing cholesterol significantly except in studies where the individuals have been highly motivated and have been unusually rigorous in banishing fat and cholesterol from their diets. This is because the body still needs cholesterol, so that it will go on making its own no matter how little you have in your diet. For many individuals, the amount their own body makes is such that no matter how hard they diet, their blood cholesterol remains above the target of 5.2 millimoles.

Drugs

There are several modern well-tolerated drugs as alternatives to the older drugs which had many side-effects. That they work in reducing cholesterol and blood lipids is certain; it is also accepted that they reduce heart disease. For those with genetic cholesterol and lipid disorders they are essential.

What is controversial is whether their use makes any difference to overall death rates in the more general population with raised cholesterol/lipids. In a nutshell, while fewer people on these drugs die from heart disease, more die from other causes – in particular 'violence-related deaths', such as car accidents, murders. This is such an unexpected finding that the first reaction of researchers was to deny it; as more trials have shown the same effect there is now what is politely termed controversy in the world of cholesterol specialists.

A resolution has very recently come from a trial which has at last shown clear benefit from drug reduction of cholesterol. In fact a 25 per cent reduction in cholesterol achieved a 42 per cent reduction in deaths from ischaemic heart disease over a five-year period – but this was in people already known to have ischaemic heart disease. The conclusions for the population at large are still uncertain.

Alternative Treatment

Nutritional medicine has long advocated eating fats in the form of mono-unsaturated fats (oily fats, etc.); this thinking has now achieved approval among the conventional medical establishment. Eating garlic and chillies is also gaining some recognition; and there is some evidence that foods like oats actually work to lower cholesterol levels within the body. Most therapies offer sensible dietary advice, which can and will reduce blood cholesterol levels and the risk of heart disease. Crank diets and fads are not sensible and will not be suggested by any reputable practitioner.

Prevention

Cholesterol and lipids are intimately linked with heart and circulatory disease. On the other hand it is unproved whether a worthwhile reduction in cholesterol is achievable by diet alone, or whether drug treatment reduces the risk of death in people who do not have cardiovascular trouble.

Dietary changes are sensible and quite easy to undertake, particularly in light of the variety of low-fat and fat-free palatable foods that are now widely available. More important, and proven, is to reduce your overall risk of heart disease by stopping smoking, moderating drinking, aiming for an ideal weight, increasing exercise and controlling high blood pressure.

Self-Help

British Heart Foundation
14 Fitzhardinge Street, London W1H 4DH
Tel: 0171 935-0185
Coronary Prevention Group
Plantation House, Suite 5/4 D&M, 31–35 Fenchurch Street, London EC3M 3NN
Tel: 0171 626-4844

ISCHAEMIC HEART DISEASE

The heart is the pump on whose actions we rely for life. We know in an intellectual way that other organs are as vital to life – the brain, pancreas, the adrenal glands. But it is the heart which we most identify with life; that steady throb, the regular pulse, even the feel of it through the chest wall. No other organ is so obviously going about its business in the same vital way as the heart. We are right to single it out, because heart disease is the biggest source of ill-health and death throughout the Western world.

When speaking of heart disease we generally have one disease in mind and that is ischaemic heart disease. The term means disease through lack of blood supply. The heart is a superb muscular pump, but it is muscle and like any other muscle it needs a large assured blood supply to function. The consequences of a diseased blood supply vary from poor heart effort, through **angina** (see page 158) to heart failure and a **heart attack** (see page 144).

The blood supply to the heart comes via the coronary arteries, literally the heart's arteries. So there are various interchangeable terms when talking about heart disease; there is coronary heart disease – really saying the same thing twice (heart heart disease), but explaining why a heart attack is also called a coronary. A heart attack is often called a myocardial infarction; myocardial for the muscle layer of the heart and infarction being an interruption of blood supply severe enough to cause muscle to die. This is often abbreviated to MI. What blocks the arteries? It is atheroma, a mixture of fat and blood clot adhering to the walls of the arteries like sludge in a pipe. From this is derived the term atherosclerosis.

Ischaemic heart disease has been known to exist for centuries, though it is unusually common in the twentieth century. Heart attacks on the other hand were unheard of before this century. Cardiovascular disease is a term which includes disease of the arteries both in the heart and elsewhere in the body. In general, the risks of ischaemic heart disease and of heart attacks are identical, allowing for a few rarities.

Risk

- 1 in 3 of the over sixty-fives have cardiovascular disease.
- Ischaemic heart disease causes 150,000 deaths per annum (267 per 100,000 of population) through heart failure and heart attacks.
- Men are at greater risk than pre-menopausal women of the same age, but the risks converage after the **menopause** (see page 86).
- Increased risk goes with age and a family history of heart disease.
- Risks are greatly increased by smoking; the more cigarettes the higher the risk.
- Risks are increased by heavy drinking (see **alcoholism**, page 268), raised **cholesterol** (see page 153) and **obesity** (see page 208).
- **Diabetes** (see page 204) increases the risk, even if treated.
- A genetic tendency to heart disease has recently been identified, the significance of which is as yet unclear
- Risk is decreased by regular exercise and by modest drinking.
- There is uncertainty about the relative importance of each of these risk factors.

Recognition

SYMPTOMS

- Angina

This is pain from the heart which follows exertion. The exertion may be running for a bus, going up a hill, excitement or even just following a heavy meal, after which blood is shunted towards the intestines and away from the heart. Angina pain is a squeezing sensation in the chest. It seems to radiate up into the jaw and it may travel down the left arm. There can be odd variations; e.g., pain in the jaw alone or pain in the left hand alone. The important thing is the relationship to exertion. Once you rest the pain ebbs away in a few minutes.

- Breathlessness

An ischaemic heart is an inefficient heart, unable to keep up with the demands made of it by the body. So breathlessness arises (see also **heart failure**, page 147).

- Heart attack

Central crushing chest pain (see **heart attack**, page 144).

SIGNS

There are usually no signs. If arteries are diseased other than in the heart there may be poor circulation and pain on walking. There may be high blood pressure, irregular heart rhythms and features of raised cholesterol. The diagnosis is really suggested by the patient's history rather than by the results of examination.

INVESTIGATIONS

- ECG (Electro-cardiogram)

This records the electrical activity of the heart. It can reveal abnormal heart rhythms and sometimes the signs of a previous heart attack. However, it can be perfectly normal despite severe heart disease. Much more diagnostic is an exercise ECG. Here you walk at speed on a mechanical treadmill; the aim is to push up heart rate to the point that angina occurs (or you are exhausted). In 75 per cent of cases of severe ischaemic heart disease typical appearances occur on the ECG during this heavy effort.

● Scans

Echo-cardiographs (see page 299) show whether the heart is beating normally and whether there are abnormal valves contributing to angina. A **thallium scan** (see page 301) is a way of seeing if the heart muscle is working where even the ECG stress test is not conclusive. There are several variations on scans each adding to the information available. It is likely that soon **MRI scans** (see page 300) of the heart will be possible; this technique gives outstanding images of stationary structures like the spine. Once it can be used in the moving heart it may allow the actual coronary arteries to be inspected without the need for angiography (see below).

● Angiography

This technique involves passing a thin catheter into the femoral artery in the groin, guiding it into the heart and then injecting a dye into the heart and watching how it flows around the coronary arteries. It sounds hair-raising but it has become routine where serious heart disease is suspected and where a decision needs to be taken about coronary artery bypass surgery.

ASK YOUR DOCTOR

● **About any unusual or recurrent chest pain.**
● **Where the nearest specialized centre is for investigation and treatment, if you do have heart disease.**

Remedy

You may have to alter your lifestyle with regard to exercise, smoking and diet.

MEDICATION

For angina at its simplest this involves using a glyceryl tri-nitrate spray (GTN), a substance which is thought to work by dilating the coronary arteries. It works within a minute or two. For many people with angina GTN is sufficient, given in a variety of forms – as tablets dissolved under the tongue, long-acting tablets, a spray or as patches worn on the skin which release the drug over twenty-four hours.

More sophisticated drugs include beta-blockers and calcium-channel blockers. Widely used drugs include atenolol, propranolol, verapamil and nifedipine. These are especially useful if, as is often the case, **high blood pressure** (see page 150) is contributing to the ischaemic heart disease.

Simple aspirin in a dose of 75mg a day reduces the risk of strokes and heart attacks by up to 25 per cent.

SURGERY

The aim of surgery is to improve circulation through the coronary arteries. One way is to dilate arteries which are narrowed by atheroma, a technique called angioplasty. This is done in a way very similar to angiography (see above) with dilation of a balloon to open up the artery. It is a good technique for dealing with just one or two narrowings or to buy time until coronary artery bypass surgery is necessary (see below).

● Coronary artery bypass graft (CABG)

This increasingly common operation replaces the diseased coronary arteries with vessels taken from the individual's own body – usually one of the leg veins or an artery in the breast. Controversial to begin with, there is now no doubt that CABG can give years of symptom-free life. It is major surgery but with a mortality of less than 1 per cent in the best centres.

Alternative Treatment

Nutritional therapists and many other therapies have long recommended a healthy lifestyle consisting of a diet low in animal fats, high in vegetable produce, exercise and relaxation. There is increasing scientific support for the claims that garlic and chillies help protect against ischaemic heart disease. There are homoeopathic remedies available, depending on the degree of disease and the symptoms, and aromatherapists claim to be able to break down fatty deposits with massage and suitable oils. Any therapy involving gentle exercise or relaxation should be useful, but always advise your therapist of your condition and consult your doctor before taking up any kind of exercise. Acupuncture might help.

Prevention

Ischaemic heart disease accounts for 40 to 50 per cent of all deaths in the Western world, not to mention the enormous toll in symptoms, restricted lifestyles and worry. Measures which might reduce that toll even by a fraction will pay off in terms of thousands of lives saved or improved. This far outweighs any gain that can be foreseen at present for preventing that other big killer, cancer. Prevention concentrates on the control of risk factors for atheroma.

SMOKING

If a manufacturer introduced a product guaranteed to kill 50 per cent of those using it they would be hounded out of business; yet this is the grim statistic attaching to tobacco. Elsewhere in this book you will read of the many diseases made worse by tobacco. It is a matter of continuing astonishment that sophisticated societies allow the free use of tobacco; the least that should be done is to ensure that users know the risks they run. On the matter of ischaemic heart disease this risk is directly related to the number of cigarettes smoked.

CHOLESTEROL

The arguments for reducing cholesterol look compelling but are based on less definite scientific proof than you might imagine (see page 153). Nevertheless it is sensible to follow a prudent diet, low in animal (saturated) fat.

HIGH BLOOD PRESSURE

Good control reduces the risk of stroke, but not of heart disease.

ASPIRIN

For those with known heart or circulation disease, taking aspirin (75 mg) a day will reduce overall mortality from cardiovascular disease by 25 per cent. People with peptic ulcers, asthma or on warfarin cannot take it.

EXERCISE

You do not need to train to Olympic standards to benefit from exercise. A brisk half hour walk three times a week is almost as good as vigorous regular exercise and will reduce your chances of ischaemic heart disease.

ALCOHOL

Excess alcohol causes high blood pressure and contributes to ischaemic heart disease. Those who take modest regular amounts of alcohol appear to have a reduced risk of ischaemic heart disease, as compared to those who are teetotal or who drink to excess. Modèst is up to 21 units a week for a man and 14 units for a woman (where a unit is a glass of wine or half a pint of beer). It is thought that the high level of alcohol consumption in France explains why, unique in Western countries, deaths from ischaemic heart disease are relatively low despite widespread smoking.

HORMONE REPLACEMENT THERAPY (HRT)

Women enjoy protection from ischaemic heart disease up to the menopause, after which their risk begins to approach that of men. There is good evidence that HRT reduces this risk again (see **menopause**, page 86)

EXPOSURE TO THE COLD

It has been shown that there is a substantial increase in deaths from ischaemic heart disease in winter, possibly through a higher average blood pressure or through greater viscosity of the blood. This may be a more important and avoidable reason for heart attacks than realized.

Self-Help

Coronary Prevention Group
Plantation House, Suite 5/4 D&M, 31–35 Fenchurch St, London EC3M 3NN
Tel: 0171 626-4844

POOR CIRCULATION

This section discusses circulation problems which are a threat to health as opposed to those which are an inconvenience. One inconvenient one is Raynaud's phenomenon, where fingers and toes are extra sensitive to changes in temperature and go cold easily. Annoying as this is, it is not a threat to health. Poor circulation caused by diseased blood vessels, so-called peripheral vascular disease, is a threat to health.

Peripheral vascular disease rarely occurs on its own; there is usually poor blood flow elsewhere, notably in the heart or brain. The risk factors for this overlap with those for other diseases, the underlying condition being atheroma, a sludge-like deposit that gradually narrows the arteries. The circulation to the legs is by far the most commonly affected.

Risk

- Poor circulation is common in the over-fifties.
- It is much more common in smokers, especially men.
- Diabetics are at a greatly increased risk.
- Increased risk if there is high cholesterol or high blood pressure.

- It is made worse by certain drugs, especially beta-blockers.
- There is a strong association with heart disease (hence the term cardiovascular disease).

Recognition

SYMPTOMS

There may be cramps in the calf or calves when walking. At first this occurs after walking long distances, but in time it happens after shorter and shorter walks. The pain is from the calf muscles starved of the blood flow needed to bring oxygen or to carry away their waste products. In severe cases you experience pain in the legs at rest; typically this is worse during the night. Any scratches to the leg are slow to heal; there may even be ulcers.

Men can have a combination of impotence and pain in the buttocks on walking.

SIGNS

The affected leg looks pale and feels cool. The pulses in the foot are very weak or absent. If a blockage has happened suddenly, the leg will feel stone cold and be paralysed.

INVESTIGATIONS

A quick test of blood flow is obtained using a **doppler scanner** (see page 299), which detects the flow of blood through the arteries. A full view of the blood flow to the legs can be obtained by an arteriogram. Here a dye is injected down the main artery in the groin and is followed by a series of **X-rays** (see page 301). This is an essential procedure if an operation is a possibility. Checks are made for **diabetes** (see page 204) and for **high cholesterol** (see page 153).

ASK YOUR DOCTOR

- **If you suddenly notice a cold, painful foot; this may be a blockage needing urgent treatment.**

Remedy

Mild cases need no specific treatment with medication. It is essential to stop smoking, and high blood pressure or diabetes should be dealt with. Exercise is encouraged, because the more you walk the more you stimulate new blood vessels to grow and to take over the blood supply to the limb.

Drugs are disappointing in this condition; even so they are widely prescribed and some people feel they are of benefit.

SURGERY

It is possible to graft in an artificial artery to bypass the blockage. This surgery can be very extensive, including grafts up into the great arteries in the lower abdomen. In selected cases it is highly successful.

Should you be unfortunate enough to have a sudden arterial blockage, it may be possible to remove the blood clot using catheters. There is a serious risk from untreatable blockages; the only remedy may be amputation of part of the foot or leg.

Alternative Treatment

Once atheroma is established there is little to do to reverse it. Improving overall health through some of the constitutional therapies is sensible; a homoeopath, herbalist, acupuncturist or nutritional therapist will offer holistic treatment, that is, treatment for the whole of you – mind, body and spirit, based on your specific symptoms and lifestyle.

Prevention

Peripheral vascular disease is rare in non-smokers. Many surgeons have great reluctance to operate on individuals who continue to smoke. This is not a case of being vindictive, but is a recognition that those who continue to smoke have a high chance of having re-blockage of the graft. In the long run, a diet low in cholesterol should reduce the frequency of the condition.

Diabetics are at greatly increased risk of poor circulation; try to achieve as good control of your diabetes as you can. Diabetics with circulation problems affecting their feet should pay scrupulous attention to any injury to the feet and have regular, skilled chiropody.

MUSCLE AND BONE

• Back pain • Fibrositis • Hip And Thigh Fractures
• Osteoarthritis • Osteoporosis • Paget's Disease
• Polymyalgia Rheumatica • Rheumatoid Arthritis
• Systemic Lupus Erythematosus

D ISORDERS OF MUSCLE and bone are on the whole the result of wear and tear. Bones in particular start to show signs of arthritis from the age of thirty onward; by the age of fifty, most people begin to notice significant joint problems. The hips, knees and neck are the joints which work under the greatest stress so not surprisingly these are the joints which give most trouble.

Back pain is in a different category and can occur at any age; the fact is that the human back is not very well adapted to the upright posture and lucky is the person who goes through life without some episode of low back pain.

Muscle is a very reliable structure which only occasionally causes trouble. Muscle works under the control of nerve fibres, and aside from muscle strain, problems with muscle power or control are more often the result of a neurological problem than a result of disease of muscle.

There are many sophisticated operations that can be done on bones and joints, this being the speciality of orthopaedic surgeons. The height of their expertise has been in the development of joint replacement surgery for hips, knees, shoulders and many small joints; joint replacement is among the great surgical advances of the twentieth century. Chronic conditions like arthritis and rheumatism are not so easily cured; doctors are required to make life comfortable, to offer hope and pain relief.

BACK PAIN

Back pain is an extremely common cause for inability to work and for chronic sickness. Yet there is no real agreement as to its cause, treatment or outlook for recovery, nor is there an understanding as to why back pain is becoming more common. In the past, the available tests did not produce enough detail to explain the symptoms experienced by sufferers of back pain. Things improved with **CT scans** (see page 298), which shed extra light on subtleties of the living anatomy of the back.

The breakthrough has come only recently with the technique called **MRI scanning** (Magnetic resonance imaging, see page 300). MRI scans show the structure of the back (and many other organs of the body) in astonishing detail. At last it is possible to look for minor maladjustment in the position of bones, joints, ligaments and discs and to see how that links up with the patient's symptoms.

There is a disc between each of the vertebrae of the back, acting as a kind of shock absorber. They are made up of a semi-fluid core contained within a tough fibrous coat. As time passes the discs become tougher, the core less fluid. Despite the common terminology, discs do not slip. What happens is that the semi-fluid core bursts through its fibrous cover and ends up pressing on one of the nerves from the spinal cord. The result is pain and disability. The pain often seems to radiate down the leg, when it is called sciatica.

Risk

- Back pain will affect up to 75 per cent of the adult population at some time.
- There is a doubled risk of back pain for those in heavy jobs or jobs involving lifting, carrying and bending.
- People in the twenty-five to forty-five age range are more at risk of a 'slipped' disc, which affects about 1 in 100 of the population per annum.
- Most acute back problems, including slipped discs, recover within four to eight weeks.
- 10 per cent of acute back problems last more than six months.
- There is a 10 per cent overall risk of back pain being a symptom of an underlying illness. Examples would be an **aortic aneurysm** (see page 135) or bone cancer from a tumour such as **breast** or **prostate** (see pages 71 and 104). These possibilities are more likely the older the sufferer.
- There is a high chance of symptoms recurring.
- Back pain is extremely common in pregnancy, caused by extra weight and softened ligaments.

Recognition

SYMPTOMS
Pain is felt over the lower back; there may be some specific tender spots where the muscles feel knotted up at the base of the spine. If coughing, sneezing and bending make pain worse or send pain shooting down the leg it suggests a disc problem, as does tingling or numbness down the leg.

Symptoms which appear gradually suggest that general wear and tear is the underlying cause. If sudden, a disc problem or other acute illness must be considered. Because of pain it may not be possible to stand straight or even to stand at all.

SIGNS
Inability to move, or restricted movement, is a key sign. Altered reflexes (see below) are another indication that there is a fundamental problem.

INVESTIGATIONS
How much restriction is there in back movements? This is tested by asking you to bend forwards and sideways. Then, lying on a couch, you will be asked to raise each leg in turn and perhaps re-tested to see leg movements when lying on your front.

The doctor will test your reflexes by tapping knees and ankles and probably running a firm point up the soles of your feet. The presence, absence or nature of the reflexes obtained give an idea as to whether there is pressure on the nerves into your legs and if so where that pressure is.

Doctors always have to be alert to a possibility of some other disease causing the back ache. This would be a reason for an abdominal examination, looking for **aneurysm** of the aorta, (see page 135), or a tumour of the stomach, pancreas, bowel or womb, breast or the prostate gland.

Investigations are of little help in the early stages of an apparently uncomplicated back problem. An X-ray is really only advisable if your back pain is persistent and especially if painful during the night. In such cases you would also have blood tests looking for inflammation or infection. X-rays only show bone, not ligament, tissue or disc damage. X-rays also present a risk of irradiation.

Scans are the best investigations, because they do show up the soft structures thought to cause back pain. MRI scans (see above) are the best available test.

ASK YOUR DOCTOR

- **About back pain which wakes you at night; this may be a feature of an infection or rarely cancer in the spine.**
- **If you notice difficulty passing urine or numbness around your anus, accompanying back pain; this is a very important symptom as it can mean that the nerves at the base of the spine are being squashed. You need immediate investigation and possibly immediate surgery to relieve pressure.**

Remedy

Certain general principles are accepted:

REST

With acute back pain, you simply have to rest. Your body will not let you do otherwise, by going into muscle spasm or by preventing you standing. Find a comfortable position for a day or two; a firm surface suits most people.

ACTIVITY

Once you feel you can, do. Current thinking is shifting away from prolonged rest, with the realization that those who make themselves move recover more quickly. So stretch your back, walk or swim. Of course you still must avoid heavy lifting or bending.

DRUGS

Try simple painkillers first, such as paracetamol. These are often combined with nonsteroidal anti-inflammatory drugs (NSAIDS) such as ibuprofen or diclofenac. If muscle spasm is a problem muscle relaxants are helpful.

MANIPULATION

Often helpful if given by a skilled practitioner, whether a physiotherapist, osteopath, or chiropractor. Some people report sudden dramatic cures, though it has been difficult to prove this in a more scientific way. Many individuals claim at least temporary relief of symptoms or reduced need for painkillers, allowing a return to more normal activity.

SURGERY

Surgery is reserved for chronic cases where scans have shown definite disc or bone problems, or for acute cases of serious spinal cord pressure (see **Ask Your Doctor**, above). In the best hands there is a 90 per cent chance that surgery will succeed. Five per cent will find little change and 5 per cent may feel worse.

The surgery done is of two general types. One is to remove the offending disc, thereby releasing pressure on nerves. The other is to fuse bones in the spine. Often the techniques are combined. The traditional methods of surgery require several weeks of recovery; there is great interest in so-called micro-discectomy, a more minor though still highly skilled procedure (see page 300). This may even become a day case operation.

PSYCHOLOGICAL COUNSELLING

In at least 30 per cent of cases no convincing physical cause can be found. Treatment of these sufferers is difficult. No one wants to accuse a sufferer of fraud, but it is a fact that low back pain is a convenient way of avoiding work and there is no objective way of proving the degree of pain claimed.

Then there are people whose pain is genuine but who act in a way disproportionate to the pain. Finally, there are those with known disease whom treatment cannot render pain-free. For all of these groups psychological assessment is useful. It may uncover factors which reduce tolerance of pain, depression or social problems. It may reveal unexpressed consequences of the pain such as social isolation from the inability to leave the house. People can be taught techniques for reducing a reliance on pain as a way of asking for help, if that is what they are doing.

Alternative Treatment

Osteopathy, chiropractic and acupuncture are all acceptable forms of treatment. Massage can be soothing, and useful when the root of the problem lies in muscle spasm. Where there is the possibility of disease or a slipped disc, massage is not advised.

Relaxation therapies like yoga, hydrotherapy, aromatherapy or visualization might be useful if the problem is related to stress and accompanying disorders. Psychological tension is to be expected in chronic back pain, all the more so perhaps when conventional medicine can offer only drugs and not a cure. So not surprisingly many chronic back sufferers go to alternative therapists.

Specialized practitioners can teach techniques such as the Alexander technique or Maitland's exercises which do seem to help prevent recurrence.

Good alternative practitioners are aware of the symptoms calling for conventional medical assessment, such as pain at night or weight loss. Acute back pain or any other worrying symptoms can be a medical emergency and must be seen by a doctor.

Prevention

LIFESTYLE

Learn how to lift things correctly. Be aware of your limits and do not be tempted to exceed them. Choose a working position that is comfortable and which supports your back. Experiment with different types of chairs and different heights of desk, as well as the position of any equipment you work with.

If you are in a heavy manual job you are at increased risk, some of which may be an unavoidable part of the job. Even so, you can be careful lifting and try not to exceed the loads which your back can reasonably bear.

POSTURE AND EXERCISE

Many physiotherapists offer excellent 'back schools'; others teach useful techniques such as Maitland's exercises. Physiotherapists, chiropractors and osteopaths are good at spotting aspects of your work or leisure activities which contribute to pain in your back, neck or shoulders.

Self-Help

National Back Pain Association
16 Elmtree Road, Teddington, Middlesex TW11 8ST
Tel: 0181 977-5474

FIBROSITIS

We all experience widespread muscular aches and pains at some time, and the term fibrositis is commonly used to refer to these pains. For most of us fibrositis is a problem for only a short period of time, but some individuals suffer chronic pain that can become debilitating. It may come as a surprise to know that fibrositis is a respectable diagnosis by rheumatologists (termed fibromyalgia). In fibrositis it is thought that there is an increase in muscle tone, linking somehow with tender nodules in a variety of muscles. It is likely that there is a psychological element in the disorder.

Risk

- Fibrositis is experienced by everyone at some point in their lives.
- The commonest cause of fibrositis is a viral illness giving generalized muscle tenderness for up to a week.
- Rarely, this condition is a feature of **thyroid disorders** (see page 211) or of **rheumatoid arthritis** (see page 181).
- Fibrositis is benign, whatever the level of pain.
- It is most common in women.
- The condition is often accompanied by non-specific symptoms such as poor sleep, fatigue, poor appetite or digestive troubles.

Recognition

SYMPTOMS

Aching may be confined to one muscle or it may move from muscle to muscle. Usually there are firm tender nodules within the aching muscles. The commonest sites of pain and nodules are in the lower neck/upper spine, elbows, knees and the crests of the pelvis. Typically symptoms come and go, moving between sites. Stress and cold make symptoms worse.

SIGNS

It may be possible to feel tender nodules at the sites given above. There may be features of **depression** (page 278) or of an **under-active thyroid** gland (page 211). There are no general signs of ill-health, nor is there any long-term deterioration; such features would lead to a review of the diagnosis.

INVESTIGATIONS

Blood tests (see page 298) are taken to check for other inflammatory conditions like **polymyalgia** (see page 179), and **X-rays** (see page 301) might be taken of tender sites. If the tests are abnormal then fibrositis is not the diagnosis.

ASK YOUR DOCTOR

- **To check you over if you think you are suffering from fibrositis; the condition can be mimicked by a number of more serious complaints. Don't expect exhaustive investigations unless blood tests suggest some other underlying problem.**

Remedy

There is no guaranteed cure but the following are useful in the treatment of fibrositis.

- It is important to keep active on the general principle that unused muscles will stiffen up and that athletes do not suffer from persistent fibrositis.
- Any painkiller may help, but try to stick to something mild like anti-inflammatories (ibuprofen). These drugs are also available as gels to be rubbed into tender nodules.
- A low dose of an antidepressant (like amitriptyline) is commonly given.
- People who suffer from this condition chronically may benefit from psychological counselling or from attending a pain clinic, aimed at helping them cope with incurable pain.

Alternative Treatment

Massage is helpful from any source: physiotherapist, masseuse or aromatherapist. These professionals can also advise on changing your posture or seating position. Acupuncture or acupressure is said to help those with tender nodules. People also turn to homoeopathy, relaxation techniques and yoga. Reflexology can be useful.

Prevention

As the condition seems to be linked to psychological problems, there is unlikely to be any preventative treatment. Sufferers should accept the benign nature of the condition. However, it is important to know that orthodox medicine accepts that the pain of the condition is real even though the cause is poorly understood. Equally you should accept that there may be a large psychological component and that attempts by doctors to deal with that do not mean that they think your problem is 'all in the mind'.

Self-Help

Arthritic Association
Hill House, 1 Little New Street, London EC4A 3TR
Tel: 0171 491-0233

Fibromyalgia Association UK
8 Rochester Grove, Hazel Grove, Stockport, Cheshire SK7 4JD
Tel: 0161 483-3155

HIP AND THIGH FRACTURES

Twenty per cent of hospital orthopaedic beds are occupied by people with these conditions. Though pure accidents account for many fractures in the young, it is clear that falls and osteoporosis are major risk factors in the elderly, ones which will be of growing importance with increased life expectancy.

Risk

- Falls become more common with age, with up to 35 per cent of the elderly having significant falls in any three-month period.
- In the elderly one in five falls will result in a fracture.
- **Osteoporosis** is the major risk factor underlying many fractures (see page 174)
- The lifetime risk of a fracture is 40 per cent of women, 20 per cent of men (this includes all osteoporotic fractures).
- Over a five-year period 10 per cent of women over seventy will have a fractured hip and of those 15 per cent will die through complications (though often these are to do with underlying conditions which have lead to the fall, such as **Alzheimer's disease** [see page 272]).
- In the year after a thigh fracture there is a greatly increased risk of death (12 to 25 per cent).
- Anything increasing the risk of falls is a risk for fractures, for example poor eyesight, unsafe stairs or uneven carpeting.

Recognition

SYMPTOMS

Pain and difficulty walking after a fall is self-evident. However, some fractures are virtually pain-free so a high degree of suspicion is needed when any elderly person has fallen and has subsequently a slight limp or even a mild degree of discomfort.

SIGNS

Usually no special skill is needed to recognize a possible fracture. In the case of the pain-free fractures of the hip, the affected leg is shorter and turns out.

INVESTIGATIONS

Such is the risk of a fracture after even a minor fall that really all cases should be X-rayed if there is the slightest doubt. Occasionally a fracture turns out to be caused by bone weakness through other disease, like cancer. This should show up on the **X-ray** (see page 301).

ASK YOUR DOCTOR

- **To advise on prevention of osteoporosis well before you reach old age.**
- **For a check if you have even slight discomfort in your groin after a fall.**

Remedy

The treatment of a fractured hip is surgical repair of the fractured bone. What is done depends on the site of the fracture. If it is on the shaft of the bone it can be repaired and held in place by a metal plate and screws. If the fracture involves the joint with the hip bone you will need a hip replacement. Either way recovery from surgery is quick, though long-term recovery takes several months depending on your overall state of health.

Alternative Treatment

Physiotherapy and massage will help individuals back to their feet and give them the confidence to walk again. There are several homoeopathic and herbal remedies which are said to enhance the healing process, particularly of bones.

Prevention

- The prevention of osteoporosis merits a whole section to itself. It will be a growing public health issue (see page 174).
- The prevention of falls and accidents is the subject of regular campaigns, reinforcing common-sense actions such as: ensuring stairs are well lit; wearing stable footwear; avoiding loose rugs and carpets; keeping homes uncluttered; and having stair rails fitted if needed.
- Many elderly people experience giddiness on standing up; this is due to poor circulation to the brain and little can be done about it. It is, however, a risk factor for falls. If you have this condition, give yourself enough time to regain your balance when you stand up, making sure you have something to hold on to before you start walking.

Self-Help

National Osteoporosis Society
PO Box 10, Radstock, Bath BA3 3YB
Tel: 01761 432472

Royal Society for the Prevention of Accidents
Cannon House, The Priory, Queensway, Birmingham B4 6BS
Tel: 0121 200-2461

OSTEOARTHRITIS

This is a classic example of a 'wear and tear' disorder. Although the name suggests a disease of bone, it does in fact involve cartilage. Cartilage covers the ends of bone, somewhat similar to the non-stick coating on a metal frying pan. By giving a smooth surface to the bone, it allows it to move easily against the cartilage of the other bones making up a joint. Cartilage is a living structure, a mix of collagen fibres for strength and complex biological chemicals which hold water and which give cartilage the ability to absorb shocks without the underlying bone splintering. With age and use the cartilage wears down, becomes thin and eventually cracks. The end result is bone-to-bone contact, causing joints to become stiff, creaky and painful.

Bone, which is also a living structure, tries to compensate by overgrowing at the joints, giving the characteristic swellings seen in fingers and knees. Skeletons of every antiquity have been found with features of osteoarthritis. It is not a modern disease; it just seems more common as people live longer.

Risk

- By 65 years of age 80 per cent of the population have X-ray changes of osteoarthritis (called OA).
- Only 20 per cent of sufferers will actually complain of symptoms of OA.
- The condition is twice as common in women.
- Joints subject to the greatest stresses (like knees, hips and the neck) develop the condition earlier.
- Activities which increase mechanical stress multiply the risk; for example, knee problems in sports enthusiasts.
- There is probably a small genetic risk.
- Any condition which interferes with joint function will accelerate OA, e.g., gout or deformity.
- Although extremely common in Caucasians it is relatively uncommon in blacks and Chinese.

Recognition

SYMPTOMS

The main features of OA are pain and stiffness of joints. Gradually (meaning over a decade or two) these symptoms worsen. In more advanced cases the joints creak and are felt to grate on movement. You may hear this when you move your neck or knees. Swellings gradually grow at the furthest joint of the fingers (closest to the nail). Swellings of the middle joints are a feature not of OA but of **rheumatoid arthritis**, see page 181. Women are particularly prone to these swellings. Eventually it can be difficult to use a joint at all and there may be constant pain.

The symptoms tend to improve with rest but the stiffness worsens overnight. Sufferers have to take things slowly first thing in the morning. Cold and damp make symptoms worse.

By no means does the appearance of OA mean a steady progression to pain and disability. For most sufferers it is more of a minor inconvenience which can be accommodated into the often sedate and leisurely lifestyle of the elderly. OA of the hip is the most disabling form since this will restrict so many activities of daily living.

SIGNS

The swellings are as described. The doctor will note the general lack of movement of the affected joints and can feel the creaking as they move. Sometimes joints feel warm and there may be obvious deformity; for example, the famous knobbly knees.

INVESTIGATIONS

These may not be needed as the condition is so obvious. Nevertheless, **X-rays** (see page 301) are often done to put on record the degree of involvement of joints and just to exclude other causes of pain, like fragments of bone inside the knee joint. Blood tests may suggest other causes of joint pain, especially rheumatoid arthritis.

Symptoms bear little relationship to the X-ray appearance. You may have a hip joint which looks unusable on X-ray, yet suffer little discomfort and vice versa.

ASK YOUR DOCTOR
- **About joints which feel persistently warm; although this can happen in OA it is not a common feature.**
- **About the local availability of orthopaedic surgery, to decide when you should be referred for an orthopaedic decision on surgery.**
- **About assessment by an occupational therapist to advise on aids to improve your abilities; for example, devices to help you unscrew jars or to pull on stockings without bending. These simple but brilliantly conceived gadgets can make all the difference to your independence.**

Remedy

LIFESTYLE
- All sufferers should try to keep active, within the limits of the disease. Go for exercise that does not jar joints, like walking or stretching exercises. Swimming is an excellent activity as it also relieves gravitational pressure on joints and is used in a medically controlled way called hydrotherapy.
- Try to reach an ideal weight. This is especially important if OA is affecting your hips and knees. This can be a difficult goal as the very disease itself may prevent you from increasing activity significantly.
- While aiming for activity in general, recognize that at times of flare-ups you will need to rest affected joints.
- Do not spurn the humble walking-stick.

MEDICATION
- If you do need painkillers use the mildest possible. Anti-inflammatory drugs are widely used and are effective but there is worry about a long-term risk of provoking stomach ulcers and possibly of causing an increase in the rate of progression of OA. Several anti-inflammatory drugs are now available in a gel form, which can be rubbed into affected joints.
- Acutely painful joints can be helped by steroid injections.

PHYSIOTHERAPY
This therapy teaches exercises for regular use at home, and puts joints through their full range of movements. Heat treatment, wax baths and electrical stimulation are all physiotherapy techniques which can relieve pain in specific joints. Hydrotherapy treatment in specially warmed pools can give great relief to hip joints.

SURGERY
- Hip replacement is now so common that we tend to forget just what a sophisticated operation it is. The artificial joints are the result of years of

experimentation on materials, cements and technical aspects of the surgery. Improvement, not to say cure, can be expected in 99 per cent of cases. There is an annual 1 per cent failure rate of artificial hips, plus they have a limited lifespan of only ten years or so. Thus a decision on surgery takes into account the individual's general health and circumstances.

- Surgery to give an artificial knee is becoming more common, though not yet quite as successful as hip replacement. The small joints of the fingers can be replaced as can the shoulder joints. Undoubtedly this kind of surgery will become increasingly routine, limited only by the economics of treating such a huge percentage of the population – a serious question.

Alternative Treatment

Many suffers say they gain relief from taking cod liver oil. A good vitamin and mineral intake is recommended, taking supplementation where necessary. Massage in any form is very helpful for individual joints. Other therapies used include acupuncture, homoeopathy, herbalism, osteopathy, chiropractic, reflexology, Alexander technique and Autogenic training.

Prevention

The one agreed and important preventable risk factor is **obesity** (see page 208), as it puts extra strain on hip and knee joints which take so much strain anyway.

A generally active lifestyle is sensible, but avoiding activities which put jarring stresses on joints – this means paying attention to well-fitting and supportive footwear, especially for sportsmen and joggers.

It seems that OA will be a price to be paid for an increasingly long-lived population but there is every indication that the technology of joint replacement will keep up with this disease.

Self-Help

Arthritic Association
Hill House, 1 Little New Street, London EC4A 3TR
Tel: 0171 491-0233

Arthritis Care
18 Stephenson Way, London NW1 2HD
Tel: 0171 961-1500

OSTEOPOROSIS

Osteoporosis is a condition in which the bones lose their density, thinning and eventually becoming brittle. Bones appear unchanging but they are living structures, the components of which are constantly being absorbed and regenerated. Unless there is an adequate supply of calcium the bone structure becomes thin and less strong. The bones themselves remain the same size but they become more likely to fracture, a consequence being the epidemic of hip fractures in our increasingly elderly population. Until very recently osteoporosis was seen not as an abnormality, but as an inevitable component of ageing. This attitude is changing, partly as hormone replacement therapy

(HRT) becomes more popular, partly as more people live longer and partly as it is realized that changes to lifestyle can make a real difference to the chances of having severe osteoporosis.

Risk

- Osteoporosis affects about one-third of women and about one-twelfth of men.
- The degree of osteoporosis accelerates after the **menopause** (see page 86). The earlier the menopause the higher the risk.
- Nearly 40 per cent of women and 20 per cent of men will eventually have fractures attributable to osteoporosis – about 150,000 per annum.
- White-skinned peoples are at greater risk than blacks.
- Smokers are affected more than non-smokers (as are drinkers).
- There is an increased risk after prolonged periods of inactivity.
- There is an increased risk in thin people.
- A diet low in calcium and vitamin D increases the risk.
- Sunshine on the skin is protective (by increasing production of the vitamin D needed to absorb calcium).
- Long-term treatment with steroids will hasten osteoporosis.

Recognition

SYMPTOMS

Symptoms are generally due to fractures of bones. The vertebrae in the back may become so weakened that they collapse on themselves. This causes severe sudden back pain, which settles after a few weeks. It may recur. The end result of successive collapses is a back that is bent (the typical dowager's hump) and loss of height.

More dramatic is the fractured hip or thigh, often after quite trivial trauma (see **fractures**, page 170). The wrist is another site where osteoporotic bone fractures easily. Pain in bone is not a usual feature of osteoporosis and should lead to a search for some other cause.

SIGNS

There are no warning signs of osteoporosis. It is by its effects that it is noticed; that is, loss of height and the appearance of an increasingly curved spine.

INVESTIGATIONS

X-rays (see page 301) taken because of a suspected fracture usually give the first clue. The bones look less white on the X-ray, meaning that the X-rays are passing more easily through the thinning structure. This is a late feature of osteoporosis because bone can lose up to 30 per cent of its substance before changes show up on X-ray.

Blood tests (see page 298) indicate calcium levels and may suggest other inflammatory conditions giving rise to fractures or bone pain.

ASK YOUR DOCTOR

- **About bone pain, especially if it continues through the night. Such pain cannot be put down to osteoporosis.**
- **For advice on preventing osteoporosis.**
- **To estimate your risks of osteoporosis, taking into account your lifestyle, smoking habits and diet.**

Remedy

The first step is to see if there are treatable causes of the condition, for example, steroid tablets or an **over-active thyroid** gland (see page 211). Otherwise, treatment is best at reducing further bone loss, less good at reversing the changes already there.

LIFESTYLE

Increase your general level of activity. Combine this with exposure to sunshine whenever it presents itself (although ensure that you wear sunscreen). Have a diet high in calcium and vitamin D; these can be found in dairy produce. Supplementary vitamin D should be taken by those who are confined to the house and so have no exposure to the sun.

MEDICATION

Calcium and vitamin D tablets are available and have been shown to protect against progression of the condition. They should be considered for anyone with a poor diet. Supplementary calcium cannot, however, replace lost bone, only protect against further loss.

CALCITONIN

Calcitonin is a hormone involved in the body's handling of calcium. Treatment does seem to be effective but there are several side-effects and it is an expensive drug.

ETIDRONATE

A phosphorus-containing drug, etidronate is given in repeated cycles of two weeks of etidronate followed by eleven weeks of calcium and so on. The drug is effective and well tolerated; its widespread use is again limited by cost.

HORMONE REPLACEMENT THERAPY (HRT)

A highly recommended treatment for women, discussed below and at length in **Menopause**, see page 86.

It is becoming clear that many men with osteoporosis are deficient in male hormones, treatable by giving testosterone. The risk/benefit equation is not yet decided, because giving testosterone increases the risk of **prostate cancer** (see page 104)

Alternative Treatment

Diets emphasizing calcium and vitamin D intake can be recommended. Magnesium also helps the body to absorb calcium. Boron reduces the body's excretion of calcium and magnesium, and is said to increase the production of oestrogen, which protects the bones. It has shown promising results in the treatment of post-menopausal women. Fluoride may also be useful for preventing and treating the condition because it stimulates new bone formation and is incorporated into the crystal of the bones to make it stronger.

Established osteoporosis is helped by supervised exercise programmes. A reflexologist or homoeopath will also offer treatment.

Prevention

The prevention of osteoporosis is an increasing challenge for public health and for those who wish to enjoy a mobile old age. The aims are simple:

- building a good bone mass;
- maintaining good bones;
- reducing the loss of calcium from middle age onwards.

BUILDING A GOOD BONE MASS

The more solid your bones by the age of thirty, the greater the 'reservoir' to protect you against loss of bone thereafter. Physical activity, and a good intake of calcium and vitamin D from childhood are the key controllable factors. It is estimated that this can increase bone mass by 10 per cent, a highly worthwhile achievement.

MAINTAINING GOOD BONES

This means keeping up a diet adequate in vitamin D and calcium, as well as continuing physical activity. Excess intake of alcohol and smoking are two avoidable factors which will accelerate bone loss in youth and in middle age. Caffeine may also rob the body of calcium, which can lead to osteoporosis.

You may have a disease such as asthma controllable only by taking steroid tablets. This will greatly increase the risks of osteoporosis and this should be taken into account by your doctors in planning treatment.

REDUCING THE LOSS OF CALCIUM FROM MIDDLE AGE

For women, HRT is the treatment of choice to prevent osteoporosis. Increasingly evidence is showing that the benefits of HRT taken for five to ten years far outweigh its drawbacks. Taking it for that length of time halves the chances of a fracture of the thigh.

Calcium (1.5 g) and vitamin D (about 400 units per day) tablets are almost as effective as HRT in preventing osteoporotic hip fractures, with the advantage that men can take them, too.

Testosterone, calcitonin and etidronate may be suitable for selected cases.

SCREENING FOR OSTEOPOROSIS

The X-ray technology (bone densitometry) is well established. Because of a national shortage of scanners screening is readily available only for those with a family history of osteoporosis or who have had fractures at an unusually young age. Anyone at special risk because of having had steroid treatment or other bone-density reducing disease should ask about screening.

Self-Help

National Osteoporosis Society
PO Box 10, Radstock, Bath BA3 3YB
Tel: 01761 432472

PAGET'S DISEASE

James Paget was an astute nineteenth-century physician, with the distinction of having not one but two diseases named after him (the other one is a kind of eczema of the nipple). In Paget's Disease, the bone becomes increasingly thickened, heavy and distorted. Although the bones look big and sturdy, their structure is weak. In most cases of this common condition there are few problems, but it can lead to pain, disability, deformity and occasionally other illness.

Risk

- Paget's disease is unusual below the age of forty.
- The condition is present in about 10 per cent of the population by ninety years of age.
- Men are more often affected than women.
- Although often seen on X-rays, only a minority of people report symptoms.
- Paget's disease most often affects the skull, spine, hips and legs.
- There is a very small risk (1 in 1000) of turning into a bone tumour.

Recognition

SYMPTOMS
The commonest symptom is bone pain of a constant gnawing character; headaches of the same nature are reported. As the disease progresses the long bones become bowed and the head looks enlarged. Deafness can result from pressure by thickening bone on the nerves of hearing where they pass through the skull. The deformed long bones of the leg are prone to fractures. Other complications are excessively rare.

SIGNS
In advanced disease the appearance is unmistakable: a stooped, heavy-headed person, bowed over and with legs curved out.

INVESTIGATIONS
Areas of typical Paget's bone are often seen on **X-rays** (see page 301) ordered for some other reason. If the individual has no symptoms they can usually be ignored. **Blood tests** (see page 298) reveal the very high levels of enzymes involved in the growth of bone.

ASK YOUR DOCTOR
- **If you feel your head is enlarging. It can happen and Paget's disease is the likeliest cause.**
- **About persistent bone pain. Though Paget's disease is a common cause in an older age group, bone tumours and infection have to be considered.**

Remedy

No treatment is called for if it is just an incidental finding on an X-ray. Where pain is a problem, simple anti-inflammatory painkillers are used first. The next option is the drug calcitonin, the synthetic form of a hormone involved in the regulation of calcium. It has to be given by injection several times a week and side-effects are common. A phosphate-containing compound (etidronate, used also in osteoporosis) is a helpful alternative. Other specialized treatments are available for severe cases.

Alternative Treatment

There is nothing obvious which can prevent the course of the disease, but pain or discomfort might be eased by any of a number of therapies, including acupuncture, massage, aromatherapy and herbalism.

Prevention

The generally benign nature of the condition makes prevention unnecessary. There is a theory that a virus sets off the disease. It is a long way from this theory to finding some means of prevention.

Self-Help

National Association for the Relief of Paget's Disease
207 Eccles Old Road, Salford, Manchester M6 8HA
Tel: 0161 707-9225

POLYMYALGIA RHEUMATICA

In a list of diseases most satisfying to treat, polymyalgia would rank high. The sufferer has an array of symptoms, hard to pin down but making their life a misery. The treatment is easy to undertake. The response to treatment seems little short of miraculous; symptoms disappear literally overnight.

As with many conditions, the Latin medical name restates the obvious in obscure terms. It means aching in lots of muscles and joints. It is a disease whose cause is unknown but which is suspected to be one of a group of illnesses where the body reacts against its own tissues. Others are **rheumatoid arthritis** (page 181), **thyroid disease** (page 211), and **pernicious anaemia** (page 199). There is considerable overlap with a condition called temporal arteritis, where the prominent symptom is a painful artery in each temple. Temporal arteritis carries a significant risk of sudden blindness.

Risk

- There are about three cases per 100,000 per annum in the population as a whole, but it is much more common in the elderly.
- There are about eight new cases per 1000 of over-eighties per year.
- In the over fifties there are about 1.3 new cases per 1000 per annum.
- Overall, polymyalgia affects about 1.5 per cent of elderly people.
- Women are affected three times as often as men.

Recognition

SYMPTOMS

Symptoms may appear either suddenly or gradually over a few weeks. The main symptom is pain and aching in the muscles of the shoulders and upper arms; the muscles often feel tender to touch. There is muscle stiffness, worse in the morning.

Often the sufferer feels generally unwell but in a non-specific way. There may be depression and weight loss and even a persistent fever. The temples can feel tender (this is often noticed when brushing the hair). This is a very important symptom (see below).

Signs
There is possibly some joint tenderness and swelling. It may be possible to feel a tender firm artery in each temple.

Investigations
Blood tests (see page 298) show that there is a high level of inflammation in the body. As this can be caused by many other conditions, a general health check is sensible.

ASK YOUR DOCTOR
- **To consider the diagnosis in any elderly person who suddenly deteriorates, with muscle pain and vague ill-health.**
- **If you feel a tender artery in your temples. This is an extremely important symptom: it may be the only warning before sudden blindness in one eye.**

Remedy

Treatment is with steroid tablets. Many doctors will prescribe on suspicion of the disease, even before the results of blood tests, especially if there is a tender artery in the temples, in the hope of avoiding sudden blindness.

The response to steroids is most gratifying for patient and doctor. Often overnight and certainly within two to four days the symptoms disappear. There then follows a gradual, careful reduction in the dose of steroids, guided by blood tests and by how the individual feels. This process will take anywhere from eighteen months to several years. There may be side-effects from the steroids – weight gain, a moon face, perhaps high blood pressure and a risk of **osteoporosis** (see page 174). These are unavoidable consequences for treatment of what would otherwise be a quite intolerable illness for the two to ten years it takes to run its course naturally, and always with a risk of sudden blindness.

Alternative Treatment

Because of the risk to sight, this is not recommended. A diet rich in calcium will help compensate for the osteoporosis caused by the steroids.

Prevention

There are no known means of prevention of polymyalgia. What is important is to bear it in mind with any elderly person with unexplained ill-health and muscles pains. Early recognition is important in order to avoid the possible complication of sudden blindness in one eye. It takes just seconds to check whether an elderly person complaining of headache has tender arteries in the temple.

Self-Help

Arthritic Association
Hill House, 1 Little New Street, London EC4A 3TR
Tel: 0171 491-0233

RHEUMATOID ARTHRITIS

Rheumatoid arthritis is a common, widely studied but still poorly understood condition in which the joints become severely inflamed. Once the cause of an enormous amount of disability, it is still a serious diagnosis but modern medical and surgical treatments allows most sufferers to lead a reasonably normal life. It is an aggressive form of arthritis. Unlike **osteoarthritis** (see page 171), which deteriorates slowly over several years, rheumatoid arthritis can progress over just a few weeks or months. That said, there is great variation in how any one individual is affected, with some having no more than a few painful joints, whereas others can be immobilized.

There has long been a theory that the disease is somehow linked with an as yet unidentified infection, which sets the body reacting against itself (a so-called auto-immune disease, see page 183). The disease affects the joints, mainly the smaller ones, like fingers, toes, elbows and knees. There may eventually be great distortion of hands and feet.

One unusual feature of rheumatoid arthritis (RA) is that it can cause a range of symptoms outside of the joints.

Risk

- RA affects 2 to 3 per cent of the population. The same risk applies worldwide.
- There are three new cases per 1000 of population per annum.
- Women are affected three times as often as men.
- RA appears most often in people in their 30s and 40s, but can occur at any age.
- A family history of RA increases the risk to 5 to 10 per cent.

Recognition

There is no typical form of onset but the following are characteristic.

SYMPTOMS

There is swelling, stiffness and pain of small joints in the hands and feet. In 25 per cent of cases there is a single swollen joint; e.g., the knee. Gradually small joints on both sides of the body become involved. Morning stiffness is usual. Suffers sometimes feel generally unwell with a vague tiredness.

Joints may eventually become deformed; the fingers and toes start to splay outwards; there are tender swellings of the middle joints of the hands (in contrast with osteoarthritis, where the furthest joints are affected). Tendons may break, giving rise to sudden deformities of the fingers or toes. There can be many associated features of RA in the eyes, lungs, blood, heart and skin.

Occasionally RA begins and progresses in a rapid way.

SIGNS

A doctor will look for the typical pattern of joint involvement and note morning stiffness. Sometimes nodules can be felt under the skin.

There are several conditions which can present with symptoms similar to those in RA which need to be considered. Often blood tests will help to differentiate these but it may be a question of waiting and seeing how the clinical course progresses. In really obscure cases a biopsy taken from a joint may be needed.

INVESTIGATIONS

The diagnosis is confirmed by **blood tests** (see page 298) which are positive for the so-called Rheumatoid factor, an immunological marker. Another blood marker, the **ESR** (see page 299), is a measure of general inflammation in the body; this is usually raised and is a useful measure of the activity of the disease. There is a typical **X-ray** (see page 301) appearance of joints affected by RA.

Although these investigations are highly suggestive of the disease, their absence does not exclude RA, which is really a clinical diagnosis; that is, one made on the basis of the patient's history and the signs found on examination.

ASK YOUR DOCTOR
(For rheumatoid arthritis sufferers)

- **If you start to have neck pain; you may be developing a slippage of bones in the neck; this can cause a potentially serious compression of the spinal cord.**
- **If you develop a sudden swollen joint and feel unwell; you may have an infection in the joint.**
- **About the side-effects of any drugs you are prescribed; some of the more aggressive treatments risk serious side-effects of which you should be aware.**
- **To be referred to a specialist rheumatologist. Such specialists build up great expertise and sympathy in dealing with RA and are well placed to judge when surgery might be needed to prevent or repair tendons threatening to break.**

Remedy

RA is a disease likely to last for many years. Many parts of the body can be affected, with symptoms ranging from the trivial (cold fingers) to the disastrous (spinal cord compression). You will need different drugs at different times, access to physiotherapy and surgery; you will probably need to make adjustments to your home, work and lifestyle. This prospect has to be accepted early on in the condition and is best coordinated by a physician you trust.

The outlook is by no means all gloom. Only 10 per cent of sufferers become seriously disabled; 40 per cent will have ups and downs but with only modest joint deformity. Another 25 per cent will have more major deformity. In at least 25 per cent of cases the disease burns itself out with no residual disability. The outlook is better if the disease appears suddenly and for men. There are other specialized pointers to the likely outcome, but the individual case remains uncertain.

RESTING JOINTS
Splints force you to rest a joint. Sometimes if you are affected in joints all over your body you will need admission to hospital for a general rest.

PHYSIOTHERAPY
Aims to keep joints mobile and to teach the sufferer to use his or her muscles and joints in the most effective way.

ANTI-INFLAMMATORY DRUGS

Aspirin was the first of these and still has a role, but is generally replaced by NSAIDs (non-steroidal anti-inflammatory drugs). There is now a wide range of these, with fewer side-effects than pure aspirin.

DISEASE-ALTERING DRUGS

You may come across gold injections, penicillamine, steroids, salazopyrine, chloroquine. Their use, side-effects and long-term effects are technical, but they can all reduce the activity of the disease. Because of their potential side-effects they are given under specialist supervision.

In really severe cases even more powerful drugs are increasingly being used; these include azathioprine, cyclophosphamide and (especially in the USA) methotrexate. As doctors gain experience with these drugs they will probably be used in milder cases.

SURGERY

The advice of a surgeon skilled in dealing with RA is invaluable in treating tendon ruptures, deformities, and planning joint replacement.

Alternative Treatment

Some people feel that their condition is affected by particular foods. Gentle professional manipulation of joints may help; for example, from an osteopath. There are homoeopathic remedies for flare-ups of pain and stiffness, as well as those which might help to alter the course of the disease. Acupuncture claims some success in treating RA, and aromatherapeutic oils may help to reduce the swelling.

Prevention

As long as the cause of RA is unknown there are no strategies for prevention. The wide range of surgical and medical treatments ensures that most people with RA can now lead a reasonably normal life. It is likely that the powerful disease-modifying drugs mentioned earlier will reduce the progression of the disease.

Self-Help

Arthritic Association
Hill House, 1 Little New Street, London EC4A 3TR
Tel: 0171 491-0233
Arthritis Care
18 Stephenson Way, London NW1 2HD
Tel: 0171 961-1500

SYSTEMIC LUPUS ERYTHEMATOSUS

A fascinating and probably under-diagnosed disease, systemic lupus eyrthematosus (also called SLE) is another of the auto-immune diseases, in which the body reacts against its own tissues. In the same way as it might react against an infection, for example, by forming antibodies which damage a wide range of organs, the body begins to attack itself. The symptoms can vary from skin rashes and arthritis through psychiatric effects to heart or kidney damage. Recognition of the disease is often delayed because there are no absolutely specific tests. SLE is a significant diagnosis because it can cause kidney failure and increases the risk of strokes.

Risk

- Lupus affects one in 1000 of the population. There are probably many more mild unrecognized cases.
- Certain groups are at much higher risk; for example, black American women have a one in 250 chance.
- Women are nine times more likely than men to have the disease.
- Lupus most commonly begins between the ages of 20 and 40 years.
- Lupus can rarely be caused by drugs, for example, hydralazine and the contraceptive pill.

Recognition

SYMPTOMS
Arthritis with fevers is probably the most common presentation, together with a sense of ill-health. In 80 per cent of cases there are skin changes; the most typical is a 'butterfly-rash' across the cheekbones; that is, a red sore rash spreading out symmetrically across the bridge of the nose and over the upper cheeks (hence butterfly). It is a feature of SLE rashes that sunlight makes them worse.

Also common are tiny tender spots on the fingertips and fingers themselves that are extremely sensitive to the cold (Raynaud's phenomenon). The sufferer often feels depressed. There may be more dramatic psychiatric symptoms such as **dementia** (see page 272). SLE is a possible reason for hair loss from the scalp (alopecia)

SIGNS
The usual ones are swollen joints plus odd widespread rashes. The lungs are often affected with gradual restriction in function.

INVESTIGATIONS
The diagnosis is difficult. It is helped by finding certain immunological markers; the best known are anti DNA antibodies. As DNA is the protein at the very heart of the cell it is not surprising that antibodies against it cause damage to many organs.

Once the diagnosis is suspected investigations look for evidence of damage to other organs. The kidneys are often involved as shown by testing urine and **kidney function** (see page 240). SLE can cause pooling of fluid around the heart (pericardial effusion) detected by **ultrasound** scans (see page 301).

ASK YOUR DOCTOR
- **About SLE as an explanation for vague ill-health and arthritis in a young woman.**

Remedy

It is important to determine how active the disease is; in particular whether the kidneys are affected, as this is the usual reason for death from SLE. Mild cases are managed with anti-inflammatory drugs to control joint pains. Severe cases are treated with steroids. Very bad cases, for instance those with kidney damage, are treated with drugs which reduce the activity of the immune system (immuno-suppressants); these include azathioprine, cyclophosphamide, chlorambucil or chloroquine. Aggressive treatment of this kind has reduced the mortality in the most serious cases of SLE.

Sufferers can count on a 95 per cent, five-year survival rate. Ninety percent survive to ten years or more.

Alternative Treatment

Dietary changes advised include increase in oily fish, and vitamin E and selenium. Some sufferers report food allergies and intolerance, which can be tested and treated alternatively. Acupuncture claims to restore the immune system, and there are many other therapies which confirm good results in treatment. It is essential, however, that conventional medical treatment is maintained throughout exploration of and subsequent treatment with complementary medicines.

Prevention

The drugs causing the condition are well known, hydralazine was commonly used to treat high blood pressure; a few older people may still be on it. Others are anti-epileptic drugs and the contraceptive pill. The focus of prevention is otherwise early detection and skilled treatment in order to reduce the risks of kidney damage.

Self-Help

Lupus UK
PO Box 999
Romford, Essex RM1 1DW
Tel: 01708 731 251

BLOOD AND THE LYMPH NODES

- Anaemia • Haemophilia • Hodgkin's Disease
- Leukaemia • Myeloma • Pernicious Anaemia
- Sickle Cell disease

THE BLOOD AND lymphatic system comprise a fluid transport system which carries oxygen and nutrition all around the body, providing a defence system against disease to the remotest cell of the body. We are familiar with the vessels that carry blood – the arteries and veins. Fluid leaks out of those vessels, permeates the tissues and is collected by the lymphatic system which has its own system of vessels that return the tissue fluid back to the main blood circulation.

The lymph nodes are collections of cells at strategic parts of the body, distributed in such a way that they can mount an early defence against invading organisms. This is why there are so many lymph nodes around the head and neck, the main site of entry of bacteria and viruses in food and in the air. The defence is undertaken by the production of antibodies together with the release of aggressive white cells which are drawn to foreign invaders.

Minor treatable disorders of the blood and lymphatic system are extremely common. Anaemia in one degree or other is often found in children and menstruating women. Enlarged lymph nodes (often called glands) in the neck are features of throat infections and even enlarged 'glands' elsewhere in the body are usually the result of a viral illness. The more serious conditions are mainly confined to an older age group. Even leukaemia, though popularly associated with children, is quite unusual before middle age.

ANAEMIA

Strictly speaking anaemia is not an illness in itself but a symptom; there are many conditions that give rise to anaemia, which means low blood count. Blood is a highly complex fluid in which there are red blood cells, whose task is to carry oxygen around the body; white blood cells involved in dealing with infection; platelets involved in blood clotting and thousands of other proteins, hormones, chemicals. Anaemia concerns the quantity and quality of the red blood cells.

Red blood cells are made in the bone marrow at the rate of two million per second. Each red cell lives for about 120 days. Given an average volume of blood of five litres, each adult has five billion billion red cells. A single drop of blood contains over five million red cells alone.

This extraordinary rate of production can go wrong in several ways. There might be a shortage of raw materials – like iron or vitamins; this leads to iron-deficiency anaemia or pernicious anaemia. The bone marrow can also fail; this serious condition happens in leukaemia and similar diseases. There can be excess blood loss, as happens with heavy periods or with slow steady internal bleeding from an ulcer. Or the blood cells may be breaking down unusually fast, a condition called haemolytic anaemia. Finally there are inherited conditions leading to anaemia such as sickle-cell disease and thalassaemia.

In working out the reason for anaemia, all of these possibilities have to be considered. The speciality of medicine which does this is called haematology; it is a highly complex job to interpret the abnormalities of blood production and composition.

Risk

- The commonest reasons for anaemia are heavy periods or pregnancy.
- Thanks to its stores of iron the body can cope with a poor diet for a long time; it can take a few years for poor diet to lead to iron-deficiency anaemia.
- Babies can go through a phase of anaemia during periods of rapid growth.
- Adolescent children growing rapidly are also at risk.
- Losing just 8 ml of blood a day (4 mg iron) can in time cause iron deficiency; this can occur as a result of heavy periods (the average blood loss in menstruation is 80 ml), bleeding piles, peptic ulcers, hiatus hernia or taking aspirin and similar drugs regularly.
- Hookworm infestation is, worldwide, the commonest reason for blood loss and chronic infection leading to anaemia.
- Sickle-cell anaemia is a risk in those of African origin, but found in many other populations.
- Thalassaemia is associated with Greeks but again is found in a wide range of populations in Southern Europe, Middle and Far East.

Recognition

SYMPTOMS

Your blood count can drop by 10 to 20 per cent without causing symptoms. Even severe anaemia can go unnoticed if it happens slowly enough, because the body compensates for the anaemia. When symptoms do occur they are non-specific, often taking the form of tiredness, or feeling faint. As anaemia becomes profound so there may be breathlessness on exertion. Depending on the type of anaemia you may notice that your nails are brittle, your tongue is sore and there are painful cracks at the corner of the mouth. Rarely you may develop difficulty swallowing, because of the growth of a web obstructing the top of the gullet.

The inherited anaemias such as sickle cell or thalassaemia give rise to poor growth, jaundice and bone pains. Though the diagnosis may be suspected on the basis of the individual's racial group, only blood tests will confirm the exact diagnosis.

SIGNS

In a mild anaemia there will be none. Later, there is pallor especially seen by looking at blood rich areas such as the nail beds and the undersurface of the eyelids (this is why doctors often take a quick look at these places). However, the clinical impression of anaemia is terribly unreliable; realistically if there is any question of anaemia you need a blood test.

INVESTIGATIONS

These aim to detect anaemia and clarify the cause. A straightforward blood count provides a lot of information – the degree of anaemia, whether iron or vitamin deficiency is likely, or the possibility of other disease or an inherited condition. More sophisticated blood tests measure iron in the blood and other vitamins.

● Bone marrow sampling

This is reserved for puzzling anaemias which appear to be caused by more than iron deficiency. The marrow is sampled using a thick needle passed into the hip bone.

● Other tests

May be needed to pin down the reason for blood loss. The need for these depends on the overall picture; an anaemic woman who has heavy periods but a good diet needs no further investigation. An anaemic woman with a good diet but who is post-menopausal needs thorough investigation for hidden blood loss; these may include a **barium meal** (see page 297), a **barium enema** (see page 297) or other tests.

All cases of anaemia should be followed up by repeat blood tests to check that there is a response to treatment.

ASK YOUR DOCTOR

● **About heavy periods; a lot can be done for these now without the need for surgery.**
● **Never ignore bleeding from the bowel, in the urine, in vomit or in phlegm. Though there are frequently innocent causes, all cases need medical assessment.**

Remedy

The treatment of anaemia is twofold: correcting the anaemia and dealing with what has caused it. Treatment of most cases is easy, just by taking iron and vitamin tablets; very occasionally iron is given by injection or even via an intravenous drip in an emergency; this is sometimes the case if a pregnant woman has become severely anaemic close to delivery or in someone with the inability to absorb iron because of disease.

The underlying cause may be dietary, corrected by advice. Bleeding from the womb, bowels or urinary tract must be dealt with as appropriate; e.g., healing a **peptic ulcer** (see page 129), controlling heavy periods. Whatever the cause it is important that it's followed up to ensure that there has been a good response to treatment. A common error is to stop treatment as soon as you feel better, which can take as little as two weeks. You feel better because your body has grabbed the new iron and poured it straight into production of red blood cells. However, your body also needs to store iron to smooth out the ups and downs of normal life and this takes much longer; thus it is important for you to continue to take iron supplements for three to six months, depending on how anaemic you were.

FAILURE TO RESPOND

Any lack of response should lead the doctors to double-check the diagnosis; perhaps there is some continuing source of blood loss, perhaps there is an inability to absorb iron through a disease such as **ulcerative colitis** (see page 132). There are also many chronic diseases in which a mild anaemia is part of the picture; these include **rheumatoid arthritis** (page 181), **systemic lupus erythematosus** (page 183), **tuberculosis** (page 229), kidney failure (page 240) In these cases the anaemia is difficult to control, as is the anaemia of inherited conditions such as thalassaemia.

Alternative Treatment

It makes good sense to have a diet high in iron and vitamins, which can be provided by soya beans, liver, red meats, spinach, lettuce and raisins. Avoid eating liver if you are pregnant because of the risk of vitamin A overdose. There are many guides to food content to help you. There is no reason to worry about developing anaemia on a vegetarian diet, as long as you take iron-rich foods; there are lots to choose from aside from red meat. It becomes more difficult if you follow a vegan diet, when iron and vitamin deficiency is a real possibility, especially for infants, adolescents and menstruating women. There are some therapies which claim to be able to enhance the body's ability to absorb iron from food. Therapies which might be useful include herbalism, homoeopathy, nutritional therapy, acupuncture, acupressure and reflexology.

Prevention

In the developed world a normal diet of meat, fish, eggs, vegetables should make serious anaemia unlikely unless there is also abnormal blood loss. Children, adolescents, menstruating women and women in pregnancy are all well-recognized groups who need extra iron and vitamins. Though diet can provide this, often iron and vitamin tablets are a convenient way of dealing with the situation especially in adolescents following a faddy diet.

- The body needs about 1 mg a day of iron; children and menstruating women need 2 to 3 mg a day. In late pregnancy you need 4 to 5 mg a day. Note: the body cannot absorb more than about 4 mg of iron per day, so extra dosage won't serve any purpose other than, perhaps, making you constipated.
- Ensure your children have a balanced diet; your health visitor can advise on this.
- The elderly on a poor diet or those neglecting themselves, for example alcoholics, can become anaemic, though this does take some time to develop. Those at risk should take iron and vitamin supplements.
- Certain racial groups are at risk of inherited forms of anaemia; screening is sensible in these cases; for example, Afro-Caribbean, Greek and southern European groups, especially in the case of children who are failing to grow properly.
- One of the aims of routine ante-natal care is to pick up early cases of anaemia; we now know that some degree of anaemia is normal in pregnancy, so not all pregnant women must automatically go on to iron treatment, but it is important to detect those who are developing severe anaemia and to treat that.

Self-Help

Sickle Cell Society
54 Station Road, Harlesden, London NW10 4UA
Tel: 0181 961-7795
UK Thalassaemia Society
107 Nightingale Lane, London N8 7QY
Tel: 0181 348-0437

HAEMOPHILIA

These are a group of conditions in which the blood fails to clot normally. The result is frequent bleeds which occur spontaneously (e.g., nosebleeds) or severe bleeding following minor knocks. The most dangerous consequence of haemophilia occurs as the result of repeated bleeding into joints; as well as being painful and disabling at the time, recurrent joint bleeds lead to long-term deformity of the joint.

When blood clots it is the end result of a series of reactions involving platelets and clotting factors in the blood. It is an intricate system; while it is vital for blood to clot, it is also vital that it does not clot at the wrong time in the wrong place. Haemophilia is the result of a failure to produce one or other of those clotting factors. The severity of haemophilia varies considerably, depending on the extent to which the sufferer is able to make the factors needed to make the blood clot.

Cases of haemophilia have been reported for centuries, the witnesses being both impressed and appalled at how blood would flow relentlessly from the sufferer until death eventually ensued. There is also a great scientific interest in these conditions because of the light they shed on the normal mechanisms of blood clotting and there is now a better understanding of the complicated and inherited genetic defects that underlie the conditions.

Haemophilia A is the commonest form of haemophilia and it is the one to which the text refers.

Risk

- Haemophilia almost exclusively affects males.
- Incidence is estimated at 1 in 5000 to 10,000 of the male population; two-thirds of these are from families known to be affected with the condition.
- About a third of known cases arise through new genetic defects.
- With modern treatment life expectancy appears normal (see **Remedy**, below).

Recognition

SYMPTOMS

In about 50 per cent of cases children are severely affected from birth; it soon becomes clear that there is a problem. Infants with haemophilia continue to bleed from the umbilical cord after it has been cut, and the trauma of birth raises large blood-filled sacs on the skull. Even gentle handling may result in bruising, and the advent of crawling causes unusual and multiple bruises. A haemophilic toddler will soon begin to experience painful bleeding into joints.

Fifty per cent of children are less severely affected; in these cases the diagnosis is suspected when there is unusual bleeding after minor surgery, on teething, or following hard knocks.

SIGNS

The combination of easy bruising and spontaneous bleeding suggests haemophilia, but only blood tests will differentiate from other conditions that can do the same, such as leukaemia or defects elsewhere in the clotting system. All health professionals are now rightly alert to battered babies and may well suspect physical abuse in a child covered in bruises; this is why blood tests are so important in such cases.

INVESTIGATIONS

Tests will show that blood fails to clot normally; further tests will indicate whether this is because of a lack of clotting factors, which is haemophilia, or a defect in the rest of the complex system of blood clotting, such as a low platelet count.

ASK YOUR DOCTOR

- If you notice easy bruising or unusual bleeding in a child; the earlier the diagnosis is made the better.
- About any family history of bleeding disorders.

Remedy

CLOTTING FACTOR REPLACEMENT THERAPY

The treatment consists of replacing by injection those clotting factors that the sufferer lacks. For most haemophiliacs this is Factor 8. In an ideal world this would be given twice a day; practicalities of cost, availability and time make this impossible for most sufferers. Instead, they or their families learn to inject Factor 8 in times of need; for example, if they feel bleeding into a joint or if they have a prolonged nosebleed. Special arrangements are made if a haemophiliac requires surgery, either using large quantities of Factor 8 or something called DDAVP, which achieves a similar effect.

Factor 8 is still largely derived from donated blood; there was always known to be a risk of infection in that blood, which was screened for viruses causing Hepatitis. During the 1980s it became clear that another lethal contaminant was present and that was the HIV virus which causes AIDS (see page 13). The tragedy that has unfurled is that 30 per cent of all haemophiliacs in the UK became infected with HIV before the problem was solved. Where once the commonest cause of death for haemophiliacs was bleeding in the brain after a head injury, it is now AIDS. Factor 8 produced by DNA technology is becoming available, which should avoid any risk of contamination by such viruses.

Alternative Treatment

None can be recommended; haemophilia is a potentially lethal condition which must be controlled by specialists.

Prevention

At present the best means of prevention is through early recognition.

- Babies born to families known to carry haemophilia are screened at birth. This will pick up two-thirds of cases.
- For the rest it is a question of taking note of unusual bruising and bleeding.

In theory it will be possible to screen for haemophilia but at present this is far too complex to do on any wide-scale basis. However, in selected cases with a strong genetic risk it is possible to test the unborn fetus for the disease by sampling the fetus's blood or tissues; this can be done from as early as ten weeks into pregnancy.

Self-Help

The care of haemophiliacs in the UK is highly organized; all sufferers have access to NHS centres where advice, monitoring and treatment is coordinated.

Haemophilia Society
123 Westminster Bridge Road, London SE1 7HR
Tel: 0171 928-2020

Macfarlane Trust (For those infected by contaminated blood products)
PO Box 627, London SW1H 0QG
Tel: 0171 233-0342

HODGKIN'S DISEASE

It was in London in 1832 that Dr Thomas Hodgkin described seven puzzling cases of death in people whose spleens and lymph glands were enlarged. It was seventy years before a scientific understanding of the underlying disease emerged; and it was not until the 1960s that effective treatment for this relatively common condition was established. The disease is now considered curable in most cases.

Hodgkin's disease is one of a group of conditions called lymphomas; these are malignant conditions affecting the lymphatic system of the body. The lymphatic system is a subtle and vigilant defence system which runs parallel to the circulatory system in our body, guarding our bodies against foreign invasion by bacteria and viruses. The spleen and lymph nodes, which can be felt most easily in the neck, armpit and groin, are part of the lymphatic system and will become enlarged in the event of infection. Lymph nodes are often incorrectly called 'glands', and swollen glands are simply enlarged lymph nodes.

The cause of Hodgkin's disease remains unknown.

Risk

- In the UK there are 2.4 new cases per 100,000 population per annum, 1500 in all. There is great international variation in the frequency of the disease.
- The condition starts most often in the 15 to 40 age range, affecting men more than women.
- Hodgkin's Disease has become more common during the twentieth century.
- There is a slightly increased familial risk of the disease.
- It causes about 360 deaths a year.

Recognition

SYMPTOMS
Typically someone notices that they have an enlarged gland (lymph node) which persists and grows. The neck is the commonest, most easily noticed site but it can be in the groin

or armpit; the swellings are usually painless. Frequently the sufferer feels vaguely unwell, tired and perhaps has itching of the skin and weight loss. A particularly noticeable feature is night sweats or unexplained fever at other times of the day.

SIGNS

The enlarged glands have a smooth 'rubbery' feel to them. By pressing under the ribs on the left a doctor might detect an enlarged spleen.

INVESTIGATIONS

A blood count is usually normal; this helps exclude other possible conditions such as leukaemia or chronic infection. The necessary investigation is a **biopsy** (see page 298) of one of the enlarged glands, looking for the typical cells that are diagnostic of the disease. A chest **X-ray** (see page 301) and a **CT scan** (see page 298) will show if there are enlarged glands scattered throughout the rest of the body, along the lymphatic system. This is important in staging the disease.

ASK YOUR DOCTOR
- **About any persistently swollen glands, remembering that enlarged glands for a week or two are features of any common infection and indeed are indications that the body is doing its job.**

Remedy

Without treatment Hodgkin's Disease was invariably fatal, but modern treatment of Hodgkin's disease by some combination of radiotherapy and chemotherapy has transformed the condition to one which is now considered curable in most cases. The combination of treatment depends on the extent of the disease as shown by staging. In general, disease confined to a few glands can be treated by **radiotherapy** (see page 301) whereas **chemotherapy** (see page 298) is needed if the disease has spread to the spleen and bone marrow or lungs.

The latest chemotherapy techniques are much less unpleasant to endure so that sufferers can still go to work and lead a normal life even while undergoing chemotherapy every few weeks for six months or more.

Survival is now expected in the great majority of cases: at least 90 per cent survival at five years in cases of early disease and over 50 per cent over five years for people with widespread disease.

Unfortunately, there is a price to pay for the treatment. As it is so often young people affected, particular care is taken to try to preserve fertility in the case of women or to put sperm into a frozen sperm bank in the case of men. There also appears to be a long-term risk of developing leukaemia and other cancers which is estimated at 1 per cent. This has to be set against the fact that even as recently as the 1960s advanced disease resistant to radiotherapy was fatal more often than not.

Alternative Treatment

As with other forms of cancer, psychological support is of the greatest importance in handling both the diagnosis, treatment and the years of follow-up.

Prevention

The cause of the disease remains unknown; a theory that it is linked to glandular fever is now discounted. The most important thing is to seek medical attention as soon as a persistently enlarged gland is discovered, especially if there is a constant feeling of being unwell.

Self-Help

The Hodgkin's Disease Association
PO Box 275, Haddenham, Aylesbury, Bucks HP17 8JJ
Tel: 01844 291500

LEUKAEMIA

Leukaemia is a term for several different cancers of the bone marrow, where the white blood cells are made. Childhood leukaemia is rare but attracts enormous publicity despite its rarity – the understandable reaction to the notion of cancer affecting children when cancer is more generally considered a disease of adult life. Childhood leukaemia is usually an aggressive disease of rapid onset, making the child very ill very quickly. The treatment of childhood leukaemia has been a modern success story; most cases are controllable if not curable.

Adult leukaemia attracts less publicity but is much more common. The treatment of adult leukaemia is quite effective. Adult forms of leukaemia tend to develop more slowly with a long period of vague ill health before a diagnosis is made.

In acute (acute means arising suddenly and of an intense or severe nature) leukaemia there is a switch within the bone marrow from making a normal varied production of cells to making a high percentage of abnormal white cells which spill into the bloodstream. The production of red cells, platelets and normal white cells decreases, giving rise to the anaemia, poor blood clotting and lack of resistance to infection characteristic of leukaemia.

In chronic (long-term) leukaemia, although the end result is the same the process is less dramatic, spread over months or years rather than the few weeks of acute leukaemia.

Risk

- There are in all nearly 7000 cases of leukaemia a year.
- Childhood leukaemia affects just three per 100,000 children per year, giving rise to 450 cases per annum.
- The peak ages of incidence are at two to five years and again from 40 upwards, becoming more common with age.
- Chronic leukaemia affects men twice as often as women.
- Known risk factors include exposure to ionizing radiation; e.g., X-rays, radioactivity and ironically chemotherapy given to control other cancers.
- There is no scientific proof of an increased risk from living near nuclear power

stations, though the suggestion lives on in popular mythology.
● There are well–recognized genetic factors accounting for certain forms of leukaemia.

Recognition

Features differ between the aggressive acute leukaemias, more associated with children, and the slower developing chronic leukaemias of adult life.

SYMPTOMS

Acute leukaemia causes a rapid collapse of the bone marrow; within a matter of weeks there is anaemia, causing tiredness and breathlessness. Lack of resistance leads to a persistent sore throat and infections such as skin boils or chest infections. Without normal blood clotting the sufferer bruises easily and may bleed spontaneously from the nose or into the urine or bowels.

Chronic leukaemia gives rise to more vague symptoms of tiredness and malaise. Depending on the type there may be some enlarged lymph glands or aching in the left abdomen from an enlarged spleen. Eventually the symptoms of acute leukaemia appear, but this can be as late as three or four years from onset.

SIGNS

There are remarkably few signs. There may well be widespread bruising and enlarged glands. The diagnosis is really made on suspicion and following blood tests.

INVESTIGATIONS

A **blood count** (see page 298) gives a quick, fairly reliable diagnosis; a bone marrow sample has to be taken to confirm diagnosis.

ASK YOUR DOCTOR
● **About persistent tiredness especially when combined with easy bruising.**
● **About your child if he or she has repeated infections over a short period of time; doctors will often take a blood test just to be sure. Remember, however, that childhood leukaemia is very rare and is unlikely to be the cause of persistent illness in children.**
● **About treatment at the best local centre. Only in specialized units can physicians gain enough experience of rare childhood illnesses to give the most up–to–date treatment.**

Remedy

ACUTE LEUKAEMIA

More than nine out of ten children with leukaemia respond to treatment and overall at least 70 per cent remain cured. The path to that result is one of harrowing, painful and demanding treatment for which the parents and the child must be prepared. The first phase of treatment has to be in hospital where high doses of chemotherapy are given intravenously until the abnormal white cells are cleared. This usually takes four weeks, during which the child is at high risk of infection. Next it is usual to eradicate the cells from the brain and spinal cord by a combination of irradiation and chemotherapy. Lastly, the individual goes on to long-term chemotherapy by mouth for up to two years.

The results in adults are less good, with about 70 per cent responding to treatment and 30 per cent achieving cure, depending on the exact type of leukaemia.

CHRONIC LEUKAEMIA

The treatment is generally less intensive than for acute leukaemia and can be achieved using drugs taken by mouth. At present, chronic leukaemia is not curable but control offers several years of a good quality of life. From the time of diagnosis the outlook is a survival rate of five to nine years, depending on the type of leukaemia.

In future, bone-marrow transplants will offer more hope of cure but at present they are difficult to arrange because of the need to find a closely matched donor. Also exciting is the use of interferon to achieve control, if not cure, in certain types of leukaemia. Interferon is a naturally occuring anti-cancer protein.

It is important to realize that this is a greatly simplified review of leukaemia; the range of leukaemias is far more complex, as are the treatment options. This underlines the point that it is essential to be in a highly specialized unit for diagnosis and treatment.

Alternative Treatment

More than most diseases acute leukaemia puts enormous stresses on the sufferer and his or her parents. There is the shock of the diagnosis; the strain and side-effects of treatment, then the endless uncertainty about whether a cure has been achieved. This has long been recognized by the specialized units which aim to maintain an open, honest and trusting relationship between the professional staff and the patients. Sufferers say that they derive much benefit from sharing their worries with other sufferers and with other parents. Many alternative therapies can address the strains on the body caused by aggressive treatment of leukaemia, and are particularly useful for rehabilitation. Homoeopathy, herbalism and acupuncture are most often used. There are also many less recognized therapies which claim to deal with all kinds of cancer. If something works for you and does not interfere with the treatment you are receiving from conventional sources, there is no reason why some experimentation shouldn't be undertaken.

Prevention

ENVIRONMENTAL FACTORS

Known risks for leukaemia include exposure to benzene and exposure to radioactivity. These risks are closely controlled by health and safety regulations. Few people realize that there is a background level of radiation in every rock in the UK, which varies from area to area and which may explain geographical variations in a variety of cancers; realistically little can be done about this.

There was an increase in the numbers of people with all forms of leukaemia in Hiroshima after the dropping of the atomic bomb, though the total number of cases was still low. Bombs have grown bigger since then.

People treated with irradiation for **Hodgkin's disease** (page 192) have about a 1 per cent risk of developing leukaemia and need careful follow-up. However, there is no evidence that procedures such as standard X-rays increase the chances of leukaemia.

GENETIC FACTORS

These factors underlie certain forms of leukaemia; we are a long way from identifying a genetic predisposition to leukaemia, let alone screening for it.

Self-Help

Leukaemia Care Society
14 Kingfisher Court, Pinhoe, Exeter EX4 8JH
Tel: 01392 64848
The Leukaemia Research Fund
43 Great Ormond Street, London WC1N 3JJ
Tel: 0171 405-0101
Each Leukaemia treatment centre will have further information about other groups and grant-making bodies.

MYELOMA

In the Walt Disney cartoon *The Sorcerer's Apprentice* Mickey Mouse tries to stop a magical broom from working by chopping it in half. To his dismay each fragment turns into another functioning broom; no matter how much he chops them up, each fragment goes to work doing the same task. This could be an analogy of myeloma.

One of the ways in which the body is protected against infection is by the action of certain cells called lymphocytes, which produce antibodies against foreign proteins. In myeloma it seems that just one of these cells goes wrong and it continues to churn out the same protein. The cell reproduces again and again, over what is believed to be many years. Eventually the bone marrow is largely replaced by innumerable clones of that same original cell, each manufacturing the same protein and together producing vast quantities of perfectly useless antibodies. This has the effect of reducing the body's ability to mount an effective antibody attack against infection.

Meanwhile, the production of red blood cells plummets and so the sufferer becomes anaemic. The excess protein clogs up the kidneys, which start to fail and there is great loss of calcium from bones leading to spontaneous fractures and collapse of bone. It is as if a factory capable of turning out sophisticated computers malfunctions, producing nothing but the buttons for setting the controls.

Risk

- Myeloma is a disease of the older population, usually over age 60.
- It appears to have become more common during the twentieth century.
- There are about 3500 cases per annum, with a prevalence of six per 100,000 of the population.
- Cases are often discovered by chance after a screening blood test.
- Myeloma causes 2100 deaths a year.

Recognition

SYMPTOMS

The features are those of anaemia, plus bone pain of a vague type and often a sudden increase of pain if a bone collapses on itself (commonly in the spine). The sufferer is prone to infections. Although the kidneys are affected it is unusual nowadays for kidney trouble to be the first indication of the condition; it is usually diagnosed much earlier than that.

The abnormally high quantities of protein in the blood make it thicker and less able to flow smoothly around the circulatory system; this gives rise to totally unspecific symptoms such as giddiness, headaches and drowsiness.

SIGNS

Apart from the pallor of **anaemia** (see page 186) and perhaps some tender bones there is nothing diagnostic on examination.

INVESTIGATIONS

The blood count shows anaemia, kidney damage and the presence of great quantities of the abnormal protein. Protein is also detected in the urine. **X-rays** (see page 301) show that many bones have punched out areas as a result of thinning. A **bone-marrow** (see page 188) sample clinches the diagnosis.

ASK YOUR DOCTOR

- **If you have symptoms such as tiredness and giddiness, with no detectable cause and often a mild depression accompanying the symptoms. Most doctors and patients like to have the reassurance of a blood test and myeloma is an example of a disease which might not be diagnosed without one.**

Remedy

Treatment is worthwhile, even though at present it is not curative. Untreated myeloma is fatal, usually within about a year. Treatment buys time but the condition eventually returns. However, the time bought is very significant, with survival for several years being common. The drug used is melphalan; localized bone disease responds well to radiotherapy. Increasingly aggressive treatments such as interferon (see page 196) or other **chemotherapy** (see page 298) agents are being used for recurrent disease. It is likely that the treatments will eventually lead to a cure for the condition.

Alternative Treatment

In our present state of knowledge myeloma is controllable but not curable. This puts a great burden of fear on sufferers from the condition, for whom support by any means must be helpful. However, beware practitioners who claim to be offering a cure; there is no evidence to support such claims.

Prevention

There is some debate over what to do in cases where the disease is detected unexpectedly at a very early stage following blood tests done for some other reason. There is an argument for treating such early disease more aggressively than is at present the case. Specialist advice should be obtained on this.

Self-Help

BACUP
3 Bath Place, Rivington Street, London EC2A 3JR
Tel: 01800 181199

PERNICIOUS ANAEMIA

Pernicious anaemia is a special form of anaemia caused by deficiency of the vitamin B12. Unlike other common forms of anaemia, treatment has to be lifelong.

B12 is a vitamin essential for the production of DNA, the crucial information-carrying molecule in the cell. Tiny quantities (2 to 3 millionths of a gram) are needed per day and this is best obtained from eggs, meat, fish. These tiny quantities are scavenged in the stomach by a protein produced in the walls of the stomach called intrinsic factor, uniquely tailored to perform this task. The complex of intrinsic factor/B12 is processed in part of the bowel and the B12 is absorbed into the bloodstream.

In pernicious anaemia there is a loss of those specialized cells which secrete intrinsic factor. This process appears to be caused by an auto-immune condition (i.e., one in which the body reacts against some of its own tissues, like rheumatoid arthritis and thyroid disease). Eventually the production of blood cells slows down; those cells which are produced look abnormal through the microscope. Left untreated, there are also neurological changes giving rise to tingling in the hands and feet and potentially paralysis and dementia.

There are several other reasons for this type of anaemia, discussed below. A folic acid deficiency is a common cause.

Risk

- Pernicious anaemia affects 1.2 per 1000 of people over the age of sixty in the UK.
- There are wide international variations in risk; e.g., the disease is rare in Africans or Asians.
- Three women are affected for every two affected men.
- The condition is rare below 40 years of age.
- It is associated with other auto-immune conditions, especially **thyroid disease** (see page 211).
- Sufferers have often become prematurely grey and have blue eyes.
- Women with pernicious anaemia have a normal life expectancy, once treated; men have a slightly increased risk of cancer of the stomach.

Recognition

SYMPTOMS

There are the usual symptoms of anaemia e.g., tiredness, breathlessness on exertion. The tongue feels sore and others may notice that you look pale and slightly yellow, due to mild jaundice. Eventually you will develop tingling in your fingers and toes and your walking may become unsteady; in really neglected cases there can be dementia, but this is highly unusual.

SIGNS
In advanced cases the individual looks very pale, because the blood count is roughly a quarter of what it should be. A blood count this low would in any other condition put you into a state of collapse. The spleen often is enlarged; there are changes in sensation in hands and feet.

INVESTIGATIONS
A routine **blood count** (see page 298) reveals profound anaemia and abnormally enlarged red cells. Other tests will show low levels of B12 in the blood and antibodies to the cells in the stomach which make intrinsic factor. A dietary deficiency in folic acid can give a similar picture and so the levels of that vitamin are routinely checked. The possibility that disease in the bowel might be affecting the uptake of B12 will be considered, and investigations may be necessary to check that out.

To prove the diagnosis it is usual to perform a Schilling test in which radiolabelled B12 is given by mouth and its absorption measured over twenty-four hours.

ASK YOUR DOCTOR
- **For nutritional advice if you are following an unusual diet: a strict vegan diet can lead to B12 deficiency. Ask what supplements you should take.**
- **About the latest guidance on taking low doses of folic acid to reduce the risk of having a baby with spina bifida, if you are pregnant.**

Remedy

Treatment is with regular injections of vitamin B12. At first these are given every few days, but they are eventually needed only once every three months or so. However, the treatment must be lifelong. There is an extremely rapid response to these injections: the blood begins to recover within forty-eight hours and the individual begins to feel better within days. Neurological problems may take several months to disappear; in some cases they never completely go.

Alternative Treatment

None recommended in this condition, though you may find it useful to know foods which are naturally rich in B12 and folic acid: these include green vegetables, meat, milk and milk products, eggs, fish. Beware of a strictly vegan diet, which can lead to deficiencies in B12 and possibly folic acid. A nutritional therapist may be able to help you with the ins and outs of this aspect of treatment. There may be some therapies which can enhance your body's ability to absorb vitamins and minerals; acupuncture is one which might be useful. A homoeopath or herbalist may recommend useful treatment of some symptoms based on your individual constitution.

Prevention

The normal dietary requirements for B12 and folic acid are met by a diet including rich sources of these; see above. Vegetarians should have adequate B12 intake from a balanced diet, but vegans may not.

People who have had their stomach or certain parts of the bowel removed will not absorb B12 and must have regular injections; this should be part of the normal follow-up.

> *Folic acid is given in pregnancy; recently it has been found that taking low doses of folic acid before pregnancy and in the first three months reduces the risk of having a baby with the distressing condition of spina bifida. In that disease the spinal cord is exposed at the base of the baby's spine, with risks of paralysis and other neurological damage. At the time of writing the recommendation is 0.4 milligrammes of folic acid a day up to the twelfth week of pregnancy. Taking folic acid is a very significant, simple preventative measure and you are strongly recommended to discuss it with a health professional if you are considering pregnancy.*

Self-Help

The Food Commission
102 Gloucester Place, London W1H 3DA
Tel: 0171 935-9078
Vegan Society
7 Battle Road, St Leonards-on-Sea, East Sussex TN37 7AA
Tel: 01424 427393

SICKLE CELL DISEASE

Haemoglobin is the molecule within red blood cells which carries oxygen around the body. This molecule has many variants which have evolved over time, one of which, haemoglobin S, is found in large numbers of people in Africa and can give rise to sickle cell disease. As long as someone has a high percentage of normal haemoglobin, as well as haemoglobin S, they will remain well and also enjoy the added benefit of some protection against malaria; in terms of genetic programming, this probably explains why this variant of haemoglobin persists.

If, however, there is a predominance of haemoglobin S, and an insufficient percentage of normal haemoglobin, there is a problem. Haemoglobin S reduces the flexibility of the normally round red cell, which instead can take up a curved shape like a sickle, hence sickle cell. The abnormal sickle cells burst more easily than normal red blood cells and it is for this reason that those with sickle cell disease become anaemic. Furthermore, their red blood cells can block up the smallest blood vessels, cutting off blood supply to small areas of bone or brain, kidney, liver, etc. This can happen at any time. People who have a sickle cell trait (that is, a mixture of normal and abnormal haemoglobin) are generally well most of the time, only running the risk of blood clots if they become low on oxygen.

Risk

- Up to 25 per cent of the African population have the sickle cell trait. In the Afro-Caribbean population the rate is one in ten, in Asians one in fifty. In a Caucasian population it is one in 1000; the condition is also found in the Middle East and parts of Southern Europe.
- In the UK there are 5000 to 6000 people with full sickle-cell disease.
- Sickle-cell disease gives rise to chronic anaemia and affected children have poor growth.
- Dehydration, infection or severe cold can set off painful clotting crises.
- Those more mildly affected – the sickle cell trait – are only at risk in situations of low oxygen, typically during anaesthesia for surgery.

Recognition

SYMPTOMS
Pains occur unexpectedly, affecting most commonly the bones or the spleen (in the left upper abdomen) but potentially including any organ of the body. There may be chronic tiredness and poor growth. Complications from previous blood clots can lead to fingers and toes of different sizes. Pregnancy is a time of particular risk to the mother as blood clots can form throughout her bone marrow and her lungs. Those with the sickle-cell trait can go through life without a problem except at times of surgery.

SIGNS
There may be features of **anaemia** (see page 186) and abnormalities of the skeleton as mentioned above.

INVESTIGATIONS
Sickle cells can be seen in the blood of those most severely affected. Carriers of the sickle cell trait cannot be detected in this simple way. Instead, their haemoglobin has to be analysed to detect the abnormal haemoglobin S.

ASK YOUR DOCTOR
- **About screening your family if you know that you are at risk; i.e., from an at-risk racial group or if you know other relatives who have had the condition.**

If you are sickle-cell positive it is most important that this goes on to your medical records.

Remedy

SICKLE CELL DISEASE
Every effort is made to avoid conditions which will make things worse, including infection, dehydration, the cold. When pains occur sufferers will need powerful painkillers. Occasionally so much blood ruptures that a blood transfusion is necessary; emergency surgery may be required to deal with an organ whose blood supply has clotted off. All this is possible in the developed world where sufferers can lead a

reasonable life; sufferers in the under-developed world are lucky to survive through to adult life.

SICKLE CELL TRAIT

For most of these people life can go on perfectly normally with just a few precautions. If you need a general anaesthetic it must be carefully controlled to keep up oxygen levels. There are also certain types of surgery which should be avoided – those in which the blood supply is cut off for a period of time. This can be disastrous in someone with sickle-cell trait as the blood supply to that area can be clotted and stopped altogether. Flying is possible as long as the aircraft is fully pressurized.

Alternative Treatment

None is applicable.

Prevention

This consists of avoiding those circumstances which might set off a sickle-cell crisis; we have mentioned dehydration, the cold and low oxygen levels. It is most important to identify those with the sickle-cell trait via blood tests and this should be extended to include all members of the family if one has been found to be sickle-cell positive.

So far no drugs to improve the disease have been discovered. One current approach is to try to stimulate the production of another type of haemoglobin, haemoglobin F, which is the normal haemoglobin in the fetus and in newborn babies, so it acts as a substitute for the abnormal haemoglobin.

It is possible to make the diagnosis of sickle-cell disease in the unborn fetus in the first three months of pregnancy, giving the option of a termination. This may become the method of choice for controlling the disease in those parts of the world where it is common and a significant cause of death in childhood.

Self-Help

The Sickle Cell Information Centre
St Leonard's Hospital, Nuttall Street, London N1 5LZ
Tel: 0171 601-7762
The Sickle Cell Society
54 Station Road, Harlesden, London NW10 4UA
Tel: 0181 961-4006

HORMONE DISORDERS

• Diabetes Mellitus • Obesity • Thyroid Disease

HORMONES ARE CHEMICAL messengers released by glands; they go to work around the body, far away from the site of the gland which produced them. They make up one of the control systems of the body, commonly called the endocrine system; the other more familiar control system is the nervous system. Hormones are in the main quite simple chemicals but the changes they cause are major. Insulin adjusts the whole complicated process of energy production throughout the body; other hormones regulate calcium balance, growth of cells, and pregnancy. Yet more hormones are involved in the menstrual cycle, digestion, kidney function, heart activity. And there are more.

While obesity does not strictly belong in a section about hormones, it is often (wrongly) considered an illness related to glands, and it has been featured here for this reason.

DIABETES MELLITUS

Diabetes is a disease in which there are higher than normal levels of sugar in the bloodstream. Sugar is one of the fuels of the body and it is carried in the bloodstream to all the body's tissues. The level of blood sugar is linked with the levels of the hormone insulin. Without insulin, sugar is not properly absorbed by the cells of the body, giving rise to an array of symptoms.

Insulin is made by the pancreas, a gland which lies at the back of the abdomen. In one form of diabetes there is a decrease in the amount of insulin made by the pancreas. This results in diabetes of dramatic onset and with rapid and serious ill-health which invariably used to be fatal. Treatment with insulin transforms the disease, allowing a full recovery and good health.

There is another form of diabetes, commonly known as maturity-onset diabetes, where the pancreas makes normal supplies of insulin but the tissues of the body become resistant to the insulin. This gives rise to less dramatic symptoms and is often found by chance. Treatment is with diet or drugs. Modern treatment of diabetes offers a return to normal life, a careful but not restrictive diet, and simple self-monitoring of the condition. It is, however, a lifelong diagnosis requiring regular medical checks to avoid possible long-term consequences, such as leg ulcers, blindness and kidney failure.

Risk

- About 2 per cent of the UK population have diabetes, though not all are diagnosed.
- Risk increases with age but the severe form is commoner under the age of forty.
- One in six diabetics needs treatment with insulin; the rest manage on diet alone or with drugs.
- There is a large increase in the chances of developing diabetes if your parents or siblings have diabetes.

- Diabetes is especially common in some population groups; for example, twice as common in Afro-Caribbeans and up to five times more common in those from South East Asia.
- Diabetes is becoming more common in countries enjoying an affluent Western lifestyle with increasing numbers of overweight people.
- Certain drugs, especially water tablets used to control blood pressure can cause diabetes; it disappears if the drugs are stopped.
- Sugar in the urine is common during pregnancy; this must be carefully investigated but is only occasionally true diabetes. Temporary diabetes in pregnant women is called gestational diabetes.

Recognition

SYMPTOMS
- Passing unusually large amounts of urine

This is very often the first symptom, though one which may only be remembered in retrospect. The increase occurs night and day; perhaps for the first time you find you need to get up two or three times a night to pass urine, and not just small amounts either. This symptom is due to the high levels of sugar in the bloodstream, some of which spills out through the kidneys, carrying fluid with it.

- Thirst

Your body is losing fluid in the urine; the natural result is to feel thirsty.

- Weight loss

In insulin deficiency diabetes your body cannot use the sugar in your blood. It is starvation in the midst of plenty. So the body turns to its other fuel supplies, especially fat which it can convert to fuel. Your body keeps going but you notice that you are losing flesh. In the other form of diabetes, maturity-onset, it is common to be overweight and to put on more weight as the condition worsens.

- Tiredness

Naturally you are tired; your body is short of energy.

- Minor symptoms

Women frequently develop severe thrush, a yeast-like organism causing a rash or itching in the groin or under the breasts. It thrives in the high levels of sugar. Other germs can also take advantage of the high sugar, giving rise to boils, spots, minor injuries that become infected easily. You may noticed blurred vision due to changes in the amount of water in the eye. Perhaps your fingers and toes become numb or tingle.

COMA

In insulin-deficiency diabetes, the body will eventually exhaust all its fuel supplies unless the warning symptoms are detected and the condition is treated. The sufferer slips into a state of confusion and severe dehydration. There may be a sweet smell on the breath (like pear-drops) and the breathing is deep and sighing. This is a medical emergency with a high risk of death.

SIGNS

Using a diagnostic strip, your doctor can detect this sugar in the urine, the most common symptom of diabetes, in seconds. This is, however, not conclusive proof of diabetes and should be confirmed by some of the following investigations.

The commonest forms of damage are: eye disease, which can progress to blindness (diabetes is the commonest cause of blindness in the UK); arterial disease showing itself as ulcers of the feet, poor blood flow or even gangrene of toes; **heart disease** (see page 157); kidney damage; and nerve damage causing numbness of the feet or impotence.

INVESTIGATIONS

Blood tests (see page 298) will be done to measure the actual amount of sugar in the bloodstream. Very high levels confirm the diagnosis. Occasionally there is a borderline result which calls for more sophisticated blood tests taken when fasting and at set times after food (a glucose tolerance test).

A general physical examination is necessary to see whether the diabetes is causing damage to the body. Occasionally examination suggests that the diabetes is in fact secondary to some other condition such as chronic disease of the pancreas.

ASK YOUR DOCTOR

- **To check your urine if you have any suspicious symptoms and routinely every year from middle age.**
- **About attending a diabetic clinic.**
- **Where you can have regular skilled diabetic eye checks; some opticians provide these, sometimes you need to see an eye specialist.**
- **How you can be taught the warning signs of your diabetes going out of control.**

Remedy

DIET

Forget about special diabetic foods or peculiar, unappetizing diabetic diets. They are no longer recommended. Instead, diabetics should eat a healthy diet which avoids refined sugar but allows natural sugar; for example, in fruit and potatoes. A dietitian will work out what each individual needs by way of energy (carbohydrate) intake, given their job and lifestyle. There are also recommended levels of protein and fat. It is important to lose weight if you are overweight.

You should end up following a diet which would actually be entirely acceptable and healthy for a non-diabetic, with just a little extra restriction of refined sugar. Diet alone controls many older overweight diabetics.

DRUGS

Used in more severe cases or where diet alone is not enough. There is a wide choice, some of which can be taken just once a day. Side-effects are uncommon.

- Insulin

There is no substitute for insulin in severe diabetes, especially in children and young adults. For older patients with poor diabetic control despite tablets, insulin may be the next step. There is often an understandable resistance to going on to insulin. There is no way of avoiding that daily injection. Clever pen-type devices have reduced the unpleasant aspects of injections, but even conventional insulin injections using a syringe should be almost pain free. You need to be taught how to self-inject; there are very few people who cannot manage to learn with help from diabetic nurses.

● Insulin by mouth

This would be a great advance; it is on the horizon and is under intense research.

● Monitoring of control

A newly diagnosed diabetic needs to check their urine for sugar frequently about three times a day. A simple dipstick is used. As the diabetes come under control you check less frequently until perhaps a random check every couple of weeks.

A more accurate measure of control is to check the levels of sugar in the blood. There are devices to help with this. Again, it needs to be done frequently at first, but can eventually be done every few weeks. Every few months you should have a more sophisticated blood test which gives a kind of snapshot of the overall level of blood sugar in the preceding few months.

At least once a year you should have a general check-over looking for the signs noted earlier. Special attention needs to be given to an eye check and a check of blood flow to your feet and to any foot problems. The foot is commonly where ulcers or chronic infections begin. Badly clipped toenails are dangerous for diabetics for this reason and you should ensure you have careful chiropody. Early eye problems can be dealt with by laser treatment.

Even with the best control diabetics run increased risks of heart attacks (a three to five times higher risk) and strokes (double the risk).

Alternative Treatment

There is evidence that guar gum reduces blood sugar. However, this is not in any way a substitute for conventional medical assessment and treatment of diabetes. A homoeopath or acupuncturist might suggest treatment which would address the endocrine (hormone) system in the body, perhaps changing the severity of the condition. There are also herbal remedies which may be useful on a daily basis. Ensure that you see a registered therapist in every situation. Diabetes becomes a medical emergency if it is not properly controlled.

Prevention

A balanced diet and avoiding overweight will reduce your chances of developing diabetes in later life. Unfortunately this runs counter to our affluent lifestyle, which is why diabetes is becoming more common.

● Water tablets given to control high blood pressure may produce diabetes, which goes if they are withdrawn.
● If you have any of the symptoms given earlier, have a test for diabetes since all evidence points to the benefit of early diagnosis and treatment.
● Drink alcohol in moderation; heavy drinkers can damage their pancreas, which will result in diabetes.

- If you are diabetic insist on regular eye checks and foot checks.
- Know as much about your condition as you can; you are in the best position to tell if it is going out of control.

Self-Help

British Diabetic Association
10 Queen Anne Street, London W1M OBD
Tel: 0171 323-1531
Diabetes Foundation
177a Tennison Road, London SE25 5NF
Tel: 0181 656-5467

OBESITY

Obesity is a condition characterized by an excess of fat in relation to size. It is rarely caused by disease, and extremely rarely caused by **thyroid disease** (see page 211). Many wish it were otherwise, but there is no escaping it. Obesity is caused by overeating. This does not necessarily mean gluttony; evidence suggests that some obese people do indeed eat modestly yet stay obese. This may have something to do with how efficiently they store energy as fat.

But these are subtleties; in reality, obesity is the end result of years of eating more than your body needs to survive. A modest excess of intake is all it takes, building up to obesity over a decade or two. The condition is widespread and increasing in affluent societies. It creates untold misery, widespread discomfort and contributes to many medical conditions of which **heart disease** (see page 157), **diabetes** (see page 204), **strokes** (see page 262) and **arthritis** (see page 171) are just a few.

Risk

- Those who are 20 per cent or more overweight risk about a 25 per cent increase in premature death. For those 30 per cent overweight there is about a 50 per cent increase in the risk of early death.
- Men who are even just 10 per cent overweight have a 13 per cent increase in early death.
- Obese women are at slightly less risk of early death than obese men.
- An affluent lifestyle predisposes to overweight.
- Obesity is related to snacking, especially on refined carbohydrate foods, and those high in saturated fats.
- Middle-aged spread is a real phenomenon, making obesity an age-related condition.
- Plump children tend to grow into plump adults.
- Heredity may play a small part but it is more likely that obese families share unhealthy eating habits.
- Lack of exercise is both cause and effect, because obese people find it harder to exercise.
- Hormone disorders causing obesity include **thyroid disease** (see page 211) and Cushing's syndrome (very rare).
- Eating may be a comfort activity at times of stress or unhappiness; many obese

people are unhappy because they are obese, and obese because they were unhappy.

● Drugs can cause obesity by stimulating appetite; for example, steroids and insulin.
● A return to ideal weight reduces substantially the risk of early death.

Recognition

SYMPTOMS

Symptoms of obesity are dependent on the overweight person. There are standard tables that give a guide to the ideal weight for your height and build. People 10 to 20 per cent above the ideal are overweight. The obese are those 20 per cent or more over their ideal weight.

A useful measure is the Body-Mass Index, (BMI). This is weight in kilograms, divided by the square of height measured in metres. Thus an 11 stone (70 kg) 5 ft 9 inch (1.76 m) man becomes 70 divided by (1.76 × 1.76) = a BMI of 22.6. Men should have a BMI in the range 20 to 25, women 19 to 24. A BMI of 30 or more indicates obesity.

Other measures include the thickness of fat in the arm.

SIGNS

There is frequently a conspiracy of silence about someone's obesity; no one comments on it; it is just part of who they are. The conspiracy is only broken when other medical problems arise. Early arthritis of the knees and hips; high blood pressure, diabetes, strokes; these are all much commoner in the overweight and the obese. All too often the individual is only advised strongly to lose weight when they have already run into one of the complications.

ASK YOUR DOCTOR

● **To weigh you and tell you how that compares to your recommended weight.**
● **To comment on any unusual diet you might be considering.**
● **His or her views on any drugs prescribed by a diet clinic.**

Remedy

Firstly, it is important to accept that there is a problem. Since obesity builds up over time, an individual has time to become used to their shape; they may even feel comfortable with their size if not with the consequences.

BEING REALISTIC

Many people underestimate their intake of food. They forget to count snacks, the odd biscuit, alcoholic beverages. These all add up.

DIET

It is fundamental to realize that once someone is overweight, they will maintain that weight even while eating normal amounts of food. This can be increasingly frustrating for someone trying to lose weight. An overweight person often exercises less, and tires easily; therefore, fewer than average calories are burned. A low-fat, low-calorie intake is necessary to lose weight permanently.

On a diet of a genuine 1000 calories a day most people will lose weight; the aim being to shed just one or two pounds per week. Your diet should be properly balanced between carbohydrate, protein and fats, taking no more than about 25 grams per day in the form of fat. It is very helpful to have regular support from a diet group, a nurse or a dietitian.

Crash diets may give spectacular results, due mainly to loss of fluid, but these are always short lived. Unless eating habits are permanently changed, that fluid will be quickly reabsorbed and you will be back at your starting weight.

EXERCISE

This is an important part of every lifestyle. Walking a mile a day is an excellent achievable target, which will make a small but useful contribution to losing weight, as well as being good for your heart.

DRUGS

This is a controversial area. Some doctors prescribe drugs which reduce appetite in order to help the individual through those difficult first few weeks. They can all cause side-effects; the older ones were addictive, so their long-term use is inadvisable. Unless there has been a change in eating behaviour, the individual will put weight back on once the drugs are stopped.

Water tablets (diuretics) have a similar short-term role in helping to shed weight due to fluid retention, showing itself as swollen ankles and breasts. They lose effect if used for long periods and can put a strain on the kidneys.

Thyroid hormone is given by some slimming clinics. It has no place in the treatment of overweight unless there is proven under-activity of the **thyroid** gland (page 211).

SURGERY

A case can be made for surgery if obesity is life-threatening. In one operation much of the small intestine is removed. This is serious surgery with a high risk of liver disease and a not insignificant risk of death. There is a safer operation (though still major surgery) which reduces the size of the stomach by stapling it. Some people have their jaws wired together for a few weeks, being fed a controlled liquid diet.

OTHER MEDICAL TREATMENT

Occasionally obesity is due to a physical illness of which an under-active thyroid gland is the commonest. A blood test will diagnose this. Other gland disorders are exceptionally rare.

Alternative Treatment

Be wary of any tablets on offer for weight loss, no matter how 'natural' the ingredients advertised. The chances are that they contain a mild diuretic which will give just a temporary weight loss. No diet should make you feel ill or involve bizarre foods. Ask your doctor or dietitian if in doubt. Acupuncture may be able to kickstart a sluggish metabolism (the rate at which you metabolize food), and some herbal preparations claim to do the same. Be cautious of extravagant claims. Many alternative therapies suggest sensible dietary tips as part of the treatment; these can only help. Don't eliminate anything major from your diet without first checking with your own doctor.

Prevention

- Overweight is a problem in most affluent societies; there is not a lot to do about that except to try to eat to satisfy hunger as opposed to eating for the sake of eating. There is some evidence that eating little and often is much healthier than three big meals.
- Excess weight can often begin in infancy. Fat babies grow into fat children who grow into fat adults. There are standard growth charts for babies which your doctor or health visitor can consult to see if a child is being overfed. If you feel your child or teenager is overweight, say something; do not rely on them growing out of it, because they might not.
- Offer fruit or vegetables as snacks in preference to sweets or biscuits, and take regular exercise.
- Enjoy food; it is one of the fundamental pleasures of life and we in the developed world are unbelievably fortunate in the range and quality of the food on offer. Moderation is the key.

Self-Help

Overeaters Anonymous
PO Box 19, Stretford, Manchester, M32 9EB
   There are many local branches of Weightwatchers and similar groups; check your local yellow pages.

THYROID DISEASE

The thyroid gland encircles the windpipe just below the Adam's Apple. Its function is like that of a thermostat of a heating system or the accelerator of a car engine, because it controls the general level of activity of the body. An over-active gland (hyperthyroidism) causes the heart to race, digestion to increase, and confers apparently boundless energy. Untreated, there comes a point where the body just cannot cope, leading to heart failure and weight loss among other things.

An under-active gland (hypothyroidism) conversely leads to apathy, fatigue, heart problems and weight gain. Thyroid problems are extremely common and can be diagnosed long before they cause the very severe symptoms they used to. Treatment is straightforward, though commonly lifelong.

Risk

- One in 3500 newborn babies has an under-active thyroid gland.
- An under-active gland is found in 1 to 3 per cent of those over 65 and six times more often in women than men.
- Thyroid problems are more common in areas of a country low in the natural iodine needed to make thyroid hormone.
- There is 3 to 5 per cent lifetime risk of developing an over-active gland.
- Over-activity is six to eight times commoner in women.
- Over-activity is greatest in the 20 to 50 age group.

- Occasionally thyroid disease forms part of a wider disease process, including **diabetes** (see page 204) and **rheumatoid arthritis** (see page 181).

Recognition

Symptoms of an Under-Active Gland
- Weight gain, decreased appetite, chronic constipation.
- A puffy appearance of the face, coarsening skin, thinning hair, deep gruff voice.
- Tiredness, apathy, poor concentration.
- Infrequent heavy periods.
- Cold hands; an overall sensitivity to the cold.
- Rarely, confusion or coma.
- Poor growth in children.

Symptoms of an Over-Active Gland
- Weight loss despite increased appetite; diarrhoea.
- A gaunt, even starved appearance; hot, sweaty, shaking hands.
- Either nervous energy or tiredness.
- A goitre (thickening) in the neck; staring eyes that stand out from the sockets.
- Aversion to the heat, general sweating.
- Infrequent periods.
- Excessive height in children.

Signs
A rapid pulse (over 100 per minute) goes with an over-active gland. In the elderly an over-active gland often makes the pulse fast and irregular. A slow pulse (below 60 per minute) goes with an under-active gland. Both forms of thyroid disease can give rise to heart failure with breathlessness on exertion, swelling of the ankles and possibly chest pain.

Investigations
Blood tests (see page 298) allow a highly precise diagnosis. Serious thyroid over-activity is really unmistakeable. About the only thing it might be confused with is a severe anxiety state. By contrast even serious under-activity is commonly missed by everyone: the sufferer, their relatives, their doctors. That is because it comes on gradually and the changes in appearance or behaviour are easily put down to the natural process of ageing.

ASK YOUR DOCTOR
- **About thyroid tests in any elderly person whose general condition is deteriorating.**

Remedy

An under-active gland is treated by daily tablets of thyroxine, the thyroid hormone. The dose is gradually built up to a correct level, as shown by blood tests. Once stabilized, treatment continues for life with occasional blood tests to check dosage.

An over-active gland is treated with drugs that rapidly reduce the levels of thyroxine made by the thyroid gland. This takes a few weeks, followed by treatment for nine to eighteen months in all. About 50 per cent of cases recur within two years, requiring more drug treatment or surgery to remove the thyroid gland. Treatment with radioactive iodine is another method of destroying much of the thyroid gland without the need for surgery.

Whatever method is used, it is vital to have regular follow up because up to 50 per cent of people will develop an under-active gland over the next few years.

Alternative Treatment

Some therapies, including acupuncture and reflexology, may be able to give treatment to address hormone problems generally. There are natural forms of thyroid gland treatment which can be offered by a registered herbalist. Ensure that all treatment is undertaken alongside conventional medical attention.

Prevention

- In the UK all newborn babies are screened for hypothyroidism by a simple heel-prick blood test (Guthrie test).
- Iodine is added to salt in order to prevent goitre, the swelling in the neck that can precede thyroid under-activity.
- Thyroid disease is common in the elderly and should be excluded by tests before putting general slowness down to age.

Self-Help

Hypothyroidism Support Group
47 Crawford Avenue, Tyldesley, Manchester M29 8ET
Tel: 01942 874740

THE LUNGS AND BREATHING

- Asthma • Chronic Bronchitis and Emphysema
- Cancer of the Larynx • Hay-Fever • Lung
Cancer • Pneumonia • Tuberculosis

T HE LUNGS ARE the first point of entry for many infections and irritant fumes. The lungs have well-developed defence mechanisms, but even so chest infections are common and more chronic disease is associated with industrial pollution. Early treatment with antibiotics has greatly reduced the ill-health caused by chest infections, leaving smoking and fumes as the greatest avoidable risks to the health of the lungs.

The risks of passive smoking are gradually becoming clearer; it probably accounts for 5 per cent of cases of lung cancer. It is also becoming clearer that the benefits of giving up smoking in terms of health risks begin within a year of giving up and that after five to ten years the individual's risk of contracting a smoking-related disease falls close to that of non-smokers.

ASTHMA

Always a common disease, asthma has become extremely widespread for reasons which are unclear. Some argue that the term is being used far more loosely, being applied to any child with a cough for more than a couple of weeks. Others believe that there has been a true increase in its incidence, blaming pollution, fumes and unspecified allergies. Since cases of asthma are being diagnosed in equally increasing numbers right across the developed world it does seem likely that there really is a true increase in incidence.

This is more than an academic issue. Asthma still carries a certain stigma; parents quite understandably will wonder what risks their child runs of serious flare-ups. Companies and governments are faced with demands to alter work or environmental practices said to cause the condition. If asthma were a precisely defined illness that all observers could agree on, these issues could be dealt with from a more consistent basis. Unfortunately that is far from being the case.

The physiological definition of asthma is a condition where the diameter of small airways in the lungs (bronchioles) narrows severely enough to cause symptoms (see below).

Risk

- More than 25 per cent of all children go through a wheezy phase.
- Only 8 per cent of seven-year-olds and under 5 per cent of eleven-year-olds remain wheezy enough to be termed asthmatic.
- Basing figures on a loose definition 10 to 15 per cent of the population suffers from asthma.
- Children with eczema have a much higher (50 per cent) risk of having asthma as well.

- Asthma tends to run in families.
- Smokers are at increased risk, as are children who are exposed to smoke.
- The role of pollution is debatable; it probably has an effect on people who are already at risk (a hereditary link, or in someone who smokes), but pollution alone has not been reliably proven to cause asthma. It can, however, make symptoms worse in someone who suffers from asthma.
- Diet may have an effect in a small number of cases.
- 5 per cent of asthmatics are made worse by using anti-inflammatory painkillers (NSAIDs).
- Since the mid twentieth century there has been a slow but definite increase in deaths from asthma; the cause is unknown.
- Deaths from asthma (in young adults) are just one per 100,000 per annum. Of the 2000 deaths per annum attributed to asthma two-thirds occur in the over sixty-fives.

Recognition

SYMPTOMS

The detection of asthma is often imprecise, dependent as much on the attitude of the doctor as on any more scientific measure. The following symptoms are suspicious:
- Recurrent wheeze

This musical sound may occur on its own or it may be provoked by exercise.
- Cough

A persistent cough is a consistent feature of asthma, though of course there are many other reasons for coughing. Coughing at night is typical, as is a cough brought on by going from the heat to the cold or vice versa, or coughing caused by exercise.
- Breathlessness

True breathlessness occurs during an asthmatic attack. More often it is a feeling of having to put effort into breathing. How often asthmatics have this symptom varies greatly; it may be once a year or every day.
- Asthmatic attack

Can be a truly frightening event, with the sufferer gasping for air and turning blue from lack of oxygen. Less dramatic, but as important to recognize, is the attack which just goes on and on, gradually exhausting the sufferer.

SIGNS

There is wheeze heard all over the lungs. There may be eczema. In a severe attack the pulse rate increases, the sufferer cannot speak because of breathlessness. Any hint of blueness is a sign of dangerous attack. None of these signs may be present at the time of examination, in which case a doctor relies on the patient's description and the investigations.

INVESTIGATIONS

It is easy to measure the efficiency with which someone can breathe air out; a simple handheld device is all that is needed. The aim is to see whether that efficiency (called peak flow) varies and if so whether standard anti-asthma treatment will improve it. In doubtful cases the individual is tested before and after exercise.

Chest **X-rays** (see page 301) are usually done. Occasionally **tests for allergies** (see page 297) are done by injecting substances under the skin. These are less popular with doctors than with patients as often they show sensitivities to all kinds of things, the significance of which in real life is variable.

The diagnosis of asthma is usually straightforward in children; in adults many other causes for breathlessness have to considered in particular **chronic bronchitis** and **emphysema** (see page 218) and **heart disease** (page 157) and of course **lung cancer** (page 224).

ASK YOUR DOCTOR

- **For an opinion on chronic cough, whether in adults or children.**
- **About wheezing which occurs when exercising. This is not normal and calls for a medical assessment.**

Remedy

Asthma treatments fall into three groups. There are first aid treatments to help reduce wheeze quickly, preventative measures to reduce the activity of the condition, and emergency treatment. The aim of treatment is to allow the asthmatic to lead a normal life including playing sports.

FIRST AID

These are the familiar puffers (inhalers), by convention coloured blue. Popular drugs are salbutamol and terbutaline. They work by relaxing the muscles that surround the airways, thus opening up the airways. Manufacturers have shown great ingenuity in developing devices that are easy to use even by three-year-olds. Below that age there is a bit of a problem. The drugs come in liquid form (salbutamol syrup) or there are toy-like devices to enlist the toddler's cooperation. They can be given through a nebulizer, which is a device that generates a fine cloud of gas easily breathed in by adults and children of any age. The use of nebulizers has been a major step forward in the treatment of asthma.

There are many variations on these drugs including forms that can be taken by mouth.

PREVENTATIVE

Other puffers, this time coloured red or brown and containing tiny doses of steroids, are used preventatively. Doses are as small as one-twentieth of a gram. Steroid inhalers have revolutionized the treatment of asthma by damping down the reactivity of the lungs and making flare-ups less frequent. There have been worries that inhaled steroids may restrict growth in children; this concern is not supported by research.

Another preventative treatment is with the drug cromoglycate. This drug is remarkably free of side-effects and is most effective in children.

EMERGENCY TREATMENT

High doses of steroids by mouth or by injection will stop many severe flare-ups. Hospital treatment will include oxygen, drugs via drips and, exceptionally, mechanical ventilation.

Alternative Treatment

Homoeopathic, herbal and aromatherapy practitioners all claim to provide useful treatments for asthma. It is possible that relaxation techniques will help reduce self-promoting panic which leads to an asthma attack. The question of allergies is a much vexed one and one which has lent itself to abuse by fringe practitioners using scientifically dubious methods of proving allergy. Conventional medicine does recognize a role for food allergies, especially in children; our recommendation is to explore conventional channels of investigation first. There is no safe role for the alternative treatment of an acute asthmatic attack.

Prevention

HOUSEHOLD

In general terms any asthmatic should give up smoking, avoid others who smoke and avoid smoky, fume-laden atmospheres. Parents with asthmatic children owe it to their children to stop smoking, too.

It is helpful to keep dust in the house to a minimum as the house dust mite has been shown to provoke asthma. Sadly some people react to loved family pets, posing a difficult dilemma especially where children are devoted to an animal but react to its fur.

Some asthmatics find that it reduces the severity of asthma at night to remove feather pillows and duvets.

DRUGS

Asthmatics should avoid aspirin and aspirin-type drugs (non-steroidal anti inflammatory agents [NSAIDs], widely used for arthritis and for minor injuries). There is a class of drugs called beta-blockers which is very commonly used to control high blood pressure but hazardous for use in those with asthma.

FOODS

Children are more likely to find that certain foods make their asthma worse but some adults do, too. The food colouring tartrazine has definitely been shown to do so in a small number of children. Alcohol makes asthma worse in up to one-third of adults.

OTHER FACTORS

Your emotional state can make asthma worse, aggression and anxiety being two emotions frequently linked with flare-ups of the disease. Many women find that asthma worsens before their periods.

Asthma is a serious diagnosis whose treatment should not be taken lightly. Yet for the great majority of sufferers it is possible to lead a normal life by taking advantage of modern medication, making some adjustments to your environment and by being aware of the symptoms of deterioration. There is a risk of death from asthma, but it can be minimized by undertaking sensible precautions.

Self-Help

National Asthma Campaign
Providence House, Providence Place, London N1 0NT
Tel: 0171 226-2260
British Allergy Foundation
St Bartholomew's Hospital, West Smithfield, London EC1A 7BE

CHRONIC BRONCHITIS AND EMPHYSEMA

Chronic bronchitis is a diagnosis based on the combination of breathlessness, wheezing, and the production of large amounts of sputum. The lungs become stiffer and less able to shift air in and out. Emphysema may be suspected in life, but it is often a post-mortem diagnosis showing that the lung structure has been replaced by large bubbles or cavities.

The lungs are a mass of tiny bubbles where inspired air passes close to blood and where an exchange of gases takes place – oxygen into the blood, carbon dioxide leaving the blood. Being tiny but numerous these bubbles add up to a large surface area – the average is seventy square metres. In emphysema these tiny bubbles break down into larger bubbles, with a resulting reduction in surface area available for gas exchange, hence causing breathlessness.

It can be difficult in the early stages to tell chronic bronchitis and emphysema apart from asthma; indeed, much treatment is identical. Unlike asthma, these diseases tend to deteriorate steadily. Another major difference concerns cigarette smoking. Although this does not cause asthma, it makes it worse, whereas it is believed actually to cause most cases of chronic bronchitis and emphysema.

Risk

- Chronic bronchitis and emphysema affect 5 to 8 per cent of men, and slightly fewer women.
- The incidence rises rapidly with age.
- In middle age a staggering 17 per cent of men and 8 per cent of women are affected by these related conditions.
- Chronic bronchitis and emphysema account for 38,000 deaths a year.
- They account for 7 per cent of the entire number of working days lost through illness.
- The risk of death from these conditions is related to the numbers of cigarettes smoked; a smoker on 25 a day has twice the risk as someone on 15 a day.
- A smoker on thirty cigarettes a day has twenty times the risk of dying from these conditions than a non-smoker.
- Giving up smoking reduces the risks but it takes ten years to do so.
- Only 4 per cent of cases are found in life-long non-smokers.
- Pollution and exposure to irritants play a part in causing or exacerbating the condition; the degree to which this is the case is uncertain.
- These conditions are more common in lower social classes.

Recognition

Neither of these conditions begins suddenly. Instead there is a gradually emerging pattern of symptoms over several years.

SYMPTOMS
The developed picture is one of wheezing, breathlessness and the constant coughing-up of large amounts of sputum. An ordinary cold, normally shaken off in a week or two, somehow lingers on, with cough and phlegm that worsens and is more prolonged with

each infection. Eventually the individual is rarely without a cough productive of sputum.

Breathlessness is the next symptom. It would be wrong to suggest that breathlessness always worsens, but in those in whom it does it can reach a point that the individual cannot leave the house.

SIGNS

The earliest signs are persistent wheezing, particularly in a smoker. In advanced disease the sufferer is breathless on modest exertion. Their chest may look 'barrel-shaped' or it may be appear fixed and move little during breathing. The muscles in the neck are tensed because they are brought into use to help breathing. Sufferers typically breathe out through pursed lips.

The lips and tongue may be blue through cyanosis (lack of oxygen) and there may be swelling of the legs through heart failure.

INVESTIGATIONS

Investigations will reveal poor lung capacity and may show strain on the heart. In flare-ups it is useful to test sputum samples to see which organisms are involved.

ASK YOUR DOCTOR
- **About any persistent cough.**
- **To advise on how to give up smoking.**

Remedy

- The single most fundamental thing is to give up smoking; unfortunately this does not reverse the damage done but it does at least reduce the rate of deterioration of the condition. If possible avoid polluted, irritant atmospheres.
- The same drugs used to treat **asthma** (see page 214) are used to treat chronic bronchitis and emphysema, though with less effect. These include drugs to open up the airways, such as salbutamol, and steroids by mouth or by inhaler to reduce inflammation.
- Infection is treated with antibiotics; it is sensible to have an annual vaccination against **influenza** (see page 19).
- If heart failure is present it is treated in the standard way (diuretics, ACE inhibitors), but it is a most serious turn of events.
- Many sufferers benefit from oxygen at home and there are also convenient portable oxygen devices. Oxygen should be prescribed only after assessment by a chest physician; this is because in certain circumstances it can actually make matters worse.
- In a severe flare-up the individual has to be nursed in hospital, where he or she can have intensive therapy to remove phlegm from the lungs and to assist ventilation.
- Once the stage of severe breathlessness and perhaps heart failure is reached, there is a 30 to 50 per cent five-year survival rate.

These are miserable conditions. Many doctors feel that they are worse than some cancers in their effects, given the constant breathlessness, the limitation of lifestyle and the steady decline.

Alternative Treatment

Aromatherapy and herbal remedies using inhaled aromatic oils may help the acute flare-ups. Exercise programmes to take you to the limits of your breathing capacity are increasingly advocated and may be available through physiotherapists. Gentle exercise like yoga or T'ai chi might be useful. Homoeopathic remedies and treatment by acupuncture are often suggested, particularly for very chronic cases.

Prevention

Once again, cigarette smoking is the major avoidable cause of these conditions. If you haven't already done so, give up smoking at the first sign of bronchitis or wheezing. The risks for non-smokers are minimal (see above). Although the role of pollution is unclear, it seems sensible to take whatever steps you can to avoid noxious atmospheres, especially in the workplace. Use masks if these are recommended for your job and check that ventilation systems are installed (there are statutory requirements for these depending on the industry).

If you are unfortunate enough to have the diseases, make sure that infections are treated quickly. Many doctors are happy to supply sufferers with antibiotics to use at the earliest sign of infection, such as increased cough and coloured sputum.

There is interest in the use of exercise programmes to improve the quality of life. Your local chest physician may be able to arrange this.

Self-Help

Action on Smoking and Health (ASH)
109 Gloucester Place, London W1N 3PH
Tel: 0171 935-3519
QUIT (Smokers quitline)
Tel: 0171 487-3000

CANCER OF THE LARYNX

Although cancer of the larynx is not very common, it has been included here because with early detection it can almost always be cured.

Risk

- There are three to four cases per 100,000 per annum (1700 to 2300 cases).
- Men are affected ten times more than women.
- Smokers are at increased risk.

Recognition

SYMPTOMS
Hoarseness is the earliest symptom. As a rule of thumb anyone with hoarseness lasting more than two to three weeks should seek medical attention. Later symptoms include difficulty in swallowing, ear pain and coughing up blood. These are all features of advanced disease.

SIGNS
An ear, nose and throat (ENT) specialist will see the tumour as a thickened area on the vocal cord. A **biopsy** (see page 298) is taken to confirm the diagnosis and probably a **CT scan** (see page 298) to see whether it has spread elsewhere.

ASK YOUR DOCTOR
- **For an ENT opinion if you are persistently hoarse, even though the hoarseness will likely prove to be completely benign.**

Remedy

As long as the cancer is confined to the vocal cord, treatment is by **radiotherapy** (see page 301) to the vocal cord. Immediately after treatment your voice will be worse but in the long run the voice returns to normal. The cure rate is better than 90 per cent.

Large tumours or those that have spread are dealt with only by extensive neck surgery including removing the larynx and with it normal speech. Despite this drastic treatment the cure rate is only about 30 per cent.

Prevention

Early assessment of persistent hoarseness is crucial. Many cases will prove to be due to a post-infectious roughening of the vocal cord or to benign nodules on the cords. Where it does prove to be cancer, the difference in outlook between disease detected early and late speaks for itself.

HAY-FEVER

In the modern, urban world the term 'hay-fever' is a bit of a misnomer; a better term might be pollen fever or atmosphere allergy, affecting the eyes, nose and the lungs. Underlying hay-fever is a reaction to irritants in the atmosphere. These can be substances to which people become allergic; such substances are called allergens. Or they can be substances which are irritant in themselves such as smoke fumes or chlorine in swimming pools.

The sufferer from hay-fever looks at the year less poetically than others. He or she can anticipate reactions to different allergens at different times of the year: tree pollens are to blame in spring and early summer, giving way to grass pollens till late summer after which spores from mould become more common. In addition you may react to animals (their skin, urine and salivary proteins) and the house dust mite. It is, however, unlikely that any one sufferer will be affected year round; most sufferers are particularly prone at one or perhaps two times of the year.

Modern treatment is very helpful, though it can involve travelling with a battery of medication – eye drops, tablets, nasal sprays and inhalers – for the relevant season.

Risk

- Hay-fever is the commonest form of allergy, with millions of sufferers.
- It is estimated to affect from 2 to 10 per cent of the population.
- Up to 20 per cent of young adults are affected.
- It is often associated with **asthma** (20 per cent of sufferers have both) and eczema by way of an atopic nature (see **eczema**, page 4)
- There is an increased risk to workers in industries generating dust and fumes.

Recognition

Symptoms

The eyes feel itchy and look red around the outside; they water easily and often run. There is a sense of needing to blink. Frequent sneezing and a dripping nose are common, as are wheezing and coughing. Often there is an irritation in the throat and ears. The nasal and chest congestion inhibit the senses of smell and taste.

Signs

The watery-eyed, sniffing patient, coughing his way into the doctor's surgery is virtually diagnostic. The undersurfaces of the eyelids are especially red and granular in appearance. With long-standing hay-fever polyps often form in the nose, blocking off one nostril; the chest may sound wheezy.

Investigations

Investigations are not usually helpful except to pin down allergies to very specific conditions; i.e., the sufferer experiences symptoms only when exposed to certain moulds or the family pet. **Allergy tests** (see page 297) involve injecting small amounts of a range of allergens into the skin and gauging reaction. Blood tests can also characterize the allergy.

ASK YOUR DOCTOR
- **About preventative treatment well before the hay-fever season.**
- **About special treatment to see you through an important event, such as an exam.**

Remedy

Antihistamine Tablets

Modern antihistamines are good at controlling the symptoms of mild hay-fever, such as itchy eyes and sneezing. They have the benefit of being non-sedative and so are safe to use when driving or operating machinery. They do not interfere with concentration. Modern antihistamines include terfenadine, cetirizine, astemizole; some are available in chemists without prescription.

Anti-Inflammatory Drops

Cromoglycate is the best known anti-inflammatory drop preparation. Drops are also useful for itchy eyes and sneezing. The disadvantage is that they need to be used several times a day.

Steroid Sprays

This is a suggested treatment for an itchy, runny nose and is considered safe to use for months on end; they cannot be used in the eyes because of the risk of side-effects. Other forms of steroid spray also reduce wheezing, used in exactly the same way as in **asthma** (see page 214).

DECONGESTANTS

These are very popular over-the-counter remedies and are good for short-term control. Doctors disapprove of their use for more than a week or so because they alter the lining of the nose in such a way that once you stop using them symptoms return more severely, leading to a vicious circle of overuse.

STEROIDS BY MOUTH

These are reserved for desperate situations where the risk of using steroids for a few days is negligible compared to the benefits.

The treatment of hay-fever for any but the most mildly affected will usually call for a combination of the above, adjusted by individual experience.

Alternative Treatment

Recommendations include foods rich in vitamin C, liquorice and vitamin B-complex tablets. Some practitioners recommend acupressure or aromatherapy. A registered homoeopath might have some success implementing a programme which will allow you to become virtually immune to the allergens currently exacerbating your condition. Acupuncture and osteopathic treatment might be useful.

Prevention

AVOIDANCE OF ALLERGENS

In an ideal world this might be possible. In practice it is impossible to escape pollen or spores in their season without resorting to extreme measures such as filtered air conditioning and tightly closed windows – a miserable option in summer. However, it can help to wear sunglasses and to stay indoors when pollen release is at its maximum, which is during the afternoon, and to keep bedroom windows closed at night.

Where a family pet is proved to be the cause a difficult decision may have to be taken.

THE HOUSE DUST MITE

This ubiquitous pest exists in huge numbers in even the most pristine homes; a gram of dust from bedding will contain up to 4000 of them. They can be controlled by enclosing bedding in plastic or in fabrics to keep them confined. Remove carpets wherever possible, as they present an ideal breeding ground.

DESENSITIZATION

This used to be a popular option, by which tolerance to selected allergens was built up by having regular injections of extracts of the known allergen. It did give relief often for several seasons. The procedure has fallen from favour for a simple reason; in just a few cases even exposure to a tiny first dose would cause anaphylactic collapse. This is a particularly devastating type of allergic reaction including a drop in blood pressure and difficulty breathing and is (and was) potentially fatal. As hay-fever never killed anyone this risk is now seen as unacceptable. Desensitization can still be given but only in specialized centres with immediate access to resuscitation equipment.

Self-Help

British Allergy Foundation
St Bartholomew's Hospital, West Smithfield, London EC1A 7BE

LUNG CANCER

Lung cancer is the single most common cause of death from cancer in the UK and across the Western world. Not only that but its frequency is rising rapidly in many countries. In another age and at another time, surely people will look back to this century and to the story of lung cancer and shake their heads in disbelief. Here is a cancer, a feared disease almost always fatal, one of the few cancers whose cause is known. They will wonder how it was that the cause, cigarette smoking, was not just known but that the habit was relied upon as a huge source of government revenue. This same observer might note with incredulity the worry bordering on hysteria over the risks of cancer from power lines, nuclear power stations and unleaded fuels: valid concerns all of them but if they have caused any increase in cancer at all it is minuscule in comparison to the Big One: cigarette smoking.

Lung cancer is mainly self-inflicted and it is one of the most cruel diseases there are.

Risk

- There are 40,000 cases per annum in the UK.
- At present men are affected twice as often as women.
- The incidence in men in the UK has fallen considerably over the last 20 years, believed to be due to a reduction in men smoking, which began 20 years ago.
- In women, the incidence continues to climb, reflecting the fact that more women are beginning or continuing to smoke, and fewer men are doing so.
- The switch to filter and low-tar cigarettes has probably contributed to the fall in death rates.
- Only 15 per cent of cases of lung cancer occur in non-smokers.
- Passive smoking is associated with an increased risk of lung cancer though the exact risk is uncertain; it may increase the natural risk by 50 per cent.
- Air pollution is another risk factor: dwellers in cities and industrialized areas have about a 50 per cent increased chance of developing lung cancer.
- Exposure to asbestos greatly increases the risk of lung cancer.

Recognition

Evidence suggests that lung cancer is a slow-growing tumour which is therefore well established by the time it produces symptoms. This goes some way towards explaining the very poor outlook, no matter how early the diagnosis is made.

SYMPTOMS

The commonest symptom is a persistent cough, often combined with pain in the chest. The fact that most smokers cough often prevents an earlier diagnosis.

Coughing up blood is a symptom which should ring alarm bells in anyone, but especially in a smoker. The amount does not matter. Even after a single episode full investigation is recommended. Other common symptoms are an aching in the chest and breathlessness.

In 5 per cent of cases there are no symptoms at all, the cancer being spotted on a chest X-ray done for some other reason.

SIGNS

The diagnosis is sought regardless of whether a doctor can find any signs; those signs which are present only serve to make the diagnosis more certain. These might include weight loss, clubbed finger nails (highly curved bulbous looking nails), swollen lymph nodes (glands) in the neck or abdomen from spread of the cancer, or tender bones suggestive of involvement with the tumour. Lung cancer can produce a number of peculiar effects thanks to hormone production by the cancerous cells, such as breast enlargement.

INVESTIGATIONS

Ninety per cent of tumours show on a simple chest **X-ray** (see page 301). Abnormal cells shed into the sputum can frequently be detected under the microscope. The other main investigation is bronchoscopy, in which a tube is passed down the main airways of the lung. This allows cancers to be seen directly and samples taken for analysis. A **CT scan** (see page 298) is helpful in some cases.

ASK YOUR DOCTOR

- **To investigate any episode of coughing blood; this is most important if you are a smoker, but anyone with this symptom needs to be checked.**
- **To discuss how you can be helped to give up smoking.**

Remedy

It is a sad, salutary and sobering thought that there is but a 20 per cent, one-year survival rate, and a 4 to 8 per cent, five-year survival rate, despite treatment. This does not give a full picture because lung cancer actually includes four different kinds of tumours, three of which have a poor outlook and one of which has an appalling one.

In most cases treatment is aimed at improving symptoms rather than achieving a cure. This is important as it makes a great difference to quality of life by relieving breathlessness or by reducing bone pain.

SURGERY

In selected cases surgical removal of the tumour does improve survival.

RADIOTHERAPY

This form of treatment (see page 301) buys time and is invaluable in relieving symptoms.

CHEMOTHERAPY

Chemotherapy does improve survival in certain selected tumours but only from a matter of weeks or months to perhaps a year or two.

This is a grim picture; yet despite the outlook much can be done to make this time more comfortable by ensuring adequate pain relief.

Alternative Treatment

Patients with cancer of any type may gain great comfort from aromatherapy, or herbalism. The holistic approach to health care, which emphasizes a positive attitude to the cancer, can only help. Many cancer patients benefit from nutritional therapy, acupuncture, healing and homoeopathic treatment. With the risk of death so high, anything that works may be a conceivable option.

It is important not to overlook the great strain that the carers experience; any therapy which gives them support is invaluable.

Prevention

Evidence suggests that within five and certainly ten years of giving up smoking, the risks of contracting a smoking-related disease fall back to that of non-smokers.

POLLUTION

The agents in pollution which may be to blame for cancer have not been identified. Country dwellers can count themselves lucky. Exposure to asbestos should be a thing of the past.

VITAMIN A

There is some recent intriguing evidence that Vitamin A may protect against developing lung cancer. The effect is small and it is not clear how this should translate into general advice.

SCREENING

Screening has been tried by offering regular chest X-rays and by sampling sputum for malignant cells. Although cancers were indeed picked up, it made no difference to five-year survival rates.

Self-Help

Action on Smoking and Health (ASH)
109 Gloucester Place, London, W1N 3PH
Tel: 0171 935-3519
Quit (Smokers quitline)
Tel: 0171 487-3000
Cancer Relief Macmillan Fund
Anchor House, 15-19 Britten Street, London SW3 3TZ
Tel: 0171 351-7811

PNEUMONIA

Pneumonia is the most common cause of death from infection in the UK; in fact, it accounts for ten times as many deaths from infection as all other causes put together. This may give a misleading picture, because serious pneumonia is much more common in those who are already ill or who have something which increases their risk (see below). Pneumonia is frequently a terminal event in **stroke** victims (see page 262). In under-developed countries pneumonia is a major killer at all ages.

The lungs are made up of a several large sections called lobes. Pneumonia means infection that has spread throughout one whole lobe (hence lobar pneumonia) or which in more serious cases involves the whole lung. The term broncho-pneumonia refers to infection in both lungs which is worse than a simple bronchitis but which has not gone quite as far as to involve a whole lobe. In practice these conditions are treated in the same way.

Risk

- One to three cases per 1000 of adult population per annum (this is probably a great underestimate).
- Most cases are the result of infection.
- A minority of cases are due to lung damage that allows infection to spread; for example, breathing in vomit or an underlying lung cancer.
- Excessive alcohol intake, cigarette smoking, diabetes, pre-existing lung disease all increase the risk.
- Mini-epidemics occur in hospitals, nursing homes and similar closed institutions.
- There is an increased risk in those with lowered immunity; for instance, those on chemotherapy for cancer or with AIDS.
- Pneumonia acquired in hospital after surgery is one of the major causes of post-operative complications.

Recognition

In most cases pneumonia begins in a rather dramatic way and the sufferer is clearly unwell. There are forms, not uncommon, where the onset is much more low key.

SYMPTOMS

Often the illness starts with an unremarkable cough and cold. Then there is a deterioration over a day or two associated with high temperatures, a rapid rate of breathing, a cough that may bring up some blood. Confusion is common in the elderly. Usually there is some degree of breathlessness and often a dull ache over the part of the chest involved by the infection.

This is the typical pattern but there can be great differences in presentation. On the one hand there may be a gradual deterioration over several days; on the other hand there are forms of pneumonia (fortunately uncommon) which can progress to collapse within hours.

SIGNS

By tapping and listening to the lungs it is possible to hear those areas which are solid with infection. Taking this together with high temperatures, rapid breathing, rapid pulse and perhaps cold sores on the lips, the diagnosis is pretty certain.

In the elderly there may be nothing more than a raised pulse rate and a slight cough with loss of appetite and perhaps confusion. A normal temperature does not exclude the possibility of infection in the elderly.

In babies and children pneumonia and other serious chest infections may be suspected on the basis of a raised rate of breathing and unspecific signs in the lungs. Hospital admission is often needed to confirm and to treat the condition.

INVESTIGATIONS

A chest X-ray is the basic investigation, but is not always necessary at the start of treatment in an otherwise fit young adult. A follow-up X-ray is always needed to ensure that the infection has completely disappeared. Where there is doubt about the diagnosis, in the very ill and in children a chest X-ray might precede treatment. Sputum samples and blood tests can pin down the organisms responsible.

ASK YOUR DOCTOR
- **About having annual vaccination against influenza; this is recommended for the elderly and those with illnesses such as diabetes, chronic bronchitis, heart disease. In such individuals influenza can lead to particularly dangerous forms of pneumonia.**

Remedy

Many cases of pneumonia in adults can be safely handled at home, with high doses of antibiotics and rest. The doctor will select an antibiotic based on the organisms that are common at the moment. After three or four days the temperature should settle, appetite return and thereafter there should be steady progress to normal, although post-pneumonia tiredness can last for several weeks.

Children with suspected pneumonia, and especially babies, require more intensive treatment in hospital with antibiotics via a drip, oxygen and physiotherapy to shift phlegm off the chest. Adults who remain unwell may also need hospital care. In the elderly, pneumonia is a dangerous disease, with as much as a 50 per cent risk of death. This could be a not unwelcome terminal event following a severe stroke or occurring in someone who has advanced cancer.

The overall risk of death is 5 per cent but most deaths by far will be in the elderly, those with other serious disease and those who have acquired an unusual type of pneumonia in hospital.

Alternative Treatment

There are some good preparations for inhalation during an acute phase; see a registered herbalist for a treatment tailored to your symptoms. There are also homoeopathic remedies. Osteopathic treatment, chiropractic and massage can help to shift phlegm on the lungs, and acupuncture may stimulate the immune system to fight the infection more effectively.

Prevention

There is always a small unavoidable risk of picking up infections that may progress to pneumonia. The following will reduce additional risks.

ANNUAL INFLUENZA VACCINATION
This is recommended for anyone with chronic chest and heart trouble, for diabetics and for those with lowered immunity. Many authorities recommend it for anyone over sixty-five. The only people who should definitely not have flu vaccination are those who have a true allergy to eggs.

HOSPITALS AND NURSING HOMES
These have a duty to be vigilant for outbreaks of infection, to encourage people to become mobile quickly after operations (this reduces the chances of chest infection due to pooling of phlegm on the lungs) and it goes without saying that they should be scrupulous about sterilizing instruments and utensils.

> *Legionella (also called Legionnaire's disease) is an unusual but not rare cause of a particularly aggressive form of pneumonia. It is now recognized that the organism lives in the heating and ventilation systems of large buildings; there are accepted design and sterilization standards which should reduce the incidence of outbreaks. Such standards cannot be relied upon outside the developed world.*

POST-SPLENECTOMY VACCINATION AGAINST PNEUMOCOCCUS

Increasing numbers of people have had their spleen removed, perhaps in treatment of **Hodgkin's Disease** (see page 192). This reduces resistance to a variety of infections, of which pneumococcal infection is a frequent cause of pneumonia. There is an effective anti-pneumococcal vaccine which gives protection for up to ten years. Speak to your doctor about having this.

GENERAL

Smoking is an avoidable risk factor. Alcohol excess is a risk factor both because alcoholics have less resistance, but also because in a drunken state there is a risk of breathing in one's own vomit. This 'aspiration pneumonia' is particularly dangerous because of the associated damage to the lungs from the strong stomach acid.

Self-Help

Advice on influenza and pneumococcal vaccination can be obtained from your doctor.

TUBERCULOSIS

One of the great success stories of the twentieth century has been the decline in the West of those infectious diseases which just 100 years ago were so common and feared. Tuberculosis (TB) is an outstanding example of this. There was a time when premature death from TB was so common that it acquired an almost romantic aura, as in *La Traviata*.

TB is now relatively rare in the developed world, although in under-developed countries it is still a major problem. It is worrying that the incidence of TB has begun to rise again in the developed world.

Tuberculosis results from infection by an extremely slow growing organism, the mycobacterium tuberculosis. The usual pattern of illness starts with a mild primary infection. The organism does not die, but remains in a dormant state which reactivates if the resistance of its host falls. There then ensues a slow secondary spread which can involve almost any organ of the body. It is that ability to lie dormant awaiting its opportunity that explains why TB is associated with poverty, poor nutrition or anything else that reduces natural resistance.

Risk

- There are 7000 cases a year in the UK, a one in 8000 risk.
- In the indigenous white population the incidence is 4.3 cases per 100,000 per annum – about 2500 cases a year.
- In Asia up to 80 per cent of children are infected.
- The risk among immigrants to the UK from Asia is up to forty times greater than in the UK-born population.

- The incidence is slowly increasing again; AIDS, which causes decreased immunity, is believed to be responsible for much of the increase.
- The poor, those living in crowded conditions, alcoholics, diabetics, and the elderly are all at increased risk.
- Worldwide, TB kills 3 million per annum.
- Increasing incidence in the homeless population. Recent research has shown a 1 in 8 risk for those sleeping rough in London.

Recognition

SYMPTOMS

The initial infection is a trivial illness, rarely causing more than a week or two of coughing and malaise. What happens thereafter depends on how the disease spreads, remembering that this may be years later. The commonest symptom is a persistent productive cough, perhaps coughing blood. There might be a recurrent mild fever and sweating at night plus a general decline in health with weight loss and, in children, poor growth.

Swollen tuberculous glands may appear in the neck. TB can also affects bones, the heart and several other organs, giving rise to an array of symptoms.

There is a more aggressive form of TB, miliary TB, which causes a severe feverish illness; this is difficult to diagnose.

SIGNS

There is rarely anything diagnostic on examination, though large persistent glands in the neck in an Asian immigrant are suspicious.

INVESTIGATION

The chest **X-ray** (see page 301) shows typical changes. Analysis of the sputum reveals the TB mycobacterium; this is the best method of diagnosis. Often the diagnosis is made by **biopsying** (see page 298) neck glands.

There is a **skin test** (see page 301), the tuberculin test (Heaf test, Mantoux test), which goes positive as a result of infection; this is useful if initial infection is suspected, less helpful in diagnosing secondary disease. Untreated TB carries about a 12 per cent annual mortality; untreated miliary TB is always fatal.

ASK YOUR DOCTOR
- **About prolonged unexplained ill-health, coughing and night sweats.**
- **About what to do if you might have been exposed to TB.**

Remedy

DRUGS

Drug treatment for TB began in the 1950s with sulpha drugs, being gradually refined to the present regime. This uses two main drugs, isoniazid and rifampicin, with others added depending on individual disease. These must be taken for six to nine months, after which cure can be guaranteed in every case. There is a small chance of recurrence which is why follow-up is recommended.

Drug resistance is a growing problem worldwide, less so in the UK where treatment is carefully organized and supervised. It arises because many people discontinue their antibiotics as soon as they feel better, which may be in as little as a fortnight.

CONTACT TRACING
This is of great importance to detect those individuals who have had that trivial initial infection and who are now harbouring and perhaps also passing on the bacterium. Contact tracing is done by taking sputum samples, doing skin tests and chest X-rays.

Alternative Treatment

There are no specific treatments for TB, which must be considered a medical problem. There are, however, many useful therapies for convalescent care, and for ensuring that the immune system is strong and healthy enough to prevent a recurrence. Acupuncture, homoeopathy and herbalism all offer viable treatment.

Prevention

TB is a disease of the poor, the overcrowded and the malnourished. It is the measures society has taken to deal with these social problems that should take the credit for the decline in TB in the developed world; medicine has had a relatively small part to play. The recent increase in TB in the UK raises questions about the direction our society is taking with an increase in poverty and poor housing, though it is perhaps too soon to draw any firm conclusions.

TUBERCULIN TESTING OF MILK
This goes on quietly and efficiently, keeping at bay this route of transmission of TB from TB infected cows. Anyone tempted to buy non-tested milk should be aware of the risk.

BCG VACCINATION
The Bacillus Calmette–Guerin (the researchers who developed it) is a vaccine which reduces the risk of contracting TB by 70 per cent for fifteen years. When TB was relatively common in the UK it made good sense to run a BCG vaccination programme among schoolchildren. The value of this is now less definite. Those at high risk should still be vaccinated; these include immigrants from high-risk countries; health workers and those travelling to areas of risk.

SUFFERERS FROM AIDS, ALCOHOLISM, DIABETES
These individuals are at greater risk and should seek advice where there is a possibility of exposure to TB.

Self-Help

Your local chest physician should be the best source of advice on TB.

THE KIDNEYS AND BLADDER

• Cancer of the Bladder • Cystitis and Urinary Infections • Incontinence of Urine • Kidney Failure • Kidney and Bladder Stones

WHEN DOCTORS ASK about your 'waterworks' they are not being patronizing. The urinary system really does consist of plumbing, pipework and storage vessels; common diseases are the result of blockage, furring up, kinks, leaks and overflowing. It doesn't take a plumber to see the similarities.

The exception to this biological pipework is the kidneys themselves, which are marvels of filtration and which can be influenced by several general diseases, in particular high blood pressure, diabetes and recurrent infection. Much of the long-term care of such diseases is aimed at preventing kidney damage. There is particular attention paid to the detection and prevention of urinary infection in childhood, which is believed to underlie much adult kidney damage.

CANCER OF THE BLADDER

Tumours within the bladder are fairly common forms of cancer and have an excellent outlook if diagnosed early. Long-term follow-up is essential to ensure the best survival. It has long been known that bladder cancer can be caused by certain industrial processes involving aniline dyes or rubber; workers in those industries should be aware of the risks and have regular screening (see below).

Risk

- Cancer of the bladder accounts for 2 per cent of all cancers and 3 per cent of deaths from cancer.
- It's a disease of late middle age; rarely occurring below forty.
- Men are affected four times as often as women.
- Cigarette smoking appears to account for up to half of all cases.
- There is an increased risk for workers in the rubber, chemical, paint and leather industries.
- Some drugs increase the risk, most commonly cyclophosphamide used in the treatment of leukaemia.
- Chronic irritation can provoke it; e.g., schistosomiasis (a disease which is a significant risk in the tropics).

Recognition

SYMPTOMS

Blood in the urine is the principle symptom in most cases (though there are many other reasons for blood in the urine). The bleeding is painless in contrast to the painful bleeding suggestive of a kidney stone or of infection. Recurrent urinary infection is a less common presentation. It is rare for there to be pain elsewhere unless the tumour has spread to bone or obstructed the kidney.

SIGNS

There are probably none at all unless the tumour has spread.

INVESTIGATIONS

Examination of urine shows blood and often infection. Malignant cells might be present in the urine. **X-rays** (see page 301) using a dye concentrated in urine (a cystogram) show up nearly all tumours as an irregular area in the wall of the bladder. The next step is **cystoscopy** (see page 299); this involves passing a thin telescopic device into the bladder. A **CT scan** (see page 298) is helpful if it is suspected that the tumour has spread.

ASK YOUR DOCTOR

- **About any episode of blood in the urine. This is a most important symptom. Although frequently the cause is infection, in an older age group it may be the first sign of a tumour in the bladder, prostate or kidney.**

Remedy

Small localized tumours are dealt with via a cystoscope simply by burning. If there are many growths then cytotoxic drugs are pumped into the bladder with the aim of killing off abnormal cells all over its walls.

There are several options for dealing with more advanced disease. Various form of **radiotherapy** (see page 301) are available; it may be possible to remove a section of the bladder including the tumour. Finally the bladder itself may have to be removed; the ureters which carry urine from the kidneys can usually be diverted into the bowel, avoiding the need to wear a urine collection bag (this operation is called a urostomy).

Careful follow-up by cystoscopy is necessary for years so that any small recurrence can be burnt immediately. The outlook is excellent for early disease confined to the lining of the bladder. Where the tumour has spread into the muscle of the bladder, the five-year survival falls to about 50 per cent, and falls lower again, to around 5 per cent, if the tumour has spread outside the bladder into the pelvis and bone.

Alternative Treatment

As with other types of cancer, alternative palliative care can be extremely helpful; although no one claims that treatments such as aromatherapy or homoeopathy actually cure cancer, the treatments offered can encourage relaxation and a sense of well-being. There is no doubt that a mind-body relationship exists, and a good state of mind can be enormously beneficial in the face of life-threatening illnesses. Following surgery or chemotherapy, many therapies will offer recuperative care.

Prevention

- Stop smoking.
- Workers in the aniline dye and rubber industries should have regular screening of their urine, looking for microscopic amounts of blood and other abnormal cells.
- Occasionally new substances are suspected of promoting cancer of the bladder. There was a scare some years ago about artificial sweeteners, but this has proved groundless. However anyone who has had cancer of the bladder should avoid those substances as there is evidence that they may promote the growth of established bladder tumours.

> *Blood in the urine should always be taken seriously at whatever age. In the great majority of cases the cause is infection or kidney stones, but the chances of a malignancy increase with age; the earlier these are detected and treated the better the outlook.*

Self-Help

BACUP (British Association of Cancer United Patients)
3 Bath Place, Rivington Street, London EC2A 3JR
Tel: 01800 181199 or 0171 613-2121
Urostomy Association
Buckland, Beaumont Park, Danbury, Essex CM3 4DE
Tel: 01245 224294

CYSTITIS AND URINARY INFECTIONS

Cystitis and urinary tract infections are so common that most women will suffer from them at some point in their lives. Urinary infections are far less usual in men. While the treatment of infections is straightforward, the treatment of cystitis is more controversial.

Risk

- At least 50 per cent of women experience cystitis at some time.
- Women are at greater risk of urinary infection because the infecting bacteria can more easily gain access to the bladder.
- Urinary infection affects about 1 to 3 per cent of children; girls are affected ten to thirty times more often than boys.
- In children there is a risk of underlying abnormality in the urinary tract in up to 2 per cent of cases.
- 20 to 30 per cent of elderly women experience recurrent cystitis and infection.
- Urinary infections are common in pregnancy because hormonal changes mean that any bacteria present in the bladder are more likely to ascend towards the kidney and cause more serious infections.

Recognition

SYMPTOMS IN ADULTS

The diagnostic symptoms are usually quite obvious. There is frequency; that is, a need to pass urine often, but with little result. There is a burning sensation on passing urine. The urine itself often looks cloudy, may smell and may have blood in it. Often there is an aching over one or other kidney and an ache low in the abdomen over the bladder.

Uncontrolled shaking, called rigors, are a particular feature of kidney infection probably through release into the bloodstream of the bacteria responsible.

Cystitis is a more vague diagnosis; however, what it lacks in precision it gains in its power to irritate and annoy. Symptoms include burning and frequency, often beginning soon after a bath or sexual intercourse.

Men experience similar symptoms, often with an ache in the perineum (the muscles between the legs). If a man also has a discharge from the penis, the likely diagnosis is sexually transmitted disease (STDs, see page 106).

SYMPTOMS IN CHILDREN

Children's symptoms are far less specific. Although there may be the typical adult symptoms, more likely an infection will be detected only after investigation. It might be suspected in a vaguely unwell child who is off food and is irritable.

SIGNS

Little other than some tenderness over the bladder and perhaps over the kidneys.

INVESTIGATIONS

A sample can be tested on the spot with a testing strip dipped into the urine. These rather clever strips detect protein, blood, sugar and other chemicals. The presence of protein and/or blood suggests an infection. It would be confirmed by culturing the urine; that is, seeing if any bacteria can be grown from it. This further test is especially important in children.

Conditions other than infection can cause cystitis. Most common is vaginitis, inflammation of the skin of the vagina which can occur around the menopause, when the vaginal skin thins. This is treated with hormone creams.

Children can have similar symptoms through threadworm infestations or simply caused by scratching themselves. Sexual abuse must be considered in cases of recurrent infection in young girls.

ASK YOUR DOCTOR

- **To consider the possibility of infection in any baby or child who remains generally unwell in the absence of other common causes such as colds and diarrhoeal illnesses.**
- **To consider the possibility of infection in an elderly woman who becomes confused. A urinary infection should always be queried in such cases.**

Do not ignore repeated minor infections. There is a small but definite risk of an underlying abnormality in the urinary tract which could be increasing the possibility of infection.

Remedy

TREATMENT

Most urinary infections can be dealt with perfectly adequately by a course of antibiotics. A urine culture can test the organisms against a range of antibiotics to see which antibiotics are most effective against the particular strain causing the infection.

Kidney infections need more intensive treatment with high doses of antibiotic or occasionally admission to hospital for intravenous antibiotic therapy.

FOLLOW-UP

A urine culture taken a couple of weeks after treatment is sensible to check that there is no residual infection. This is especially important where there has been blood in the urine or after a kidney infection.

Children are a special case. There used to be a rule of thumb that any infection in a boy should be investigated, but that girls were allowed two infections before investigation. This has recently become more controversial, with some specialists advising that any infection in either sex should be investigated; others say that urinary infection in children is more common than once thought and less likely to be associated with abnormalities than supposed. Seek your doctor's advice.

FURTHER INVESTIGATION

This involves imaging of the urinary tract; that can be done in children by an **ultrasound** (see page 301) examination looking for normal 'pipework' and kidneys. In adults, the search would be for an underlying abnormality such as a **kidney stone** (page 243), bladder stone, or tumour (although these are a very rare cause of urinary infections). **Cystoscopy** (see page 299) is a method of looking inside the bladder using a thin tube and is done where a bladder tumour is suspected or where there may be inflammation of the bladder.

Alternative Treatment

Over-the-counter remedies for cystitis usually contain potassium citrate; this works by reducing the acidity of the urine, thus relieving the burning sensation; the bacteria responsible also grow less well in the more alkaline urine that potassium citrate causes. Many sufferers get some relief from drinking cranberry juice; a Swedish study has proved that some element of the juice prevents the bacteria from sticking to the sides of the bladder and urinary tract, eliminating the cause of the infection or irritation. There are several homoeopathic remedies which may help, and some herbal preparations to be taken orally or applied to the affected area.

The medical profession has not had great success treating cystitis and this has lead to energetic self-help by individual groups. Among their excellent advice is to empty the bladder immediately before and after intercourse, to avoid bubble baths, to empty the bladder regularly, to drink plenty of fresh water, and to avoid vaginal deodorants and douches.

Prevention

Every infection carries a risk of damage to the kidneys. It is accepted that repeated urinary infections in childhood can lead to damaged kidneys in later life, with a risk of kidney failure or of high blood pressure. The risk is very low in cases of recurrent cystitis;

the risk is higher (though still remote) in cases of true infection. This is why there is such emphasis on detecting and following up urinary infections in children and recurrent infections in adults.

The usual prevention is to take a regular low dose of an antibiotic for several months at a time. There are operations that can correct anatomical abnormalities in children which are allowing urine to reflux up into the kidney from the bladder. There is now more caution about doing such operations, with the realization that many children outgrow a period of reflux. Careful follow-up is essential.

Urinary infection during pregnancy is treated vigorously as it may cause damage without the usual symptoms.

Self-Help

Cystitis and Candida
75 Mortimer Road, London N1 5AR

INCONTINENCE OF URINE

Urinary incontinence is a common problem, although it has, in the past, been considered a natural result of the ageing process. There are signs of a change in attitude to this idea. Women and men in their middle years are increasingly willing to talk about incontinence, which appears to be a problem shared by a large percentage of the population. The knowledge that help can be offered through specialized incontinence clinics has made it less difficult to bring the problem to the attention of your GP.

The kidneys make urine continuously at an average of 1 ml per minute, or 1.5 litres a day (though it can be normal to make 300 to 3000 ml a day). It passes down to the bladder through the ureters. Urine is stored in the bladder, held in by a muscular valve called a sphincter. As the bladder stretches so the desire to pass urine grows. In the very young and the very old that desire immediately leads to relaxation of the muscular valve as a reflex action. One of the tasks of childhood is to develop the ability to control that urge. The ability deteriorates again in old age.

Incontinence can result, therefore, from malfunction at several levels: in the bladder and its nerves; in the sphincter and its nerves; or in the higher functions of the brain.

Risk

- Reliable figures are sparse but incontinence probably affects 5 per cent of women in their sixties and 7 to 10 per cent above that age, rising to perhaps 25 per cent or even more by age 85. Figures for men are even less reliable: a random survey conducted in England showed that 2 to 3 per cent of elderly males suffered from regular incontinence, rising to 20 to 25 per cent of those who lived in old age homes or in hospital.
- It is likely that many more people experience occasional incontinence.
- Because of the damage to the pelvic floor muscles, incontinence is often worse in women who have had more than one pregnancy.
- There is a higher risk in obese women (see **obesity**, page 208), and those with a persistent cough.
- Incontinence is a risk after prostate surgery in men.
- Incontinence can be the result of neurological disease affecting the nerves controlling the bladder; e.g., **multiple sclerosis** (see page 255).

Recognition

Symptoms

There may be a loss of urine after coughing, sneezing, laughing – events which increase pressure on the bladder. As incontinence worsens, urine can leak with much less pressure; standing upright can be enough to cause it. Such symptoms suggest a mechanical problem with the neck of the bladder.

- Opposed to this are symptoms of urgency; finding that when you need to go you have to go. This 'urge' incontinence is a feature of persistent irritation of the bladder or its outlet due to infection or age changes.
- There may be the features of **dementia** (page 272), suggesting that the control of urination by the brain has deteriorated

Signs

- Asking the sufferer to cough often demonstrates the problem. In women this may also indicate a vaginal prolapse (weakening of the walls of the vagina). Clothing and bedding may be obviously urine stained.
- Incontinence in a young person should always lead to a search for neurological disease which can affect urination; e.g., **multiple sclerosis** (see page 255).

Investigations

The basic investigations test for infection, checking for **diabetes** (see page 204) and kidney function. A common next step is to perform urodynamic studies, that is to measure pressure of urine flow and rate of flow. This gives important information about whether the incontinence is due to a problem in the bladder, or whether the problem lies in the valves or nerves controlling outflow.

ASK YOUR DOCTOR

- **About sympathetic local facilities to sort out your incontinence. Don't be shy about discussing the condition; it is far more common than you might imagine.**
- **About the risks of incontinence before any surgery to your bowel or urinary tract; though it may be unavoidable you can at least prepare yourself.**

Remedy

Surgical

In women stress incontinence is commonly due to a prolapse; this can be surgically repaired, thereby restoring the correct anatomy to the outlet from the bladder and restoring continence, much as readjusting a washer in a tap will stop leakage. A variety of other operations and devices are possible to deal with the problem in children or in adults left incontinent after surgery or with neurological disease.

Medical

In post-menopausal women the lining of the urethra (the tube which acts as an outlet from the bladder) becomes irritable and predisposes to an urge incontinence (see above).

Hormone replacement therapy (HRT) can relieve this; HRT can be taken as tablets or as a cream or pessary. There are a number of drugs which tighten up the muscles controlling the outlet from the bladder, thereby restoring continence. These include terodilin and oxybutinin. They are very useful in women, less so in men; side-effects such as a dry mouth limit their use.

PHYSIOTHERAPY
This aims to tighten up the muscles around the outlet from the bladder; the pelvic floor muscles are the sling of muscles which support the pelvic organs. They are responsible for our ability to stop and start the flow of urine. When stressed or damaged, as they may be following childbirth, their power is diminished and urine may leak. By concentrating on exercising these muscles you can increase their resting efficiency. Series of exercises may be suggested, including some which incorporate the use of vaginal weights. Women should exercise their pelvic floor on a daily basis, regardless of whether or not they have had or intend to have children.

TRAINING
Ensure a regular routine for passing urine. This may only be feasible in a controlled setting such as a hospital or nursing home.

DEVICES
Where all else fails there remains the option of permanent catheterization for both men and women, the urine draining continuously into a bag. Men can use a drainage sheath fixed over the penis; this is often the most practical solution for a man with nerve damage due to an accident or neurological disease. Catheterization increases the risks of infection.

Alternative Treatment

Some women with urge incontinence (the feeling that you just have to go) suffer from an anxiety problem for which alternative treatment is well worth pursuing. Acupuncture and hypnosis have been reported to help.

Prevention

Correct management of childbirth is the most important way of reducing the risks of urinary incontinence through prolapse. That is why women are told not to push before full dilation of the cervix, so as not to weaken the muscles supporting the womb and the walls of the vagina. After childbirth, perform exercises to tighten up the pelvic floor.

Urodynamic studies have made the diagnosis of the cause of incontinence much more precise and will be used more often in younger people suffering from the condition.

Urinary infections should be suspected if anyone suddenly develops incontinence, especially an elderly person. Infections are easily treated.

In cases of damage to the spinal cord, it may be possible to stimulate electronically the nerves which are damaged, in order to control incontinence.

Self-Help

Association of Continence Advice
The Basement, 2 Doughty Street, London WC1N 2PH

Tel: 0171 404-6875
Incontinence Advisory Service
The Dene Centre, Castles Farm Road, Newcastle Upon Tyne NE3 1PH

KIDNEY FAILURE

The kidneys are remarkable organs through which 1800 litres of blood pass each day. The kidneys filter that blood through an intricate system of filtration units called nephrons, of which there are about one million in each kidney. Blood is a complex compound of water, red cells, white cells, and many types of proteins, together with chemicals such as potassium, sodium, calcium, sugar: all are essential in one way or another to the working of the body. Blood also contains a substance called urea which is a waste product from the breakdown of protein. Each nephron allows urea and other waste products to filter through together with just enough water to dissolve them, while also managing to retain essential water, proteins and minerals. The end result is concentrated urine containing waste material.

This description presents the kidneys as being like biological colanders; i.e., what doesn't leak out is retained. The process is more complicated than this. Imagine a waste disposal unit into which you just dumped everything off the table, dirty crockery, crumbs, bits of paper and all. And imagine if your waste disposal unit carefully segregated all that material so that you ended up with one sack full of ground-up useless rubbish and the other contained every single item that could be reused right down to that sugar you spilled. The kidneys undertake just such a function in the body.

The disposal of waste material is so fundamental to life that it has to be exact. There is generous excess capacity in the kidneys, so much so that it is no problem to live with one kidney and even that kidney can lose 50 per cent of its function before problems begin.

Kidney failure (renal failure) is an extremely complex subject with many possible causes. Broadly speaking it results from two kinds of illness. Acute kidney failure is a consequence of some sudden event which has a catastrophic effect on blood flow to the kidneys (e.g., severe blood loss after a car accident). This topic is not dealt with here, as its treatment is undertaken according to the cause.

Chronic kidney failure is the end-result of gradual disease of the nephrons. We'll discuss this here.

Risk

- Chronic renal failure affects 50 to 80 new sufferers per million each year.
- Important known risk factors are diabetes, high blood pressure, recurrent urinary infections and obstruction, but in most cases of failure the cause is unclear.
- Kidney function can deteriorate over several years before the features of failure emerge.
- More than 80 per cent of people on dialysis (see below) survive for more than five years.
- After kidney transplantation five-year survival is 80 per cent, and 60 per cent survive for ten to 30 years.

Recognition

In the early stages there are usually no symptoms. By the time the following symptoms emerge kidney failure is already well established.

SYMPTOMS

At first there is just a vague feeling of being unwell, not pinned down to anything specific. You find you need to pass urine more frequently, feel tired, off your food, a bit nauseous and your skin may itch. As the failure worsens you may notice impotence, odd sensations in the hands and feet, breathlessness and swelling of the ankles. Underlying these symptoms is the gradual build-up of waste products within the body, plus high blood pressure, anaemia, hormone disturbances and upsets to the balance of body fluids.

Severe failure is accompanied by confusion, muscle twitches, persistent hiccoughs and finally, epileptic fits and loss of consciousness.

SIGNS

There are unlikely to be any signs at first. Pallor from anaemia is the next most common sign. There may be the features of underlying disease such as **diabetes** (see page 204), and **high blood pressure** (page 150).

INVESTIGATIONS

Investigations are essential for proper diagnosis. Blood tests measure high levels of urea, which is no longer being excreted in urine. There will be anaemia, and abnormalities in sodium and potassium levels. The urine contains protein and often blood. Scans will show perhaps shrunken or non-functioning kidneys. Sometimes only a **biopsy** (see page 298) from one kidney gives the diagnosis. There are many other subtle changes in body function and chemistry.

ASK YOUR DOCTOR

- **About urinary symptoms such as frequency (feeling the need to urinate often with little result) or finding you need to pass more urine than usual. Have a blood pressure check every year or two and be alert to the symptoms of diabetes.**
- **For a referral to a specialized kidney physician, if he or she finds evidence of kidney disease; this is not a disease for a general medical practitioner.**

Remedy

EARLY DISEASE

Mild kidney failure is managed by correcting any underlying cause and by adjusting the diet to reduce the work the kidneys are required to do. So high blood pressure (both a cause and an effect of kidney failure) is treated as is diabetes and recurrent infection. Through diet or drugs it is possible to correct disturbances of blood biochemistry which left alone would lead to further complications. Sufferers should follow a low-protein diet with a careful balance of fluids.

Anaemia (see page 186) is a major problem; the kidneys normally produce a hormone called erythropoietin which stimulates the formation of red blood cells. It is now possible to give erythropoietin by regular injection; this is very expensive.

DIALYSIS

Dialysis is the artificial filtration of blood, which aims to remove waste products and to maintain a correct fluid balance. It is a superb modern technology which has prolonged the lives of thousands of sufferers. There are two types of dialysis. One uses an artificial dialysis machine, through which the sufferer's blood is pumped. This needs to be done two or three times a week. Many patients can do this at home. The other method is called peritoneal dialysis, in which a chemically balanced fluid is poured into the abdomen for a few hours every day via a permanently inserted catheter. The fluid is made up in such a way that it draws out waste products from the bloodstream via the fine membrane that lines the abdomen – the peritoneum. While this takes place sufferers can go about their normal activities. The fluid is drawn off after a few hours and the process repeated several times a day.

The main risk of dialysis is infection. Dialysis is not a cure for kidney failure but it does buy time, while awaiting a kidney transplant.

KIDNEY TRANSPLANTATION

It has taken forty years of experimentation for kidney transplantation to become routine. The operation involves the connection of the blood supply to a donor kidney, and then attaching it to the ureter through which urine drains into the bladder. The main problem is rejection of the donor kidney by the body and in order to prevent this the individual has to remain on anti-rejection drugs such as azathioprine and cyclosporin. If rejection does occur re-operation may be necessary.

Alternative Treatment

None is recommended; kidney failure is a medical emergency. There are some therapies, however, which can enhance recuperation, providing better overall health and well-being. These include homoeopathy, acupuncture and nutritional therapy, among others.

Prevention

- The known major risk factors for kidney disease are diabetes, high blood pressure, recurrent urinary infection and obstruction to urine outflow. It is especially important to diagnose these problems in children, in particular cases of urinary infection. These conditions and their symptoms are covered elsewhere in this book.
- Exposure to certain chemicals such as lead or mercury can lead to kidney damage; workers in those industries should follow safety guidelines on exposure.
- A large number of drugs can cause kidney damage of which the most common are anti-inflammatory drugs used in arthritis, including aspirin. People who need to take this kind of drug for years on end should have kidney tests from time to time.
- There is a shortage of kidneys for transplantation, which may be resolved as people become more willing to release organs for transplantation following sudden death and accidents. On the not very distant horizon is the prospect of animals genetically engineered to make their kidneys suitable for transplantation to humans and less likely to be rejected. Pigs are being bred for this purpose now.

- There remains a large number of cases of kidney failure where the cause is unknown and so unpreventable in our current state of knowledge.

Self-Help

National Federation of Kidney Patients' Associations
6 Stanley Street, Workshop, Nottinghamshire S81 7HX
Tel: 01909 487795
National Kidney Research Fund
3 Archers Court, Stukeley Road, Huntingdon, Cambs PE18 6XG
Tel: 01480 454 828

KIDNEY AND BLADDER STONES

The pain and misery associated with kidney stones (renal colic) has been recognized for centuries; there are descriptions of what we now know to be renal colic going back to the ancient Greeks and Romans. Stones in the bladder used to be more common in previous centuries, so much so that surgeons who were skilled at removing stones travelled from town to town in order to keep up with the demand for their services. Their operations were dubbed 'cutting for the stone'; it is surely a reflection of the intense pain caused by bladder stones that people were willing to undergo such excruciating and no doubt dangerous surgery in order to end the agony.

Nowadays the diagnosis is readily made and effective painkillers are available, as are operations to remove stones if they do not pass naturally. However, most stones do pass from the kidney, down the ureter into the bladder and then out with the urine.

Risk

- There is one chance in fifty that you will develop a kidney stone in your lifetime.
- These odds are much higher in developing countries, where stones are believed to result from a poor diet.
- Risk increases in hot, dry climates, due to dehydration.
- Risk is increased by recurrent infections in the bladder or kidney.
- Risk increased by gout or drugs which cause gout.
- Diets high in calcium (found mainly in dairy produce) or oxalate (found in rhubarb and spinach) probably increase the risk.
- Office workers have a higher risk than manual workers, for unknown reasons.
- There is a 60 per cent chance of having a second stone within ten years of the first.
- The risk of kidney stones is increased by any abnormality of anatomy of the kidneys or bladder.
- A few uncommon biochemical conditions predispose to forming bladder or kidney stones.
- In most cases there is no clear cause.

Recognition

SYMPTOMS

Fortunately, as long as they are not causing some obstruction, most stones cause minimal symptoms; there may be a vague ache in the kidneys or bladder, perhaps repeated infection, or blood in the urine. When they do cause obstruction (by passing from the kidney down the ureter to the bladder) there is intense pain.

A kidney stone gives rise first to a feeling of pressure over one kidney, rapidly increasing to a severe pain, with nausea and restlessness. The pain seems to spread from the back towards the lower abdomen and comes in waves every few minutes, tending to reduce after an hour or two. Sufferers say it is the worst pain experienced outside of childbirth (which for men means pain beyond anyone else's experience). This is called renal colic.

A bladder stone gives rise to infection and, if causing obstruction to the outflow of urine, painful swelling of the bladder.

SIGNS

Severe renal colic is pretty much an unmistakable condition. The restless, pale, vomiting sufferer distinguishes it from other severe abdominal pains. Mild attacks from small stones may be confused with recurrent backache or mild cystitis.

INVESTIGATIONS

Simple on-the-spot testing of urine usually reveals blood and protein. Ninety per cent of stones show up on an **X-ray** (see page 301) of the abdomen. If doubt remains then X-rays of the urinary tract are done, by injecting a dye into the bloodstream which is concentrated in the kidneys (an intravenous urogram). **Blood tests** (see page 298) and analysis of any stone passed help decide whether there is some underlying biochemical disorder such as high blood calcium.

ASK YOUR DOCTOR
- **About any episode of passing blood in urine, whether accompanied by pain or not.**

Remedy

Immediate treatment consists of injections of high doses of painkillers. What happens next depends on the size of the stone and whether it is moving on or has stuck fast. Small stones (that means those less than 0.5 cm) usually pass, causing pain but little trouble. Larger ones may stick or simply cause too much pain to pass. They can be dealt with by a variety of means.

SONIC SHATTERING

Called lithotripsy, this modern technique focuses a series of shock waves of ultrasound on to the stone, thereby shattering it. The small fragments pass out in the urine. This apparatus has transformed the treatment of stones. It is also possible to pass a thin tube directly into the kidney or ureter and pull out the stone. The same goes for stones in the bladder. Thanks to lithotripsy it is now unusual to resort to a full-scale operation to open up the kidney or bladder to remove the stone.

Alternative Treatment

There are some herbal remedies aimed at reducing stone formation; the composition of these should be discussed with a kidney specialist as their value depends on the chemistry of the stones you form. Homoeopathic treatment may be useful, particularly in addressing the cause of the stones. Acupuncture and reflexology also offer various treatments which may be successful.

Prevention

People who have had one kidney stone have a high chance of developing another. Ideally they should keep up a high fluid intake; enough to pass 2 to 3 litres of urine a day, which requires 3 to 4 litres a day of intake, and more in hot conditions where water is lost through perspiration.

The uncommon biochemical disorders such as high blood calcium have specific treatments beyond the scope of this book but which require restricting the intake of calcium or vitamin D. Rarely, drugs are given to reduce levels of the calcium or other chemicals making up the stones.

General physical activity helps to reduce levels of calcium in the bloodstream and may make a difference to people who would otherwise form calcium stones.

THE BRAIN AND
NERVOUS SYSTEM

- Head and Brain Injury • Brain Tumour • Epilepsy
- Headache and Migraine • Multiple Sclerosis
- ME (Myalgic Encephalomyelitis) • Parkinson's
Disease • Stroke • Subarachnoid Haemorrhage

T HE STRUCTURE OF the human brain and nervous system is unimaginably complex. The brain is made up of ten thousand million nerve cells, supported by a similarly huge number of additional cells. Each nerve cell tangles and intertwines in thousands of cross connections with other nerve cells and it is through this dense web of interconnections that arise memory, intelligence, thought, insight, emotion, knowledge and understanding: everything that makes up consciousness.

The input and output are carried by tracts of nerves which go to the major sense organs: the ears; eyes; nose; etc.; and which reach the rest of the body via the spinal cord and the peripheral nerves.

There is a great amount known about the nervous system in terms of its anatomy, the structure of nerve cells and the chemical transmitters that pass information from cell to cell. However, the processes of the nervous system remain in many ways unclear. It is rather like being able to describe a computer in great detail; the circuitry, the materials used, the varying electrical flow. We can know all that and yet understand not a thing about the document that is being word-processed by that computer or the calculation being carried out.

The brain runs on sugar and works through electricity. It needs a high fuel input and an assured blood supply or it suffers irreversible damage. Nerve cells cannot be replaced. What you are born with, you have to manage with; so a brain injury wipes out cells permanently. Specific functions are localized in different parts of the brain; for example, sight is handled at the back of the brain, movement somewhere near the temples. Damage to one area affects the functions of that area but, thanks to its interconnections, the brain can often recover to some extent from even major injuries such as a stroke, given time.

The cause of many neurological conditions remains unexplained. In terms of ill-health the greatest challenges are to understand what causes strokes and to understand the processes of ageing that lead to **Alzheimer's disease** (see page 272). Breakthroughs in these areas alone would reduce a great amount of morbidity and death in the community.

HEAD AND BRAIN INJURY

The results of a blow to the head may range from simple bruising to major brain damage. The reasons for head injuries vary by age; children are most affected by accidents, young people by car crashes or sports injuries, older people by falls. The damage, if any, is not always obvious, so that people with a head injury are commonly admitted to hospital for a few hours' observation.

The damage caused by a head injury is due to violent shaking of the brain which can tear nerves and blood vessels, producing bleeding in and around the brain. Modern brain scans can show damage precisely, removing much of the uncertainty about the extent of damage which used to surround brain injuries. Of all deaths caused by trauma, 50 per cent are due to head injury.

Risk

- In the UK, 100,000 to 170,000 people are admitted to hospital each year following head injury; that is about 200 to 300 per 100,000 of population. Of those, about 5500 die.
- 50 per cent of those who die have been injured in a road traffic accident.
- About one in 1000 of the population suffers after-effects of a head/brain injury.
- The greatest risks of serious head injury are: road traffic accidents; sports injuries, e.g., boxing; alcohol-related accidents; assaults; accidents at work.
- In the elderly, head injuries may cause problems months after the incident.

Recognition

SYMPTOMS

Mild effects include confusion, headache, and perhaps loss of memory for events just before or just after the injury. Symptoms of more serious damage are loss of consciousness, paralysis of limbs, increasing nausea, double vision. These all suggest that pressure is building up inside the skull because of bleeding or swelling of the brain.

In the elderly a minor fall can lead to a blood clot on the brain which takes months to show up as confusion, epileptic fits or paralysis.

SIGNS

There are standard scales for classifying the degree of consciousness or the depth of unconsciousness of the patient. This is important in itself, because the deeper the coma at the beginning the lower the chances of full recovery. It also establishes a baseline against which to measure any deterioration. There is a risk of epilepsy occurring years after a serious brain injury.

There may be no witnesses to a head injury, so that doctors have to think about other possible causes of an unconsciousness; for example, drugs, infection, strokes or heart attack.

INVESTIGATIONS

These might include skull **X-rays** (see page 301), **CT Scans** (see page 298) and **blood tests** (see page 298). The reasons are respectively to spot fractures, to see blood clots which are putting pressure on the brain and to see that the person is breathing adequately.

ASK YOUR DOCTOR

- **In the case of a deteriorating older relative, mention any recent falls.**

Remedy

Except for the most trivial knock, any case of head injury should be regarded as carrying the risk of brain damage. This is why so many are kept for observation in hospital overnight, looking for confusion or coma, double vision or limbs which become weak or paralysed. The investigations will show up complications: a fractured skull may need surgical repair. Large clots of blood pressing on the brain can be drained. The seriously damaged patient is supported with drips, antibiotics and possibly artificial respiration.

It is not possible to repair damaged parts of the brain itself. However, the undamaged parts can partly take over the functions of the injured parts; for instance, in controlling limbs and speech. This may take one or two years of frustratingly slow progress, calling for great understanding and support.

In cases of severe injury as well as physical changes there are psychological changes; these are the hardest of all for friends and relatives to cope with. The personality changes; there may be wild swings of mood, irritability and aggression. Concentration is often poor and basic skills have to be relearned such as using a knife and fork.

Skilled therapists teach walking, use of the hands, speech and generally rehabilitate the sufferer. It is not an easy road because the sufferer may no longer be the loved personality remembered by the relatives.

There is a theory that children born with brain damage (cerebral palsy) will respond to flooding with stimuli, physical contact and speech. By extension this has been used for cases of brain damage. It calls for tremendous commitment from friends; if such a network can be set up it must be worth the effort.

Alternative Treatment

Post-operatively, and in the stages of recuperation, there are many therapies which may be able to help you regain health more swiftly. Of these, homoeopathy and acupuncture are the most highly thought of. The manipulative therapies, like osteopathy, chiropractic and massage, among others, may help to regain some movement in limbs. Pain may be relieved by other therapies; relaxation therapies are useful for carer and injured.

Prevention

Be alert to the hazards for children in the home and in play areas. Encourage cyclists to wear helmets and all car occupants to wear seat belts. If you follow a hazardous sport or occupation use all the safety measures available.

No one has any excuse anymore to drink and drive; less obvious but as important are the risks drunken pedestrians pose to themselves and to other road users. An overall reduction in the speed of traffic would lead to a fall in all accidents, including head injuries.

A life without risk is an impossible goal but basic precautions can reduce the toll of head and brain damage.

Self-Help

Headway (National Head Injuries Association)
King Edward Centre, King Edward Street, Nottingham NG1 1EW
Tel: 0115 924-0800

BRAIN TUMOURS

This a particularly feared diagnosis, no doubt because we recognize that it goes right to the heart of our personality, emotions and every human function. At all ages people worry that headaches mean a brain tumour. It is rarely so, but it often takes painstaking investigation before someone is completely reassured that they do not have a brain tumour.

Risk

- Brain tumours can occur from infancy to old age.
- They are commonest in the forties.
- They make up about 10 per cent of all cancers.
- There are about thirty brain tumours per 100,000 population per annum; of these, about a third are benign.
- Two-thirds of all brain tumours are malignant but many have spread from cancers elsewhere in the body.
- Brain tumours account for 1 to 2 per cent of all deaths.
- Certain forms of tumour are more common in higher social groups.

Recognition

SYMPTOMS
There are no symptoms which are absolutely diagnostic of a brain tumour. It is the combination of signs and symptoms which is important.
- Headache

This steadily worsens, is more painful at night and first thing in the morning. It is important to realize that headaches are extremely common at all ages; the vast majority are completely harmless.
- Nausea or vomiting

Increased pressure within the brain stimulates the brain centres that control nausea. The resulting nausea or vomiting comes out of the blue, not being linked with food or eating.
- Effects on eyes or limbs

The same increased pressure damages parts of the brain that control movement and vision. Possible symptoms include weakness or paralysis of arms or legs, lack of coordination. There can be partial loss of vision in one or both eyes.
- General symptoms

There is a gradual change in personality, with moodiness, loss of memory or outright dementia. Epilepsy may occur if the tumour irritates the electrical activity of the brain.

SIGNS
The pattern of weakness of limbs and changes in vision pin-points the likely site of a tumour.

INVESTIGATIONS
The increased pressure within the skull causes changes in the back of the eyes which can be seen by using an **ophthalmoscope** (see page 301). A **CT Scan** (see page 298) is the

best way of detecting a brain tumour, although a scan cannot tell if the tumour has spread there from elsewhere or is a pure brain tumour. So a general check is needed including chest **X-ray** (see page 301).

ASK YOUR DOCTOR

- **About perplexing changes in behaviour in someone who seems otherwise well.**
- **To check your child for a tumour if they become clumsy and moody, and suffer from headaches.**

Remedy

If the tumour has spread from another site, like the breast, then very likely there has been other general spread throughout the body. Treatment is then really just to relieve symptoms, probably with radiotherapy. Otherwise an operation is required to diagnose the exact nature of the tumour and to plan treatment.

Benign tumours, called meningiomas, can be removed with a very high probability of complete recovery. In the case of malignant tumours it may be possible to remove them partially, so relieving symptoms for a while. **Radiotherapy** (see page 301) also shrinks them as do certain steroid drugs. Even so the outlook is not good; about 50 per cent are fatal within a year. There are less aggressive types where 50 per cent five-year survival is possible.

Alternative Treatment

None recommended for treating the tumour itself; however, post-operatively there are many therapies which can enhance rehabilitation. Homoeopathic treatment, herbalism and acupuncture are most useful perhaps. If the tumour is malignant, and spread from another part of the body, there may be therapies that will address the primary cancer itself.

Prevention

At present there is no known way of preventing primary brain tumours. The only scope for prevention is by way of avoiding those cancers which commonly spread to the brain; for example, the lung or breast. Of these, lung cancer is the most easily prevented by giving up smoking.

Self-Help

Any of the cancer support groups may help; see other cancer entries for details.
British Brain and Spine Foundation
Royal College of Surgeons, 35–43 Lincolns Inn Fields, London, WC2 3PN
Tel: 0171 404-7777

EPILEPSY

Epilepsy is an illness which has inspired awe down the centuries. There is something inherently disturbing about a condition which can suddenly turn an apparently normal individual into someone shaking on the floor, only for that same person to return to normal in minutes or hours. It is unrealistic for a sufferer to expect to lead a completely normal life; the uncertainty of having another fit and attitudes of society will not allow this. Yet it should be possible in most cases to find a fulfilling job and to lead a careful but mainly normal life.

Epilepsy is a result of malfunction in the complex electrical activity of the brain. For some reason, a mass of neurones, the cells which make up the brain, all begin to fire at once. Depending on the function of those cells, that causes either a series of jerking movements of arms and legs or sudden loss of consciousness. In the minutes or seconds just before a fit the individual may sense that something is about to happen. This is known as an aura. The aura may even consist of smelling an unusual smell, a feeling of déjà vu or seeing something strange.

A significant number of people have a single fit only. In children this is most often a so-called febrile fit, one which happens when the child has a high fever. About 10 to 15 per cent of all children experience a febrile fit; only a small minority will go on to develop true epilepsy. In adults even a single fit should be taken seriously and investigated. There is controversy on whether a single fit should be treated; in the UK treatment is unusual whereas it is commonly recommended in the USA.

'Fits' or 'Convulsions' are interchangeable terms.

Risk

- Epilepsy is a common disorder; 2 to 3 per cent of the population suffer from epilepsy at some time.
- About 4 to 10 out of each 1000 people have active epilepsy.
- A number of people will grow out of their epilepsy – up to 80 per cent, depending on the type.
- Epileptics have a two to three times increased risk of premature death, including a significant risk of sudden unexplained death.
- Anything causing brain damage increases the risk of epilepsy; e.g., strokes, head injury, birth injury.
- Anyone with a very high temperature may have an epileptic fit; children are at risk at lower temperatures than adults.

Recognition

SYMPTOMS

The classical epileptic fit is unmistakable. The sufferer falls to the ground and lies rigid for some seconds. Then their arms and legs begin to jerk rhythmically for up to a few minutes. During this stage they may be incontinent of urine or faeces and may bite their tongue. The fit dies away leaving the sufferer drowsy or unconscious; this may last for a few hours.

In children, epilepsy can take the form of a brief 'absence', during which the child is unresponsive and blank for a few seconds. This can be very hard to distinguish from plain lack of attention. It is often only after repeated attacks that the diagnosis is suspected. This is called petit-mal.

In a baby a fit takes the form of generalized shaking and the eyes go glassy. Often the child is very hot, a so-called febrile fit or febrile convulsion. These are extremely common, affecting up to one in seven children and do not usually lead on to true epilepsy.

Not every fit is dramatic; it may simply consist of dizziness, confusion and brief loss of consciousness.

Signs
An eye-witness account of a classical fit is the best way of diagnosing epilepsy. There will be nothing to find on examination unless the sufferer has some other illness causing the epilepsy, like a stroke or a brain tumour.

Investigations
Include a **brain scan** (see page 300) to detect tumours and an **EEG** (electro-encephalogram, see page 299) to detect abnormal electrical activity in the brain; this is especially reliable in detecting petit-mal, which causes a characteristic brain rhythm.

ASK YOUR DOCTOR
- **About unusual lapses of attention in a child.**
- **To supply you with emergency drugs to cut short attacks in a child who has frequent febrile fits.**
- **If you have any suspicion of having had a fit, as there are legal consequences for driving, work, etc.**

Remedy

In 25 per cent of cases of epilepsy a cause is found which may have a specific treatment; for example, **alcoholism** (see page 268), uncontrolled **diabetes** (see page 204), **brain tumour** (see page 249). The rest are treated using any of a wide range of drugs. The aim is to return the individual to as normal a life as possible, although this may fall short of stopping attacks altogether. For those who have frequent attacks despite therapy, a sheltered life may well be the only option, but this is relatively uncommon.

During an attack
The only action needed is to ensure that the person does not harm themselves or choke. Otherwise just wait for the fit to finish. Most do within one to ten minutes.

Prolonged fits (status epilepticus)
These are a medical emergency; the longer the fit goes on the more the risk of brain damage through lack of oxygen. Call for immediate medical help.

General
Epilepsy is a diagnosis that will always change someone's life, though this may be in minor ways. Certain sports are unwise; for example, sub-aqua diving or mountaineering. It is necessary to make the home safer to avoid injury during an attack. Certain

occupations are barred, like working with dangerous equipment or driving a public service vehicle. For many people the major restriction is on driving a private car; there are strict rules which, in essence, ban an epileptic from driving unless free of fits for a year or more.

Alternative Treatment

Any of the relaxation therapies may be useful on a day-to-day basis. During a fit, some sufferers claim that Edward Bach's Rescue Remedy is useful, applied to the temples, or a drop on the tongue. Babies and children with a fever can take the homoeopathic remedies aconite or belladonna, which may help to prevent febrile convulsions.

Prevention

- Alcohol abuse is the major avoidable cause of epilepsy. Both heavy drinking or sudden abstinence can bring on a fit.
- The younger the child the more important it is to control fevers, by giving paracetamol, removing hot clothing and by bathing in tepid water if necessary.
- Anyone on anti-epileptic drugs (anti-convulsants) should have blood tests regularly to check that the dosage is right. Some epileptics avoid taking their medication because of side-effects, like drowsiness, at the cost of more frequent fits. New drugs with fewer side-effects appear steadily, so it is worth discussing modern treatment with your doctor.

Self-Help

British Epilepsy Foundation
Anstey House, 40 Hanover Square, Leeds LS3 1BE
Tel: 01532 439393; Helpline 01345 089599

HEADACHE AND MIGRAINE

Headaches are one of the most common of symptoms; at the same time they create tremendous anxiety. There is a widespread fear that headache means brain tumour, though in fact this is rarely so. Most headaches have a benign explanation, even in childhood.

Risk

- Up to 90 per cent of people, if asked, report having had at least one severe headache in the previous year. Few of these are brought to medical attention.
- Blood pressure does not cause headaches unless it is exceptionally high.
- The longer you have been having headaches, the less likely that there is a serious cause.
- Primary brain tumours affect about five people per 100,000 per annum.
- More frequent, though still uncommon (25 per 100,000), are tumours which have spread to the brain from cancer elsewhere.
- The contraceptive pill causes headaches in some women.

Recognition

Symptoms

Headaches are variously described as a band around the head, a pressure feeling on the top of the head, pain radiating up into the head from the muscles of the neck. It may be accompanied by nausea, flashing lights before the eyes, temporary blindness, difficulty concentrating and difficulty in using arms or legs. None of the symptoms in themselves can pinpoint the reason for the headache.

Headaches which are worse first thing in the morning, which wake you during the night or which come on suddenly and severely are of a more serious nature, as is any hint of epileptic fits.

Signs

Doctors look for neck stiffness, very high blood pressure, pressure changes at the back of the eye, seen by looking into the eye, and evidence that bright lights hurt the sufferer. They may discover muscle weakness and irregularity of the pupils of the eye. If these features are present it does make a serious cause more likely, such as **meningitis** (see page 25) **subarachnoid haemorrhage** (see page 266) or **brain tumour** (page 249).

Investigations

Further investigations might include a **brain scan** (see page 298) and an **EEG** (see page 299), which records the electrical activity of the brain.

ASK YOUR DOCTOR

- **To check a relation or friend if they start to have severe headaches, especially if there is a change in personality; this does suggest a brain tumour.**
- **To change your contraceptive pill if you suffer migraines.**
- **About the latest treatments for migraine.**
- **To double-check the tablets you take; consuming too many painkillers can actually cause the very headaches for which you take them.**

Remedy

Headaches with a serious underlying cause have specific treatments. The vast majority of the rest are either tension headaches or migraine in one form or other. It may be reassuring simply to know that there is no serious underlying cause and for many people that is the only treatment they want – reassurance.

Migraine sufferers can now choose from several remedies. Simplest are painkillers of varying strength combined with an anti-sickness drug. These are best taken early in an attack. Ergotamine used to be prescribed widely; its use was always limited by the risk of side-effects but it still has a role in severe migraine unresponsive to other treatment. Beta-blockers are helpful where migraine is made worse by tension. A newish drug, sumatriptan, can be given by mouth or by injection and appears to be highly effective in stopping an attack.

Sufferers from tension headaches are in some ways more difficult to treat because frequently nothing can be done about the cause, which tends to be stress-related. Painkillers and mild sedatives are worth trying.

Alternative Treatment

Feverfew is a herbal remedy for migraine which has been shown to work in controlled trials; it should be taken regularly as a preventative measure in migraine sufferers. Any alternative treatment which reduces stress may help headaches; yoga, hypnosis, aromatherapy, massage and others are worth a try. An acupuncturist, osteopath, chiropractor or reflexologist would address the root of the problem, and there is some evidence that chronic headache sufferers obtain sizeable relief. Depending on your symptoms, there are good homoeopathic and herbal remedies available. See a registered practitioner who will tailor treatment to you.

Prevention

Pizotifen and beta-blockers are two of a small number of drugs which, taken daily, reduce the frequency of migraines. Some migraine sufferers find they are sensitive to specific foods which they should avoid; chocolate and citrus fruit are two common culprits.

Stress is the plague of modern life for which there is no prevention. However, it may be possible to build allowance for stress into your schedule; for example, by allowing short breaks for time out in the day. It is better to explore these options than to take tranquillizers.

Self-Help

British Migraine Association
178a High Road, Byfleet, Surrey KT14 7ED
Tel: 01932 352468

MULTIPLE SCLEROSIS

The cause of this common disease of the nervous system is still unknown. Multiple sclerosis damages muscle control and sensation in various parts of the body, although it may be years before this results in any serious disability. At the beginning, symptoms may be so non-specific that the diagnosis is frequently delayed.

What happens in multiple sclerosis? Nerve fibres are surrounded by an insulating sheath, just as electrical wires have a plastic coating. The disease destroys this insulating layer but in a patchy way and scattered through the millions of nerve fibres in the body. There is a chance of recovery in the insulation, which explains why the symptoms come and go.

Naturally, it is the worst cases that we remember, but for many sufferers MS follows a relatively mild course even after decades – perhaps some clumsiness, some odd sensations and some muscle weakness. It is quite unpredictable how the disease will progress in any individual case. The fact that many sufferers remain mildly affected justifies taking an optimistic outlook at the beginning. With this in mind neurologists often avoid giving a diagnosis, even though they suspect the condition; not all patients appreciate this but it is done for the best of motives.

Risk

- There are about three new cases per 100,000 of population per annum (1600 per annum).

- At any one time there are sixty to 100 active cases per 100,000 population; that is, about 80,000 sufferers.
- There is a one in 800 lifetime risk of contracting the disease.
- The children of sufferers have between a one in twenty and one in fifty risk of the disease.
- Six out of ten sufferers are women.
- It begins most commonly between 20 to 35 years; only rarely does it begin after sixty.
- It is rare in tropical countries, common in temperate countries. Why is unknown.
- It may be related to having measles or other viral illnesses in childhood.

Recognition

SYMPTOMS

There is no single symptom which clinches a diagnosis of MS. Instead it is the pattern of symptoms affecting different parts of the nervous system at different times which is important. The following are commoner symptoms:

- Eyes

Blurred vision, double vision or temporary blindness in one eye are highly suspicious of MS. Typically the symptoms appear rapidly then gradually recover over a few weeks.

- Limbs

There may be an odd numbness in one limb, difficulty walking, with weakness or unsteadiness of arms or legs.

- Other

Difficulty in passing urine, impotence, pain or numbness around the face.

In 80 per cent of cases these and other symptoms disappear quickly, leaving little or no trace. It may be up to ten years before any further symptoms appear, though more commonly there are other symptoms within a couple of years. In 10 per cent of cases symptoms worsen and spread right from the start. Even so it is unpredictable how quickly the disease will progress.

The late stages of the disease can include inability to walk or to use the arms, poor vision, incontinence of urine and a host of more subtle but nonetheless upsetting symptoms. In really advanced cases the sufferer relies on others for all their care and attention. Mental alertness and memory are on the whole not seriously affected until late in the disease. Depression, not surprisingly, is common.

SIGNS

In a first attack there is frequently little hard evidence on examination; the reflexes might be a bit brisk, muscle groups may be a bit weak. The back of the eye seen through an **ophthalmoscope** (see page 301) looks swollen, but even this suspicious sign is not absolute proof of MS. As the disease progresses signs of paralysis become more definite.

INVESTIGATIONS

Modern investigation allow doctors to be more certain about the diagnosis sooner. An **MRI** scan (Magnetic Resonance Imaging, see page 300) shows up the damage done by the loss of the insulating tissues around the nerves.

ASK YOUR DOCTOR

- If you suspect you have this condition, and you feel you really want to know the diagnosis. It is natural to want to know as early as possible if you may have MS. Yet doctors will rarely be pinned down. The outlook is just too uncertain to give such a devastating diagnosis. Your doctor may even try to talk you out of having a specialist opinion if your symptoms are mild. You can insist, but think first whether you really want to know if you have MS when it may be years before you have any more problems.
- If you can see a neurologist, if symptoms become persistent. This is really to confirm the diagnosis in case you have one of the few conditions giving similar symptoms but which are treatable; for example, pernicious anaemia (see page 199).

Remedy

Even though there is no cure for MS there are useful treatments for symptoms. Steroids are most often used, by mouth or by injection, to bring flare-ups under control. There is great current interest in using drugs which alter the immune system, including beta interferon. These expensive and sometimes toxic treatments need refining but the early results are promising.

There is a choice of drugs to help stiff muscles, tremors and incontinence. It is important to treat infections early, especially urinary infections which are common.

In severe disease 24-hour nursing may be needed.

Alternative Treatment

There is little evidence that alternative therapies can change the course of this disease, or, indeed, present a cure. What they can do, however, is ensure that your body is fit and well, in order to experience fewer symptoms. There is a strong mind-body relationship and certainly if you feel a treatment is doing you some good, there is every chance it will be. Some of the more popular therapies for MS include acupuncture, constitutional homoeopathic treatment (tailored specifically for you and your symptom pattern), aromatherapy, yoga, hypnosis and manipulative therapies like osteopathy and chiropractic. As they do in every case where conventional medicine can offer little respite from the illness, charlatans abound; ensure that you are treated only by registered, trained practitioners, who are recommended to you.

Prevention

In the present state of knowledge, with the cause unknown, there are no preventative avenues. All this may change if the disease is proven to be related to childhood viral illnesses, as some research is suggesting.

Self-Help

Federation of M.S. Therapy Centres
4 Murdock Road, Bedford MK4E1 7PD

Tel: 01234 325781
Multiple Sclerosis Society of Great Britain and Northern Ireland
25 Effie Road, Fulham, London SW6 1EE
Tel: 0171 736-6267

ME (MYALGIC ENCEPHALOMYELITIS)

Also known as chronic fatigue syndrome or ME, Myalgic Encephalomyelitis is the cause of deep divide in the medical profession. On the one side there are sufferers who form articulate, convincing, well-organized and active pressure groups, pushing for recognition and research into the condition. On the other hand, the conventional medical scientists, while not denying that there is a condition of severe chronic tiredness, are deeply sceptical of many of the claims being made and remain to be convinced that there is a physical basis to this condition, as opposed to its being a focus for psychiatric symptoms.

It has long been recognized that viral illnesses are often followed by a period of great tiredness and lassitude, which may persist for months or occasionally for years. Glandular fever is the best known example of an infection renowned for this after-effect.

Over the years, different names have been used: neurasthenia was the nineteenth-century term, Da Costa's syndrome another, post-viral fatigue another. Several times this century there have been 'epidemics' of an unusually debilitating illness which leave sufferers in no doubt that something odd had happened to them, but which other observers have labelled as group hysteria. What has happened to make the subject more respectable has been a shift of emphasis from studying 'outbreaks', with their strong hysterical overtones, to studying individual cases which arise out of the blue and which are presumably untainted by copy-cat motives.

Thus arose chronic fatigue syndrome. The term myalgic encephalomyelitis, which means inflammatory pains in muscles and mild mental confusion, harks back to the characteristics of an outbreak at the Royal Free Hospital in London in 1955, when muscle aches and pains were prominent. In fact ME is not a medically accepted name, though it has become popularly used. Doctors prefer the term chronic fatigue syndrome, because this term is purely descriptive and carries no implication about any on-going inflammation of muscle and brain, which the term ME does.

Risk

- Post-viral debility lasting two to four weeks is common.
- It is well recognized after glandular fever.
- To qualify for ME you must show symptoms for at least six months.
- Reliable figures for numbers suffering from ME are not available. One Australian study suggests 37 per 100,000 population.
- 20 to 25 per cent of people surveyed entirely at random report that they suffer from 'fatigue'.
- There is a high incidence of depression and neurotic behaviour in sufferers from ME.
- Most sufferers are from higher social classes.
- Young adults or older children are most often affected.
- Female sufferers outnumber male by a two to one ratio.

Recognition

There are no objective tests for ME. Therefore diagnosis relies entirely on the sufferer's own report of their symptoms. This is not in itself unusual in medicine; no one can see a headache or feel someone else's dizziness.

SYMPTOMS

Tiredness is the major symptom. This may be constant or it may be that the individual tires very easily on exertion. Other common symptoms can include difficulty in concentration, muscular aches, mood swings, abdominal pains.

SIGNS

There are no signs specific to the condition. A doctor may note that the individual has a depressed mood, and that he or she finds exertion an effort. It is a characteristic of the condition that despite reports of joint pains, abdominal pains, sweats and temperatures there are no objective signs.

INVESTIGATIONS

There are none which are accepted to have scientific validity, though ME groups claim that there are subtle changes in cell metabolism. It is important for physical disease to be excluded since chronic fatigue/ME is a diagnosis of exclusion. There is no evidence that sufferers are more likely to have had glandular fever, which in any case leaves diagnostic immunological markers in the blood.

ASK YOUR DOCTOR

- **For a second opinion, if you have had a diagnosis of ME. It is essential that you have conventional examination and testing, looking especially for thyroid disorders (see page 211), depression (see page 278).**

Remedy

ME is not a fatal illness and patients appear well in terms of weight, appetite and general appearance. Recovery is slow; in one study 90 per cent still felt unwell after three years.

GENERAL PRINCIPLES

Rest but not idleness, plus exertion within the limits of your ability have long been accepted in treating post-viral debility. These same principles apply to chronic fatigue/ME.

ANTI-DEPRESSANTS

A low dose of an anti-depressant has been shown to help. There is no generally agreed dosage or choice of anti-depressant or length of treatment. Up to two-thirds of sufferers from ME have symptoms of **depression** (see page 278) or **anxiety** (see page 275): whether this is cause or effect is arguable.

Diet

A well-balanced diet seems sensible, though there is no evidence that sufferers are actually deficient in anything.

Alternative Treatment

Some sufferers have found acupuncture helpful. Homoeopathy, herbalism, aromatherapy and others among the more recognized therapies recommend various treatments. Beware of unregistered, untrained practitioners. Diseases where conventional medicine can offer little solace are a fairground for cranks of all description. Many therapies will improve your sense of well-being, if not your physical health, but choose your therapy and practitioner with care and ask your doctor about any claims being made.

Candida

Candida is a respectable fungus which is a normal inhabitant of the digestive tract. Infestation with candida is said to underlie cases of ME and eradication is to be achieved by means of live yoghurt, anti-fungal drugs and restrictive, starch-deficient diets. In rare cases candida does indeed cause widespread infection but this has only been found in people seriously ill with depressed immune systems. In any case it is detected by conventional tests. The proof of the involvement of candida in ME is not based on any such evidence and should be regarded with scepticism.

Prevention

As long as controversy reigns about the nature let alone the cause of ME, rational prevention is unlikely.

Self-Help

ME Action Campaign
PO Box 1302 Wells, Somerset BA5 2WE
Tel: 01749 670799

Myalgic Encephalomyelitis Association
PO Box 8, Stanford-le-Hope, Essex SS17 0HA
Tel: 013756 42466

PARKINSON'S DISEASE

Parkinson's disease is a common condition mainly affecting the elderly. It causes general slowing-down of activity, a characteristic tremor of the hands, and stiffness of movement. About 80 per cent of cases are true Parkinson's disease, where there is a specific abnormality in the brain. The other 20 per cent are due to a variety of causes, some reversible. This is called Parkinsonism.

The chemical changes in the brain underlying the condition are quite well understood; there is a loss of cells which produce a chemical called dopamine, although why this should happen is unknown. Drug treatment works by boosting levels of dopamine again.

The early symptoms are easily confused with general effects of ageing so it may be a year or two before the diagnosis is definite.

Risk

- Unusual before fifty years of age, Parkinson's disease then becomes increasingly common.
- It affects 1 to 2 per cent of those 70 years and over.
- There are about 100,000 sufferers at any one time.
- Parkinson's disease and Parkinsonism can be caused by certain drugs used to treat mental illness; e.g., phenothiazine sedatives such as chlorpromazine.

Recognition

SYMPTOMS

At first there is just a slight tremor of one limb, usually the arm. When it is not being used, the hand shakes in a regular rhythm a few times a second. The tremor stops while the hand is being used. Eventually both hands shake in this way.

The limbs are stiff; if you try to move them there is a resistance that cannot be relaxed. No longer do the arms swing when walking, but they are held stiffly at the sides. The muscles of the face become stiff also till there is a fixed, unexpressive, unblinking, rather mask-like expression. The sufferer finds increasing difficulty with any kind of fine movement; typically their handwriting becomes small and increasingly indistinct as they become less able to start and to control those skilled movements. Similarly when walking; instead of striding out they have to begin with a series of shuffles which builds up to more normal walking. Falls are common because of the unstable gait. Speech becomes slow and monotonous, due once again to increasing stiffness of the muscles of speech.

Many other symptoms can develop as the disease progresses, such as difficulty swallowing, constipation, depression, sweating and dribbling from the mouth. Mental function remains little changed until the disease is well advanced, when dementia is possible. The disease runs its course over ten to fifteen years.

SIGNS

It is easy to miss early Parkinsonism because the changes are so mild. The doctor may just form an impression of someone whose expression is a little fixed, whose walk is just a little stiff and who stands with a stoop. Tremors are common in the elderly and on their own would not make the diagnosis, though they raise a suspicion. It is often a case of waiting and seeing how symptoms progress.

There are a couple of other conditions to think of. An **under-active thyroid gland** (page 211) gives a similar immobile look as does **depression** (page 278). Both these conditions are treatable. It is important to check whether the sufferer is on any medication which might cause Parkinson's disease or make it worse.

INVESTIGATIONS

There are none which are of routine value unless a neurologist suspects one of the rare neurological conditions which can cause Parkinsonism.

ASK YOUR DOCTOR
- To consider the diagnosis in the elderly with vague limb pains and stiffness.
- To arrange an assessment by an occupational therapist who can advise on disability aids and lay-out of the home.

Remedy

The treatment is something of an art; a neurologist's opinion is sensible at the beginning of the illness and if there are dramatic changes in how drugs seem to be working.

DRUGS

L-Dopa is a replacement form of dopamine, an amino acid required by the body, and is very helpful in relieving symptoms. It works best at decreasing stiffness, less at reducing tremor. The dosage has to be carefully worked out to avoid unpleasant side-effects of nausea and confusion. Unfortunately L-Dopa tends to lose its effect after a few years and so many neurologists keep it in reserve until the symptoms are bad.

A relatively new drug, selegiline, may reduce the rate of progress of the illness.

SURGERY

Neurosurgeons have tried transplanting cells into the brain to replace those which are no longer making dopamine. The initial improvement was exciting; the long-term results have been disappointing.

Alternative Treatment

Massage and guided exercise may help relieve stiffness. Gentle manipulation by an osteopath or chiropractor may also help. Acupuncture is used throughout the disease, ostensibly to slow its progress, and to relieve symptoms.

Prevention

The drugs which can cause Parkinsonism as a side-effect are well known. They are phenothiazines, used to control major psychiatric illness, and certain anti-sickness drugs which can cause it, if taken in excess. Sometimes the use of these drugs may be unavoidable, in which case the doctor needs to be on the look out for Parkinsonian side-effects and stop the drug if these occur. Older treatments for high blood pressure could cause Parkinsonism; for example, methyldopa, reserpine. They are rarely prescribed now.

Self-Help

Parkinson's Disease Society
22 Upper Woburn Place, London WC1H 0RA
Tel: 0171 383-3513

STROKE

Stoke is one of the major causes of death and disability in all Western countries. It results when the blood supply to part of the brain is cut off. This can happen in a variety of ways. A tiny blood clot may block off a blood vessel. The walls of an artery or vein may burst. Occasionally a stroke is due to a growth in the brain.

'Cerebro-vascular accident', abbreviated to CVA, is the medical term for a stroke. The term 'stroke' is, however, a vivid description of what happens. At a stroke, something goes seriously wrong with brain function. At one extreme there can be a sudden collapse and death, at the other extreme slurred speech or a little dizziness, returning to normality after a few minutes.

Stroke covers this whole range, though strictly speaking a stroke is a CVA which lasts more than twenty-four hours. CVAs lasting less than twenty-four hours are called 'transient ischaemic attacks', or TIAs.

Risk

Despite the frequency of strokes and despite enormous research, there is a surprising lack of agreement about what factors increase or decrease risk. The following facts are generally agreed.

- Strokes are the third commonest cause of death after cancer and heart attacks.
- Each year in the UK there are about 100,000 strokes and at least 50,000 TIAs (probably a great underestimate).
- Strokes account for some 65,000 deaths per annum (12 per cent of all deaths).
- They are commoner in men.
- Strokes are rare before 40 years, then increasingly common with age.
- After 65 years there is a 1 to 2 per cent annual risk of having a stroke.
- Of the many conditions which may increase the risk of stroke the most important are **high blood pressure** (see page 150), **diabetes** (see page 204), smoking, other circulation and **heart disease** (see page 157), obesity and high cholesterol levels.
- Strokes are gradually becoming less common; why is uncertain.
- The contraceptive pill carries an extremely low risk of causing a stroke, except in smokers over 30 years of age, when that risk increases.

Recognition

SYMPTOMS

The commonest symptom is sudden weakness of a limb; in bad cases both the arm and the leg on one side are affected. The weakness may progress to complete paralysis over the next few minutes or hours. Often speech is affected, ranging from slurred but understandable speech to an inability to say anything meaningful at all.

Other possible symptoms are sudden numbness of one side of the face or a limb, loss of vision, giddiness and unsteadiness. There is often a minor headache at the same time. A severe headache, together with neck stiffness suggests a **subarachnoid haemorrhage** (see page 266).

The sufferer may fall unconscious or may remain quite clear-headed with any variation in between. Unconsciousness for any time at all carries a worse outlook for survival and recovery. By definition, in the case of a TIA, these symptoms will disappear after twenty-four hours; of course, at the outset it is unknown whether the individual is having what will turn out to be a TIA or a completed stroke.

SIGNS

There is usually little difficulty in recognizing a stroke, so the job of the doctor is to decide what part of the brain is involved, whether there is a treatable cause and what if any immediate treatment is needed.

Weakness of the left side of the body is the result of a stroke affecting the right side of the brain. Often the sufferer's vision is affected, with loss of part of their field of vision. This also gives a clue as to where the stroke has happened.

The subtleties of localization are beyond the scope of this book but suffice to say that there may be long-term changes in sensation and thought which are important to discover to achieve good rehabilitation.

INVESTIGATIONS

The immediate investigations are aimed at finding treatable causes, so include tests for blood pressure, diabetes, infections, heart or circulatory disease. **CT scans** (see page 298) have revolutionized the assessment of a stroke, making it possible to find the site of the stroke and to see whether something unexpected was the cause, such as a tumour or an abscess.

ASK YOUR DOCTOR

- **About any episode of paralysis especially if combined with slurred speech. Even if this only lasts a few minutes it should be brought to medical attention, because there may be a treatable cause which would prevent a full-blown stroke.**
- **About any irregular heart rhythm you may experience. Some can be treated to prevent a stroke.**

Remedy

Treatment falls into two broad areas: immediate treatment to cope with the immediate effects; and longer-term care once the severity of the stroke is established.

IMMEDIATE

A mild stroke needs nothing more than rest and observation, while any treatable conditions such as high blood pressure are brought under control. A severe stroke may require intensive nursing care, with special emphasis on feeding (because swallowing may be affected), physiotherapy (to avoid stiff, contracted muscles) and regular turning to avoid bed sores.

LONG TERM

Stroke rehabilitation is a lengthy, demanding process. Most recovery occurs in the first six months or so but steady improvement can continue for up to two years. During all this time the sufferer needs encouragement to walk, talk, read, think, manipulate, look and experience. The remaining undamaged parts of their brain are literally having to relearn the abilities lost with the damaged brain. Think of the intensive efforts we put into teaching children; just such efforts may be needed with adults after a stroke.

There is no denying the tremendous strain this can put on relationships; following a severe stroke the whole personality may alter, swinging rapidly between laughter and tears, calmness and aggression, and all the while dependant on others for basic care. In many parts of the country there are 'stroke clubs' where patients and carers can have support, or day hospitals which allow the carer time off.

The continuing medical risks after a severe stroke are of chest infection or urinary infection.

Even with the best treatment 20 to 30 per cent of victims die within a month of the stroke. Ten per cent will have another stroke within the year. Longer term there is 30 to 40 per cent three-year survival. Of those who do survive a stroke about one-third are left with severe disability, another third with more minor disability and one-third make a full recovery.

Alternative Treatment

Stroke is a medical emergency, and any victim must seek immediate conventional treatment. However, any therapy that comforts the sufferer or the carers is recommended; in particular, aromatherapy or massage might be useful. There are a number of other therapies which can help with rehabilitation. Acupuncture, osteopathy, reflexology and acupressure are popular choices, and any of the therapies which improve overall health, like nutritional therapy, or in some cases homoeopathy and herbalism, are often suggested.

Prevention

INDIVIDUAL TREATMENT

Some sufferers have specific medical conditions, the treatment of which will reduce the risk of having another stroke. High blood pressure, diabetes, high cholesterol are three common factors treatable by drugs or adjustments to lifestyle

- Stop smoking

Smoking increases the 'stickiness' of blood, adding to the risks of another blood clot flying off into the brain.
- Circulatory disorders

Many older people have an irregular heart rhythm, atrial fibrillation, which carries an increased risk of stroke. If so, it may be worth having anti-coagulation therapy to reduce the chances of a stroke. Taking a low dose of aspirin every day is a less hazardous alternative, especially used in treating TIAs. This is an area where specialist views are changing; ask your doctor for up-to-date information.

A circulatory disorder underlies **subarachnoid haemorrhage**, a particular form of stroke which may be preventable (page 266).
- Carotid stenosis

Quite commonly there is a narrowing (stenosis) of one of the large arteries in the neck (carotid artery) which carries blood to the brain. There is a risk of a blood clot forming on the narrowing; just a tiny fragment breaking off is all it takes to cause a stroke. These narrowings make a typical noise in the neck which can be heard through a stethoscope; otherwise specialized scans show it up.

It is possible to deal with this narrowing surgically. There is enormous controversy within the medical profession on whether this major surgery is worth the risk. Current research suggests that it is, but only in centres specializing in it, with highly experienced surgeons and carefully selected patients. Otherwise treatment would be with aspirin or anticoagulants.

GENERAL PREVENTION OF STROKES

This is a major challenge for all Western societies. As strokes are so common, measures which achieve even a small reduction in risk will prevent thousands of strokes.

- Control of high blood pressure

This is the single most easily detectable and treatable risk factor for stroke. It is estimated that the risk of having a stroke is halved if someone with high blood pressure has it brought properly under control. This holds for all ages, including the elderly.

There is a general move to encourage lower-fat diets with the aim of reducing levels of cholesterol in the population as a whole. On present evidence this will reduce the risks of having a stroke (or a heart attack), so it is sensible for anyone who has had a stroke to follow this advice. For a fuller discussion of the pros and cons see high **cholesterol,** page 153.

Self-Help

The Stroke Association
CHSA House, 123–127 Whitecross Street, London EC1Y 8JJ
Tel: 0171 490-7999

Disabled Living Foundation
380-384 Harrow Road, London W9 2HU
Tel: 0171 289-6111

RADAR (Royal Association for Disability and Rehabilitation)
12 City Forum, 250 City Road, London EC1V 8AF
Tel: 0171 250-3222

SUBARACHNOID HAEMORRHAGE

This is a particular form of stroke, notable because it is fairly common in young people. Just like other strokes it is caused by interference with blood flow to the brain. The cause is an artery within the brain which has a weak wall. The weak wall bulges out in the way that the wall of a damaged car tyre bulges as a result of the pressure within. This is known as an aneurysm. Eventually the wall bursts, allowing blood to pour out around the brain.

Risk

- There are about 15 cases per 100,000 per annum; that is about 8000 a year.
- Aneurysms are found in about 1 per cent of post-mortems; therefore, only a small number actually rupture.
- 50 per cent of sufferers die immediately or within a month.
- Many of the survivors have a degree of disability similar to that seen following a **stroke** (see page 262).

Recognition

SYMPTOMS

There is a sudden very severe headache, usually at the back of the head. Sufferers describe it as being like a blow to the head. There may be drowsiness or rapid loss of consciousness. Epileptic fits are common.

SIGNS

The sufferer is clearly in great pain; they may find bright light painful. They may have a stiff neck. It is the speed of onset and the degree of upset that distinguishes this condition from a severe **migraine** (see page 253), although in milder cases it may be impossible to be sure without investigations. **Meningitis** (page 25) of rapid onset can also give a similar picture.

INVESTIGATIONS

If possible a **brain scan** (see page 300) will be undertaken, which will show up the blood within the skull. Failing that it is possible to take a sample of the fluid which surrounds the brain, looking for blood-staining; this is known as a lumbar puncture. Special **X-ray** (see page 301) techniques can locate the aneurysm; this investigation is done if there is a chance of surgery to clip the aneurysm.

ASK YOUR DOCTOR

- **About any case of severe headache with neck stiffness and aversion to light.**
- **About the onset of unusual headaches; these may be a warning of a leaking aneurysm.**

Remedy

Unfortunately, 25 per cent of sufferers die immediately. The rest need careful nursing care until a decision can be made about whether to operate on the aneurysm. In the operation a clip is put around the base of the aneurysm, preventing further bleeding. If investigations reveal other aneurysms it is usual to clip these in order to prevent a future leak. Even so, another 25 per cent of sufferers will die during the first month.

Prevention

There is no feasible way of screening for aneurysms; prevention is a matter of dealing with any which are found while investigating someone who has already had a subarachnoid haemorrhage.

Self-Help

Stroke Association
CHSA House, 123–127 Whitecross Street, London EC1Y 8JJ
Tel: 0171 490-7999

PSYCHIATRIC DISORDERS

• Alcohol Abuse and Alcoholism • Alzheimer's Disease and Dementia • Anxiety • Depression • Drug Abuse • Eating Disorders (Anorexia and Bulimia) • Phobias • Schizophrenia • Suicide

THEORIES ABOUT HUMAN behaviour and thought have taxed the greatest minds. At one extreme theories attribute most human behaviour to inborn instinctive patterns. At the other extreme there are theories which consider that every human being has exactly the same potential as any other and that heredity does not enter the equation. At some other point sit theorists who say it is all a matter of disordered brain chemistry. As usual, one suspects that the answer is some combination of all three.

It is interesting that drug treatments for psychiatric problems work regardless of the theories of psychological causes, so they are invaluable for the treatment of serious mental illness. When it comes to preventing mental illness, it becomes slightly more complicated. So much distress is associated with lifestyle, relationships, working habits, diet and stress, to name but a few, that it is difficult to see how it can be feasible to practice prevention. It does appear to be human instinct to sympathize with people in distress; the sympathetic listening ear seems to be the best method of preventing small disturbances growing into major ones.

ALCOHOL ABUSE AND ALCOHOLISM

There is no one definition of what constitutes alcohol abuse. One school of thought claims it exists when the habit interferes with the ability to function in work and relationships. Another approach to the problem is to examine the physical effects of a person's alcoholic intake. Some people fall into a pattern of heavy drinking that stops short of actual physical dependency; others are clearly physically addicted to alcohol.

As with many other aspects of our society, consuming alcohol is an activity in which most people indulge in quite harmlessly; that said, alcohol abuse underlies much crime, driving accidents (in both drivers and pedestrians) loss of time from work, family breakdown and violence.

Alcohol consumption is measured in units of alcohol. One unit equals a glass of wine, a single measure of spirits or half a pint of beer. Safe limits for men are up to 21 units a week, for women up to 14 units a week; the reason for the difference is that women's livers also have to cope with the breakdown of the female hormones and therefore have less spare capacity to cope with excessive intake of alcohol.

Risk

It is difficult to acquire accurate figures.

- Roughly 5 per cent of men and 2 per cent of women are heavy drinkers.
- Two per cent of the population are problem drinkers.
- About 0.5 per cent are addicted to alcohol.
- Twenty per cent of male admissions to hospital are due to alcohol-related problems; e.g., accidents caused by drunkenness.
- Taking cirrhosis of the liver as a marker of alcohol abuse, the incidence is steadily rising in most countries, with France at the top of the league.
- Certain occupations carry a higher risk: journalists; workers in the alcohol industry; salesmen; doctors. This may be as much opportunity as anything else.
- Heavy drinkers are at increased risk of liver disease (10 to 20 per cent of alcoholics develop cirrhosis of the liver), pancreatitis and gastric bleeding. The risk is greater for steady heavy drinkers as opposed to 'binge' drinkers.
- Modest drinking (14 to 21 units a week) appears protective against heart disease.
- Up to 10,000 deaths a year are thought to be directly due to alcohol abuse.
- There is a greatly increased risk of suicide in alcoholics.

Recognition

SYMPTOMS

Heavy drinkers drink much more than others at social gatherings. They experience indigestion, frequent minor accidents. They lose time from work. When abuse becomes alcoholism, there is craving for alcohol constantly, often first thing in the morning which sets a pattern for the day's drinking. Having a drink becomes a priority activity in the day. They are frequently drunk and home life begins to suffer. The liver is strained attempting to rid the body of what would otherwise be poisonous amounts of alcohol.

Remarkably, 50 per cent of heavy drinkers are able to draw back from over-indulgence and revert to acceptable levels of intake. The others drink steadily every day; they suffer the need to drink. Missing a drink brings on the withdrawal symptoms of shaking (DTs, see below), confusion, sleeplessness, sweating, hallucinations, vomiting, diarrhoea and a vague sense of fear. Epileptic fits can occur. Impotence is common.

The progression from regular heavy drinking to alcoholism is estimated to take ten years in men, three to four years in women.

SIGNS

Alcohol abuse can present as depression, physical deterioration through lack of nutrition, impotence, epileptic fits (10 per cent of alcoholics) and gastric problems. Other serious features are burning feet (through vitamin deficiencies), hallucinations and memory loss. The signs of alcohol abuse can be a flushed face, particularly around the nose, a tremor, and red palms. In cirrhosis of the liver there are many red veins on the face and chest, jaundice, a rounded face and an enlarged liver and spleen.

INVESTIGATIONS

Blood tests (see page 298) can detect alcohol in the blood; liver tests will prove abnormal.

ASK YOUR DOCTOR
- **About the effects of heavy drinking either in yourself or in a relative.**
- **About how to change drinking habits that have become out of control.**

Remedy

RECOGNIZING A PROBLEM

This is the fundamental step. It may come from the drinker themselves, aware of how their life is deteriorating. It may come from their spouse or partner, concerned by behavioural changes. It may be necessary to confront the drinker with the effects of their habit.

PSYCHOLOGICAL SUPPORT

It's important to identify what the individual feels they are gaining from heavy drinking. It may be that they are using drink in their business activities; they may need guidance on alternative ways of spending leisure time; there may be personal or family tensions for which drink is seen as an answer. Very simple techniques are used to learn how to refuse an offered drink without giving offence; advice is offered on ways of relieving stress other than through drink; there is help to learn how to avoid friends who encourage drink. Each individual accepts simple goals for their drinking and behaviour.

Group therapy is widely used on the basis that it gives mutual support when things are going badly and encouragement when they are going well. Not everyone wants to confess their thoughts to a group, but those who do seem to gain from the experience. These groups are run by psychiatric units, charities and alcohol abuse teams.

Alcoholics Anonymous is one form of group therapy, but with added goals of complete abstinence from drink and with an ideological fervour not everyone can take. Those who commit themselves to it do find it an immensely helpful organization, as is its associated body, Al Anon, which provides help for the partners of heavy drinkers.

DRUG THERAPY

This is appropriate for those who are truly addicted to alcohol, for whom even cutting back on drink means withdrawal symptoms of hallucinations, tremor, fear, among others. At its simplest, drugs are given in substitution for alcohol during the three to seven days of withdrawal, drugs such as diazepam or chlormethiazole. It is usual to combine these with high doses of vitamins because many addicted drinkers are seriously vitamin deficient.

The 'DTs' (delirium tremens, or shaking confusion) is the most serious form of withdrawal symptom. Popularly portrayed in films as a 'long night of the soul', it is a much more squalid affair of overwhelming fear, fever, confusion and heart rhythm abnormalities. It should be regarded as a medical emergency rather than a sign of spiritual rebirth (though that may follow) and is best dealt with in hospital where sufferers may even need support in intensive care.

There are drugs which, taken daily, make the sufferer extremely ill when any alcohol is ingested. Atabuse (disulfiram) is one such drug; this sort of treatment is usually offered only to difficult cases.

Alternative Treatment

Dietary therapy will ensure that a proper diet is maintained. Because alcohol supplies calories (albeit empty ones) many alcoholics are not hungry and don't eat otherwise – an increasingly dangerous situation. There are homoeopathic remedies which can discourage alcohol craving. Finding other forms of relaxation, like yoga, T'ai chi, dance or music therapy, massage or aromatherapy to replace alcohol is a good idea.

Prevention

PERSONAL CONTROL

Almost 95 per cent of drinkers handle alcohol sensibly, with due allowance for weddings, wakes and away-wins. Drinking is such an integral part of our social life that it is unrealistic to label it a bad thing, except where it poses a threat to others (see below).

- Be aware of the limits of safe drinking. Exceeding these limits (see above) does not mean instant death, but it is associated with increased risks of disease.
- Do not drink every day: give your liver a rest a couple of days a week.
- The greatest threat to your health is through prolonged heavy drinking, and not the occasional binge. Bingeing is, however, a great strain on the liver and is much more dangerous than regular drinking within the safe limits. Do not kid yourself that you can handle your heavy drinking; really your liver might be coping for the time being, but there will eventually be a price to pay.
- Be prepared to accept comments about drinking; if your friends or partner think you are drinking too much try to accept that there may be a problem. Similarly, if your doctor thinks drink may be contributing to indigestion or finds abnormal blood tests, be prepared to lower your intake. All the evidence shows that early advice about drinking has better results than trying to deal with established problem drinking.
- Think whether alcohol problems might exist in any situations of family breakdown, crime, depression, absence from work, falls in the elderly, and be prepared to ask questions about drinking. But do not be moralistic in your approach; many heavy drinkers will accept reasoned advice about alcohol abuse, while those who are alcoholic are usually only too aware of the misery they have brought on themselves and others. Offer regular sympathetic support through one of the agencies mentioned below.

SOCIAL RESPONSIBILITY

- Society has decided that drinking and driving is permissible to a degree, although there are those who would argue that drinking and driving should be banned altogether, given that alcohol is involved in up to one-third of all fatal accidents.

Self-Help

Alcohol advice centres exist in many towns and can be accessed directly or through your doctor or social worker.
Alcoholics Anonymous
PO Box 1, Stonebow House, Stonebow, York YO1 2NJ
Tel: 01904 644026

Al-Anon (For Relatives and Friends of problem drinkers)
Room 338, 50 Wellington Street, Glasgow G2
Tel: 0141 221-7356
Al-Anon
61 Great Dover Street, London SE1 4YF
Tel: 0171 403-0888

Women's Alcohol Centre
66 A Drayton Park, London N5 1ND
Tel: 0171 226-4581

Richmond Fellowship
(Counselling, Day Centres, Homes)
8 Addison Rd, London W14 8DL
Tel: 0171 603-6373

ALZHEIMER'S DISEASE AND DEMENTIA

The name Alzheimer's disease has gradually come to replace the term senile dementia; dementia is still a respectable medical designation. Dementia is a generalized deterioration in an individual's memory, behaviour and ability to understand. At the same time the demented individual is fully conscious and may appear entirely well until his or her behaviour is examined.

The demented individual moves in a world of bewilderment, far removed from the benign forgetfulness we all experience as we grow older. There are many possible causes of dementia but most cases are the result of Alzheimer's disease, of small strokes affecting the brain. Alzheimer's disease is a post-mortem diagnosis based on examination of the brain which shows loss of nerve cells and abnormal tangles of nerve filaments. The cause is unknown.

It is said that Alzheimer's disease is a growing epidemic. There is some truth in this but only because as a population we are living longer, and it is just a fact of life that the longer you live the more likely you are to develop dementia. Reassuringly, the great majority of people even in their eighties and nineties do not have dementia to any significant degree.

Those who do put an enormous burden on their relatives, one which spreads to neighbours and community services. All too often those relatives are of an age when they are less able to cope with the demands of looking after a demented person. It is convention to speak of senile dementia if someone is seventy years of age or older and of pre-senile dementia in those younger than that, but there is no difference in these conditions except that those below the age of 70 are a little more likely to have one of the treatable causes of dementia.

Risk

- Dementia affects 2 to 3 per cent of the population aged 65 to 75, rising to about 20 per cent in those over 80.
- Alzheimer's disease accounts for 70 per cent of all cases of dementia.
- There are an estimated 650,000 sufferers from dementia.
- Most people with dementia die within five years of the diagnosis, through general deterioration.
- There is no evidence to link aluminium to dementia, as was once proposed.

Recognition

Unlike most illnesses, the sufferer does not realize there is a problem themselves except for flashes of insight at the beginning of the decline.

SYMPTOMS

At first there is an apparently innocent forgetfulness for dates, places and activities. Things are mislaid; the sufferer needs frequent reminding about events. Soon there is evidence of worsening memory: day-to-day affairs are neglected; food is prepared and left uneaten; things turn up in odd places – shoes in the fridge is a typical example. Left to themselves the sufferer becomes dishevelled and dirty; they may be found wandering in the street and leave lights, taps and cookers on. At some point they become a danger to themselves.

Within this picture there are often periods of normality when there may be a distressing awareness of the sad state they are entering. The completed picture is of someone unable to recognize even close friends and relatives; they are unaware of their environment.

SIGNS

Doctors will make formal tests of memory, asking for significant information such as names, birthdays and daily activities, among others. There are simple tests of arithmetic and recall. A gradual decline into dementia is almost certainly due to Alzheimer's disease. A decline marked by sudden changes is most likely due to minor strokes which progressively destroy the brain.

INVESTIGATIONS

In a small number of cases there may be a treatable cause for the dementia, which is why the diagnosis should not be made without some basic tests. The commonest treatable causes are a severely **under-active thyroid gland** (see page 211), deep **depression** (see page 278), certain benign brain tumours called **meningiomas** (see page 250), **alcohol abuse** (see page 268), a blood clot on the brain, and syphilis (see **STDs**, pages 96 and 106). How far to investigate will depend on the age and general condition but anyone under 70 should have a full assessment including **brain scan** (see page 300).

> ## ASK YOUR DOCTOR
> - **For an assessment of anyone whose behaviour is causing concern. The basic tests are very straightforward and give you time to make plans for coping. Many people worry about their own minor lapses of memory; these are rarely of any significance in the absence of other features of deteriorating personality.**
> - **If you are very concerned about forgetfulness; the results are likely to be reassuring.**

Remedy

DETECTION OF TREATABLE DISEASE

Ideally all demented people should have a full battery of tests looking for those relatively unusual treatable conditions such as brain clots, hypothyroidism and depression. In practice scarce resources limit those tests to the younger patients. However, any dementing elderly person should have at least a full physical assessment, basic blood tests and thyroid function tests. A review of medication is useful as occasionally drugs can give rise to confusion.

SOCIAL SUPPORT

There is a range of social helps which can reduce the burden of caring for a demented person. Day centres give regular relief and time out for the carer. The sufferer can be given respite care admissions to an old people's home every few weeks or months. Finally, they may be admitted to permanent nursing-home care. It is important to remember that in the final stages of Alzheimer's disease and dementia the sufferer has no awareness of environment. Because the claims on the time and energy (and usually emotions) of the carer will become excessive, it often becomes essential that care be taken over by a nursing home. Under no circumstances should any carer or family member feel guilty about such a step; it will cause no distress to the sufferer.

DRUG THERAPY

Sedatives are helpful for agitated sufferers who might otherwise spend time wandering, or being aggressive to fellow inmates or to their carers. There is scope for abuse of these drugs, with a fine line to be drawn between drugging the sufferer into apathy and giving just enough to make the task of the carers possible.

If the cause of the dementia is multiple small strokes, taking daily aspirin may reduce the frequency of strokes and therefore the speed of decline. There are no drugs that have been proven to alter Alzheimer's disease itself, though candidates for 'wonder drug' do pop up regularly with extravagant and so far unproved claims.

Alternative Treatment

The best that can be offered is a caring atmosphere and regular stimulation. While there is still awareness in the sufferer, any of the relaxation therapies may be helpful to keep them calm. Try aromatherapy or massage in particular. An acupuncturist might help.

Prevention

While the cause of Alzheimer's remains unclear scientific prevention is not possible. Minor strokes are related to high blood pressure, the control of which lessens the risk of **stroke** (see page 262). At any age it is important to keep contact with reality through daily papers, TV, meeting people, reading and generally using the mind.

Many demented people cope, if not ideally, as long as they remain in familiar settings and with some regular supervision. In fact even quite severe dementia can go unnoticed until some event which upsets the routine such as removal to unfamiliar surroundings or the illness of a spouse who used to do everything for them. There is much to be said for allowing the mildly demented person to try to cope in their regular routine for as long as they are not a danger to themselves or others, even though there is a great temptation for a well-meaning outsider to 'reorganize' their life.

It is easy to forget the burdens on the carers, often themselves in late middle-age with worries, responsibilities and disabilities of their own. There is a generation of these, usually women, coping with frustration, despair and aggression from their demented relatives. This is a burden which society itself could not cope with and it is a pity that relief for these carers is so patchy and dependent on local facilities. It is increasingly recognized that it is far better to try to give carers regular relief than to find that they become unable to cope, resulting in a crisis emergency hospital admission for the demented person for whom they care.

Self-Help

Alzheimer's Disease Society
Gordon House, 10 Greencoat Street, London SW1P 1PH
Tel: 0171 306-0606

Carers National Association
20/25 Glasshouse Yard, London EC1A 4JS
Tel: 0171 490-8818

ANXIETY

Most of us experience a feeling of anxiety in our day-to-day lives. Entangled with anxiety is stress and worry. Experts differ on how these are related: one way of looking at things is that moderate stress is healthy, working as a motivating force, but excess stress causes the state of anxiety.

Worry is a form of anxiety which focuses on one or two specific topics, perhaps money problems or some task to be completed. Anxiety refers to more generalized concerns. Persistent feelings of fear or worry need to be dealt with, because they can lead to debilitating physical and psychological symptoms, such as insomnia or digestive problems. Anxiety and **depression** (see page 278) are often part of the same disease; some sufferers exhibit more anxiety than depression and others the reverse. It is common to experience symptoms of both.

Risk

- Anxiety severe enough to cause physical symptoms is evident in up to 15 per cent of the population.
- More severe anxiety states are found in 2 to 5 per cent of the population.

- Anxiety underlies up to 25 per cent of consultations with family doctors.
- There is probably a genetic element to anxiety, as shown by the increased chance of identical twins both sharing anxiety states.
- Anxiety arising in middle-age is most likely to be part of a depressive illness.

Recognition

Anxiety often occurs in the absence of obvious cause, and severe anxiety of this kind is abnormal and disabling. There is free-floating anxiety (anxiety states or anxiety neuroses), or anxiety which attaches to a specific focus e.g. your health, as in hypochondria where you constantly worry about minor symptoms. There can be situational anxiety, often as a phobia such as agoraphobia or social phobias (see page 287).

SYMPTOMS
The symptoms of anxiety include a rapid pulse, breathlessness, tremulousness, a dry mouth, a feeling of tightness in the chest, sweaty palms, weakness, nausea, diarrhoea and abdominal pain, insomnia, fatigue, headache, and loss of appetite. Disorganization and a short attention span are also common symptoms.

SIGNS
The anxious person may show clear signs of their anxiety; they may be obviously over-breathing. The muscles of the forehead, neck and shoulder will feel tense or tender. Your doctor will ask questions designed to pinpoint depression or another mental illness and look for features of alcohol or drug abuse, especially in an anxious young person.

INVESTIGATIONS
Anxiety may also be a symptom of various other disorders including **hyperthyroidism** (an **over-active thyroid gland**, see page 211), menopausal hormonal disturbances (see page 86), drug withdrawal, **schizophrenia** (see page 290), **depression** (see page 278), post-concussional syndrome, and **dementia** (see page 272).

ASK YOUR DOCTOR
- **To explain the options for treatment, including non-drug treatment.**
- **About a child who seems to have an unusual degree of anxiety; this is unusual and may be a pointer to physical/sexual abuse, drug abuse or a psychotic illness such as schizophrenia.**
- **To refer you for counselling if you find ordinary events increasingly difficult to bear.**
- **For advice, if you are anxious or depressed for unknown reasons.**

Remedy

PHYSICAL
Many people with anxiety have specific fears about their health; e.g., a fear of cancer or of heart disease. It helps to perform a physical check-up to dispel these fears.

PSYCHOLOGICAL

Your doctor can talk you through the symptoms you are experiencing, explaining how they link up with anxiety. By practising over-breathing you can see for yourself how that results in dizziness and a light head. Visualizing things that make you anxious shows you how that leads on to symptoms of anxiety which, if recognized early enough, you can control.

It often takes an outsider to point out the stresses in your life. It can be eye opening to talk through your typical day, making clear where an unhealthy balance of stress and relaxation exists. Counsellors are available to talk through your anxieties and suggest ways in which to cope.

DRUG THERAPY

The hazards of benzodiazepine tranquillizers such as Librium or Valium have been greatly overstated; they are invaluable when used in short courses to control otherwise overwhelming anxiety. Although they do have a potential for dependence, this is unlikely to happen if they are used for a course of a few weeks. Many people find that simply knowing they have a tranquillizer available enables them to cope without taking the drug. Common prescribed drugs are benzodiazepines and anti-depressants with a mild sedative effect such as dothiepin.

Beta-blockers are drugs which reduce the heart rate and reduce anxiety without affecting concentration. They are non-addictive and especially useful where palpitations and tremor are the dominant symptoms.

Alternative Treatment

Finding methods which reduce stress and increase the ability to relax are essential to dealing successfully with anxiety. Yoga, dance therapy, T'ai chi, hypnosis, meditation and massage will all help you to relax. Many alternative therapies have a spiritual element, which can be invaluable when there is confusion causing anxiety.

Bach flower remedies can be very useful for controlling anxiety; in particular Rescue Remedy, which comes as a tincture or cream. Aromatherapy, herbalism and homoeopathy also offer specific measures for control.

Prevention

Arguably stress and anxiety are necessary motivating forces in society and to abolish them completely is likely to be achievable only by reducing society to a series of bland encounters. Some people appear naturally more 'highly strung' than others and evidence suggests that there is a genetic component to anxiety, about which nothing can be done.

Worry about money, work, relationships is an unavoidable feature of most societies. Certain events can be predicted to cause anxiety: childbirth; having a young family; work; illness; retirement and bereavement. Ideally those faced with these events should be able to turn somewhere for support. Often health visitors and local counselling groups are the first port of call. There are many groups available to help people in just such circumstances such as mother and baby groups, bereavement counsellors and counsellors specializing in marriage difficulties.

Most of us do manage to prevent anxiety growing out of hand; we recognize the warning symptoms of stress and can make a conscious effort to relax. Skilled counsellors take this further and teach the cues of rising anxiety such as over-breathing or sweating;

then you learn how to focus on other things to take your mind off the anxiety. An allowance for frustration can be built into your schedule; talking about how you feel is helpful and most societies have discovered some drugs to control the effects of anxiety such as alcohol, tobacco and caffeine.

Self-Help

PAX
4 Manorbrook, London SE3 9AW
Tel: 0181 318-5026

DEPRESSION

Like **anxiety** (see page 275), depression is an integral feature of human life. All of us feel depressed at times in our lives, so an allowance for this feeling must be made. Yet there is a stage beyond which depression becomes no longer reasonable but an illness, and a dangerous one at that. Depression can overshadow every aspect of life; such a depressive illness is as real as a broken leg and as painful as a heart attack and should be taken as seriously and urgently as any serious physical illness. Depression is part of a syndrome which can often include anxiety; its causes are numerous and sometimes biochemical, but it is also linked to emotional trauma or fear. Its symptoms are wide-ranging and often frightening.

Risk

- Severe depression affects about one in any two hundred people at any time; of those, between 5 and 10 per cent will eventually commit **suicide** (see page 292).
- More minor depression affects 5 to 10 per cent of the population at any one time, with twice as many women affected as men.
- Risk of depression is greatest after stressful events such as bereavement, job loss or moving home.
- Ten to 20 per cent of women experience mild depression after childbirth; severe depression after childbirth affects one in 500 to 1000 women and is a medical emergency.
- There seems to be a genetic risk of depression, as close relatives of depressives have a 10 to 15 per cent risk of severe depression, rising to 67 per cent in identical twins.
- Women are at greater risk, especially divorced women.
- Depression can accompany other mental illness such as **schizophrenia** (see page 290) and **Alzheimer's disease** (see page 272).
- It may be both cause and effect of **alcoholism** (see page 268) and **drug abuse** (see page 282).

Recognition

SYMPTOMS

In mild depression there are still moments of pleasure. You worry and fear the future, you may feel helpless and unwanted, gloomy and sad but you can still cope with life despite your unhappiness.

As depression deepens so the world looks more unwaveringly black. You doubt the motives and love of those close to you; you may despise yourself and disparage your achievements; the future holds nothing for you but more loss, grief and despair. Your sleep is poor. You may think you have some incurable illness that doctors are hiding from you, even believing that something physical within you is literally destroying you from the inside. You stop eating, you become apathetic, spending time crying and contemplating suicide. Physical symptoms might include backache and headaches, palpitations, digestive disorders and physical feelings of panic. There may also be lack of libido and a feeling of extreme despair, irritability and irrational behaviour.

In some forms of depression anxiety is a great feature and here the individual is consumed by agitation.

SIGNS

A depressed person is likely to appear sad and worried; there will be extended crying spells and possibly weight loss. On probing it emerges that they are sleeping badly, waking in the early hours and lying awake. It may be clear that they have delusions of illness and of persecution by those around them.

> *Mothers suffering from severe depression after childbirth (post-natal depression) are seriously ill, often convinced their baby is abnormal or that the rest of their family is unwell; there is a high risk of such women killing themselves or their children in the belief that they are putting them out of some unspeakable misery.*

INVESTIGATION

There is no test for depression, but it is sensible to check thyroid activity, as a severely **underactive thyroid gland** (see page 211) can mimic depression. In the elderly depression can be a feature of early senile **dementia** (see page 272); the depression follows from lucid moments when the person is aware of how their mind is disintegrating.

ASK YOUR DOCTOR

- If you are concerned about your health or your well-being. Unfortunately, depressed individuals find it difficult to discuss depression. Other symptoms, such as abdominal pains, headaches, neck pains, are accentuated. Depression can indeed make you physically ill and most doctors are trained to recognize the symptom pattern. However, because of reluctance to talk on the part of the sufferer, an estimated 50 per cent of cases of depression go unrecognized.

Remedy

PSYCHOLOGICAL HELP

The mild depressions which accompany the ups and downs of life are best treated by sympathy, talking through your worries and by encouraging an optimistic outlook. Depression is a serious illness and sufferers should not, under any circumstances, be requested to 'snap out of it'. It is often difficult to understand from an external point of view, but what a sufferer needs most is compassion and understanding.

A counsellor can listen to your worries, and pick up clues as to their cause. A seemingly undirected conversation will present a good counsellor with plenty of information about you and the root of your depression. An outside counsellor is much more useful than someone you know; it's easier to reveal deep-seated emotions and problems to a person you know you never have to see again. A trained counsellor will be able you to encourage you past the roadblocks you've put up throughout your life. The human mind has many methods for resisting painful truths. It will deny, distort, reject and ignore emotions which engender too much pain. A counsellor can gently ease you past the pat explanations for problems so that you are actually relieved to share the burden.

PSYCHOANALYSIS

Is a formulaic method of discovering and interpreting human emotion; Freudian psychoanalysis is the most widely known but is just one of many theories of human emotion. Whatever interpretation is used, it is helpful just to have someone understand and analyse your problems.

DRUG THERAPY

More and more cases of depression are given biological or biochemical causes; because of this drug therapy can be helpful in dealing with severe, prolonged depression. The depression that follows bereavement or stress should not be treated with drugs; time and sympathy should suffice. But when weeks are passing and the individual remains apathetic, crying, sad, here anti-depressants are invaluable. The older types (tri-cyclic anti-depressants such as amitriptyline) are effective and very widely used, taking two to three weeks for their effect to build up. They have side-effects such as drowsiness or dry mouth which make them unacceptable to some people. More important, they can be dangerous in overdose because they can interfere with the electrical activity of the heart.

For these reasons many doctors are using new generation anti-depressants such as SSRIs or Selective Serotonin Re-uptake Inhibitors, this referring to the biochemical pathways that these drugs block. Prozac is one especially well known brand but there are several others. These SSRIs are safe in overdose, but much more expensive than the older tri-cyclic anti-depressants and so tend to be used in cases where there is a suicide risk. Even more recent are drugs called Monoamine Reversible A Inhibitors (MARIs) which also appear to be effective but safe in overdose and with fewer side-effects.

Anti-depressants are not wonder drugs, nor do they work in all cases – about 30 per cent of patients do not respond. They are not a substitute for psychological support but can lift mood enough so that the sufferer can begin to accept psychological support and start to think positively about their situation.

ELECTRO-CONVULSIVE THERAPY (ECT)

ECT has an image problem – not surprising, given the fact that it constitutes the passage of a high voltage of electricity across the brain with the aim of causing an epileptic fit (the patient is kept under sedation during the treatment). There is little known as to why it works, but it does appear to, and it is a last-resort treatment for people who are so depressed that they will undoubtedly kill themselves, or who are in what is called a depressive stupor, so depressed that they remain mute and motionless.

It is true that ECT has been used indiscriminately in the past and it is also true that it can leave people with memory problems, though it is controversial how much of this is caused by the treatment and how much the result of pre-existing personality traits. About 20,000 people are treated with ECT each year in the UK.

Alternative Treatment

Arguably all psychological therapy began as alternative therapy; there is no medical monopoly on insight or sympathy or interpretation. Almost all therapies work on a holistic basis; that is, they treat a person as much more than a body or a set of symptoms. Everything from your sense of well-being, lifestyle, sleep habits, concerns, diet, stress levels, etc. will be discussed in a first consultation with a therapist and sometimes the very act of focusing on your life can put it into perspective. Again, a sympathetic ear can be the best medicine. For that reason, many cases of mild depression can be relieved in the hands of a good, trained practitioner. There is a sound mind/body relationship. If you think something is helping, it probably will.

Alternative practitioners might suggest Bach flower remedies, nutritional therapy (in particular, treatment with amino acid supplementation), acupuncture, shiatsu, massage, and any of the gentle relaxation therapies, like yoga, T'ai chi or aromatherapy.

> *Severe or prolonged depression is a potentially dangerous condition, carrying a serious risk of suicide. Sufferers should always be offered a conventional psychiatric assessment.*

Prevention

RECOGNIZING RISK

We have listed several life events following which depression is to be expected, such as childbirth or bereavement. Many groups exist to offer help in these circumstances, preventing a slide into depression that can easily happen. It is less easy to prevent depression arising from adverse circumstances of life. Life is endlessly disappointing and maturity is partly to do with reaching some balance between life as we would choose it to be and life as it is. Most people can find some hobby activity or organization through which they can find the self-esteem to protect them from at least some of life's unhappinesses and it is therapeutic to encourage those who appear socially isolated to participate in society.

SYMPATHY

The value of sympathy is not to be underestimated. There may be nothing else to offer someone whose life is indeed unfulfilling or whose marriage has fallen to bits but a sympathetic ear and the opportunity to talk.

SUPPORT

Severe depression is recurrent in probably all cases, though years may pass between relapses. Sufferers may benefit from knowing that there is a support group to turn to when they or their partners feel depression is recurring.

Drug Therapy

Depression is often part of a manic-depressive illness, the sufferer swinging between depression and manic over-activity and anxiety. These people are often extremely useful and productive members of society in between their bouts of profound gloom or exhausting hyperactivity; once it is established that they suffer from manic-depression it may be best for them to stay on lithium, a drug which smooths out swings in mood.

Biochemical Prevention

Depression has long been thought to be caused by imbalance of brain chemistry; the latest anti-depressants work by blocking naturally occurring chemicals in the brain. Despite extravagant claims, the day of the 'happy pill' is yet to dawn but is no longer inconceivable.

Self-Help

Your doctor will have access to the local support groups run by psychiatric social workers or by psychiatrists.
Depressives Anonymous
36 Chestnut Ave, Beverley, North Humberside HU17 9QU
Tel: 01482 860619
Mental Health Foundation
8 Hallam Street, London W1N 6DH
Tel: 0171 580-0145

DRUG ABUSE

In its broadest sense drug abuse includes alcoholism and cigarette smoking as well as actual illegal drugs. However, it is the abuse of illegal drugs such as cocaine (which is injected), crack (a form of cocaine that can be taken by mouth), LSD, and opiates such as heroin and morphine, which will be discussed here. There has to be some element of dependency on or excessive use of a drug for it to be considered abuse. It is a well-publicized problem; indeed drug dependency is considered to pose one of the major threats to social stability and underpins much random crime by those who need to steal to maintain their habit.

Risk

- Undoubtedly many teenagers and young adults experiment with 'soft drugs', such as marijuana and ecstasy (a short-term psychedelic drug).
- Peer pressure is a powerful influence, as it is in smoking and alcohol.
- The progression from soft to hard drugs is not inevitable; the reasons why some people become addicted to much more dangerous drugs are unknown, but there seem to be personality types who are attracted to drugs.
- Intravenous drug addicts are at high risk of infections, including hepatitis B, and HIV.
- Overdose of any narcotic drug, cocaine, crack or solvents can cause death through convulsions, liver and kidney failure or through inhaling of vomit while unconscious.
- Two to 3 per cent of morphine/heroin addicts die each year as a result of their habit.

Recognition

SYMPTOMS

Suspicion may be aroused by someone with erratic behaviour, swinging rapidly between hyperexcitability and apathy. Solvent abuse (glue-sniffing) leads to rashes around the face. Slurred speech, giddiness and euphoria should all raise a suspicion of drug abuse, as should otherwise unexplained profound changes in motivation and behaviour in a young person.

SIGNS

Injection sites are commonly on the arms but can include any accessible vein. Often old infected veins are hard. The individual can be irritable and excitable; after an overdose they can fall into confusion or coma. Convulsions are a by-product of glue-sniffing, crack, cocaine and heroin abuse. Sniffing cocaine can lead to a hole in the soft central division between the nostrils. Long term, there may be signs of **hepatitis** (see page 21) or **AIDS** (see page 13).

ASK YOUR DOCTOR
- **About blood tests for any intravenous drug abuser; there is a very high risk of hepatitis B or HIV.**

Remedy

WITHDRAWAL OF DRUGS

This is a time-consuming task, requiring great patience on the part of the therapist. Constant support is required for the addict. Less harmful drugs, like methadone, can be substituted in order to wean an abuser off potent drugs like heroin. The substitute is then withdrawn.

DETOXIFICATION

This means withdrawal of drugs suddenly and completely. It is reserved for cocaine, amphetamine and heroin addicts. Detoxification throws addicts into a potentially dangerous state with some combination of heavy sweating, yawning, restlessness, running nose, then diarrhoea and vomiting, stomach pains and muscle cramps. The symptoms can be so distressing that they work as a future deterrent against drug abuse.

DRUG MAINTENANCE

Some addicts, unable to come off completely, are supplied with drugs through the NHS and with clean needles and syringes to reduce the chances of infection through sharing needles.

DRUG OVERDOSE

An overdose of narcotic drugs; e.g., heroin can be reversed by injection of an antagonist called naloxone. There still follows a need for careful intensive therapy while the individual recovers and goes through detoxification (if they stay in hospital that long). Overdoses of solvents or cocaine are treated by controlling convulsions and supplying fluids through a drip while the individual recovers.

Alternative Treatment

There are several clinics for drug addiction working outside the NHS. Most of these supply treatment of the highest calibre but it is best to check with your doctor or a local psychiatrist with expertise in drug abuse about a clinic's reputation.

There are a number of alternative therapies which can provide comfort throughout periods of detoxification, and some will encourage the body to heal more quickly following a period of abuse. Homoeopathy, acupuncture and herbalism are all potential ports of call.

Prevention

Here is a goal that preoccupies parents, relatives, police and social workers worldwide. The main preventative strategy has been to warn young people of the dangers of drug abuse. Therapeutic drugs with the potential for abuse are prescribed with increasing care; an example is benzodiazepines (e.g., valium) whose potential for abuse is greatly overstated but which nevertheless are now prescribed more cautiously and in shorter courses.

Probably many young people go through a stage of experimentation with drugs, when too heavy-handed an attitude could push them towards more dangerous drugs as a protest. Be alert to the features of drug abuse in your children. Talk about drug use as you may talk about alcohol or sex; that is, as attractions your children are bound to be exposed to but in the hope of giving them a balanced and responsible approach.

Convincing prevention programmes are hampered by the fact that society tolerates certain drugs like alcohol and tobacco, whose effects on health can be enormous, but bans other drugs whose harmfulness is far more controversial. Not surprisingly, an increasingly affluent society experiments with marijuana and cocaine as 'social' drugs on the basis that their harmful effects are probably less than the known harmful effects of alcohol and tobacco. What is not known is whether starting on such drugs will lead to addiction with inevitably harmful drugs such as morphine or heroin.

Self-Help

There are too many local groups to mention. The following offer information and may be able to put you in touch with help in your area.

Action on Addiction
York House, 199 Westminster Bridge Road, London SE1 7UT
Tel: 0171 261-1333

Drugcare
29 Upper Lattimore Road, St Alban's AL1 3UA
Tel: 01727 834539

ADFAM (for relatives of drug addicts)
5th Floor, Epworth House, 25 City Road, London ECIY 1AA
Tel: 0171 638-3790

ANOREXIA AND BULIMIA

These two related eating disorders seem to have become far more common in the course of the last twenty years. The reason for this is debatable, but is probably related to the increasing emphasis on slimness as an ideal body type for women (and to a lesser extent men).

Risk

- Anorexia affects 1 to 2 per cent of older girls and female students.
- Anorexia is far less common in men, affecting about one in 1000.
- There are probably many more people who diet to below average body weight but who fall short of true anorexia.
- Anorexia usually begins in the mid-teens, after the age of 30.
- There is a 2 to 5 per cent risk of suicide in chronic cases of anorexia.
- Most anorexics recover eventually, but in about a third of cases they remain significantly underweight
- Anorexia is more common in people from middle-class homes and in certain occupations such as ballet dancing or modelling.
- It is common for anorexics to have gone through a period of obesity in childhood.
- Bulimia affects about 1.5 per cent of the population; another 5 per cent suffer from episodic bulimia.
- Bulimia is commonly associated with anorexia.
- Bulimia also carries an increased risk of death through associated alcohol or drug abuse.

Recognition

SYMPTOMS OF ANOREXIA NERVOSA
The sufferer has at the same time a fear of becoming fat and a desire to be ever more thin. Weight falls to at least 25 per cent below the standard weight for age and height. Women often stop having periods; they avoid food and what food they do eat is usually very low in calories. Occasionally there will be vomiting to expel unwanted food. There is a distorted body image; emaciated victims are convinced that they are fat. It is common to binge eat from time to time. They feel the cold and are often light-headed through lack of nutrition and low blood pressure. Many anorexics exercise obsessively, despite the often persistent feeling of faintness.

SIGNS OF ANOREXIA NERVOSA
There is progressive weight loss going well beyond slimness. Sufferers sometimes become covered with a fine overgrowth of hair (called lanugo). Blood pressure is low, pulse rate is low. Discussion brings out their distorted view of their weight.

INVESTIGATIONS
As weight loss can be a feature of many diseases it is important to perform screening **blood tests** (see page 298) checking especially for an **over-active thyroid gland** (see page 211) or for malfunction in the pituitary gland.

Symptoms of Bulimia

By definition the symptoms are of bouts of over-eating (binges) after which the sufferers make themselves vomit. Often they also take laxatives, diuretics and other drugs in an attempt to lose weight. Periods are usually present but may be irregular.

Signs of Bulimia

The sufferer may be anorexic but can equally be of normal weight or overweight. Chronic vomiting leads to erosion of the teeth, which are worn away by the powerful stomach acid. Chronic vomiting also causes loss of potassium, leading to muscle pains and weakness. The sufferer is usually unhappy, leads a disordered life, often abuses alcohol or other drugs and may show signs of self-mutilation.

Investigations

As with anorexia, it is important to check out other possible conditions which cause vomiting such as kidney disease, digestive problems, pregnancy.

ASK YOUR DOCTOR

- **If you are concerned about your own weight or that of someone close to you. It is usually a relative or parent who first alerts a doctor to a case of eating disorder and who accompanies the patient to the doctor. Relatives may be able to give some insight into tensions that underlie the condition; this is helpful because the sufferers themselves are usually uncommunicative.**

Remedy

Intervention is valid on several grounds. Sufferers of eating disorders are unhappy people; a suicide risk has been mentioned. Secondly, there is also the physical result of malnutrition by way of fatigue and dizziness, which may affect performance at a time of critical school or university exams. The behaviour of sufferers often shows up tension within the rest of the family which should be sorted out.

Treatment of these eating disorders is not yet established; cases should be referred to specialized centres familiar with the latest research.

Mild cases can be handled by regular supervision by experienced therapists. A target weight is agreed. This may well be below a desirable weight but is at least above the starvation level. Then the individual works towards that weight, possibly with rapidly absorbed liquid food supplements initially. The therapists and relatives remain vigilant for signs of any abuse of laxatives or self-induced vomiting.

In the case of bulimia, the best approach seems to be one that identifies what makes the sufferer binge and teaching them to handle that stimulus. The sufferer is also given a set diet that they should not exceed or eat less than.

Serious cases may need to be admitted to hospital in order to restore dietary balance and to correct the effects of starvation or vomiting on the heart, kidneys and bones. There are a few drugs which improve bulimic behaviour and anti-depressants can help in anorexia. In extreme circumstances the sufferer may have to be force-fed under a court order; this lifesaving measure would be used rarely because it jeopardizes the trust between sufferer and therapist, and does not, in the end, address the real cause of the problem.

PSYCHOTHERAPY

This is widely practised but no one method has been shown to be better than another. There is a particular association between bulimia and sexual abuse. The families of anorexics are said to show unusual rigidity and overprotection.

> *Recovery tends to be a slow affair, spread over several years, but most do recover, though studies suggest that many anorexics and bulimics do not return to entirely normal eating practices.*

Alternative Treatment

The strain on the body caused by eating disorders can be addressed by alternative therapies, but they do not seek to provide a cure for the conditions themselves. Both bulimia and anorexia are fundamentally emotional (psychiatric) in nature and should be dealt with by trained professionals.

Prevention

In the present state of knowledge the best prevention is early detection of the conditions, so that help can be offered before the sufferer has developed serious ill-health. No doubt if society were to adopt role models that were not thin attitudes would change, but there seems little prospect of that. There have been recent moves to restrict advertising which promotes thinness as being desirable, or which seems to be promoting unhealthy eating patterns.

Self-Help

Anorexia Anonymous
24 Westmoreland Road, Barnes London SW13 9RY
Tel: 0181 748-3994

Eating Disorders Association
Sackville Place, 44–48 Magdalen St, Norwich NR3 1JE
Tel: 01603 621414

PHOBIAS

A phobia is a fear which is out of proportion to the threat. While many people have a fear of spiders, those with a phobia will be terrified that one might suddenly appear, are reduced to panic at the sight of a spider and become sweaty and anxious at the very thought. Other common phobias are fear of flying, fear of heights and agoraphobia (a fear of going outside the home into crowded places). The range is much wider; people have phobias about being in restaurants, needing a toilet when out, winds and lightning.

There are two broad theories of phobias. One school of thought says that a phobia is the result of a bad experience with the object of the phobia – a near-drowning which leaves you with a fear of the water, a fall from a tree that leaves you with a fear of heights. Probably many phobias do start in this way. Once anxiety begins it feeds on itself so that, according to this theory, when you approach water you feel increasingly anxious, which makes a feeling of anxiety more likely the next time you go near water. This is the behavioural theory. There is also some evidence that training in the form of a mother–child or teacher–child relationship might encourage a phobia. A mother who shrieks at the sight of a cat instils at an early age an irrational fear of cats in her child, who is too young to react logically but who will have, because of this, an over-riding bad feeling about them; she may not even remember why.

Allied to this there seems to be some biological rationale behind a phobia such as fear of spiders and snakes, open spaces, illness; this fear was presumably protective to the species in prehistoric times. Support for this comes from the fact that such phobias are found in all cultures.

More psychoanalytic theories say all that is simplistic nonsense. You may think it is water you fear but in reality, they say, you fear what water represents. Water might represent a loss of self, perhaps a hidden desire to return to the womb. For obvious reasons these two groups of theorists tend not to communicate!

Of course the rest of us know that there is an element of truth in both of these approaches. Phobias can exist on their own or as part of a broader psychiatric illness such as schizophrenia, alcoholism and anxiety states.

Risk

- Severe phobias affect 1 in 500 adults.
- Up to 1 per cent of the population have some significant phobia.
- Milder phobic symptoms affect about 20 per cent of the population.
- Agoraphobia is one of the commonest phobias.
- Most phobics are women.

Recognition

Phobics recognize their problem and may seek advice when their phobia is affecting their lives.

Symptoms
Accompanying the phobia is anxiety and perhaps other neurotic traits such as panic attacks, faintness when exposed to the stimulus and a feeling of depersonalization.

Signs
The doctor should be alert for signs of associated disorders such as alcohol abuse, depression, and drug abuse.

ASK YOUR DOCTOR
- **If you feel that a phobia is beginning to dominate your life; no matter how bizarre the object of your fear the chances are that you can be helped.**

Remedy

BEHAVIOUR THERAPY

The most effective treatment for single phobias is desensitization. This means being gradually exposed to the feared object or activity. For example, someone with a fear of insects would begin by just thinking about them. Once they can handle that anxiety they might look at pictures of insects in books; then touch the pictures. Soon they can look at dead insects, then live ones. This is a process of desensitization and effects a cure in most sufferers.

SUPPORT

This is critical; self-help groups reassure sufferers that their preoccupations are not so unique.

MEDICATION

Is useful to treat overwhelming anxiety and any associated depression. Anti-depressants and benzodiazepines are widely used.

Alternative Treatment

Support groups are extremely helpful. Hypnosis and relaxation techniques can be very effective as are herbal remedies or aromatherapy to reduce anxiety. Some sufferers believe in things like past-lives' therapy, on the assumption, no doubt, that their phobia is the result of an experience in a previous life. Different things work for different people, and as long as a therapy is undertaken at the hands of a recognized and registered therapist, and the treatment works, there can be little argument against it.

Prevention

Phobias are probably no more preventable than anxiety in general; they are part of our life. Some carry biological advantage; e.g., a fear of heights, a fear of certain animals. What is most important is the realization that phobias are not unusual and that effective treatment is available. The earlier treatment begins the less likely the phobia is to become deeply entrenched.

Self-Help

Open Door Association
447 Pensby Rd, Heswall, Wirral, Cheshire L61 9PQ

PAX
4 Manorbrook, London SE3 9AW
Tel: 0181 318-5026

Phobic Action
Claybury Grounds, Manor Road, Woodford Green, Essex IG8 8PR
Tel: 0181 506-0600

SCHIZOPHRENIA

Schizophrenia is a mental illness in which there is a breakdown of reason, personality, and thought processes; it is often associated with self-neglect. It is probably the disease which most people have in mind when speaking of madness. The sufferer changes from a familiar figure into a barely recognizable person who hears words no one else can hear, has visions no one else can see; who harbours fears and emotions beyond all reason.

Schizophrenia does not mean a split personality; it does not mean someone who is eccentric, free thinking, visionary or awkward, though the term has been abused in that way. Nor is it a romantic illness, although sufferers may have startling use of language and produce striking art.

There is now little doubt that the disorder results from some combination of heredity and upbringing, even if argument continues about the influence of each.

Risk

- About 1 in every 200 adults is suffering from active schizophrenia at any one time. In the population as a whole about 1 in 100 persons is currently suffering or has suffered from it.
- While schizophrenia can occur at any age it is commonest from the teens to the late forties. Men are more likely to develop it when younger and women when older.
- The risk of developing the disease is greatly increased if a near relative, a brother, sister or parent has had schizophrenia. Studies suggest that there is a 14 per cent risk if either parent has had the disease and as much as a 46 per cent risk if both parents have been schizophrenic.
- Schizophrenia occurs all over the world; there are areas where it is especially common, such as Northern Sweden and the west of Ireland, or where it is rare, such as in Papua New Guinea.

Recognition

Symptoms

The existence of the illness was first agreed in 1896 and the term schizophrenia was first used in 1911. Apart from these facts just about everything else about the illness is the subject of argument and controversy, including the symptoms. However, most psychiatrists would accept the importance of the following symptoms.

- Hallucinations

These are experiences no one else shares. The sufferer may hear voices giving a running commentary on their behaviour; frequently a schizophrenic may say that voices are controlling his or her behaviour. Tragedies result when the voices order a schizophrenic to kill their spouse or to murder their own children. Schizophrenics may have visions and feel things that no one else is aware of. As a result of a hallucination their behaviour may change; after all, you too would stop walking if you saw a tiger lying across the pavement.

- Delusions

This means a belief totally out of keeping with reality, as judged by others sharing the same culture and with access to the same information. For example, it is now inconceivable to believe that our planet Earth is held up on the arms of the giant Atlas. Yet a schizophrenic might claim not only to know that Atlas is indeed holding up the Earth, but also to discuss with him how much his arms ache. It is a particular feature of such delusions that they are completely resistant to normal logic. Show a photo of Earth floating in space and it will be explained away by some bizarre twist of reason.

● Feelings of passivity

The schizophrenic's behaviour appears outside their control. Thoughts, voices and visions tell them to do things, to sit, to stay silent, to fight. When these influences are quiet the sufferer may just lie about, neglecting themselves, not washing, eating nor caring for themselves or others.

● Disorders of thought

Schizophrenics imagine their thoughts are being broadcast to the world; that what they are thinking everyone knows about. On the other hand a schizophrenic may feel that thoughts are being put into their own minds from some outside body; another person, a piece of furniture, the television, and that they have no control over this.

● Other features

Schizophrenia of gradual onset may just show itself as a withdrawal from the world, self-neglect, neglect of responsibilities, depression, increasingly vague and inappropriate behaviour. Sometimes it shows itself more dramatically as increasingly bizarre speech and actions more and more out of keeping with previous patterns of behaviour.

> *Other possibilities always need to be borne in mind. Dementia due to brain disease can cause peculiar symptoms; severe depression may cause delusions of suffering from serious disease; drugs and alcoholism can alter behaviour causing swings of mood and self-neglect.*

SIGNS

At what point is individualistic behaviour truly odd? When do beliefs become more than just eccentric? How to recognize when ordinary 'normal' adolescent moodiness has gone beyond understandable limits? Such questions bedevil discussions on schizophrenia. Yet most psychiatrists would agree that a combination of symptoms from the above selection is highly suggestive of schizophrenia.

ASK YOUR DOCTOR

As a relative of a sufferer:

● **About the chances of cure and outlook for behaviour and work.**
● **About how to obtain help in flare-ups.**
● **How to ensure that the sufferer takes the medication needed.**

Remedy

About 40 per cent of sufferers from schizophrenia make a complete recovery and remain well more than five years later. They return to their former lives, jobs and relationships.

It is a past episode like a case of pneumonia. Another 40 per cent remain permanently damaged mentally. They may require regular supervision. Sometimes they can cope with an undemanding job, but frequently they remain a burden on others. Schizophrenia is an important cause of permanent disability in the community.

For about 20 per cent of schizophrenics the illness fluctuates and they have repeated episodes of serious illness.

DRUG TREATMENT

The treatment of schizophrenia was revolutionized in the 1950s by the discovery of a group of drugs which rapidly brought symptoms under control. These drugs are still widely used; chlorpromazine is the best known. There have been a few new drugs and they can also be given as a regular injection every two or three weeks. Thanks to these drugs, schizophrenics could eventually lead more of a normal life in the community. This has been one of the major reasons for the trend towards closing the large psychiatric hospitals, once the depository of those for whom nothing could be done.

PSYCHOTHERAPY

This has been disappointing in schizophrenia, really because the thoughts and feelings are so illogical in their nature that talking about them gets nowhere. For the 60 per cent who do not make a full recovery, regular support is important to spot the earliest signs of a flare-up.

Alternative Treatment

There is no appropriate alternative therapy for curing schizophrenia, although some may be offered. Relaxation therapies like yoga, T'ai chi or visualization may be useful. Acupuncture or acupressure may address fundamental imbalances within the body.

Prevention

Unfortunately, there is no evidence of useful preventative measures.

Self-Help

National Schizophrenia Fellowship
28 Castle Street, Kingston upon Thames, Surrey KT1 1SS
Tel: 0181 974-6814

SANE
2nd Floor, 199–205 Old Marylebone Road, London NW1 5QP
Tel: 0171 724-8000

SUICIDE

For many people each year suicide is the desperate response to what they see as insurmountable problems in their lives. Suicide is one of the most common reasons for early death and has been on the increase for many years. Society now looks at suicide from the point of view of the individual rather than regarding it as a crime, as was the case until relatively recently.

There are important differences between those who simply attempt suicide and those who plan it carefully with a view to success, although the two groups share an increased incidence of psychiatric disturbance.

Risk

- In the UK 1 per cent of deaths are due to suicide, two-thirds of these are men.
- The overall risk of suicide is eight per 100,000 population, or about 4500 per annum.
- The elderly, especially elderly men, are most likely to commit suicide.
- Risks are increased by serious illness, recent bereavement, social isolation, alcoholism, being single or divorced and previous psychiatric problems.
- Suicides among teenagers have increased threefold since the 1960s, for unknown reasons.
- Of the severely depressed, 5 to 10 per cent will eventually commit suicide, as do similar percentages of alcoholics and schizophrenics (see pages 268 and 290).
- There are high rates of suicide in those with access to drugs; these include doctors and dentists.
- About 100,000 people attempt suicide each year, as seen in hospital admissions. Most of these are young women. This figure represents 2.5 per cent of all hospital admissions.
- One per cent of women aged 15 to 30 attempt suicide each year.
- Attempted suicide is the most common reason for admission to hospital in people under 50 years of age.
- It is estimated that 50 per cent of suicide attempts go unreported.
- Of those who attempt suicide 1 to 2 per cent succeed in committing suicide in the year following the attempt and 10 per cent will eventually commit suicide.

Recognition

SYMPTOMS

The individual may be known to have problems of depression, alcohol or drugs or relationship difficulties and may have talked about suicide. Young women often take an overdose as a spur-of-the-moment gesture without any obvious warning of their intentions.

SIGNS

In general, the more care a person takes in arranging suicide and the more violent the means the more likely that their intention was indeed to kill themselves. Even so every case of attempted suicide deserves psychiatric assessment as there will be those who have serious on-going worries which may lead them to attempt suicide in future.

ASK YOUR DOCTOR

- **If you believe someone is a serious suicide risk. That person may have a treatable condition such as depression underlying their suicidal intent.**
- **If you feel life is becoming too much for you; don't hesitate to voice your concerns to a doctor, friend or telephone helpline. Do not assume people know how badly you feel unless you give them a clue.**

Remedy

The immediate priority is to deal with the effects of whatever method has been chosen to attempt suicide. If tablets have been swallowed it is vital to identify these and to know how many have been taken. Fortunately, many commonly prescribed sleeping tablets and tranquillizers are safe in overdose unless combined with alcohol; it is a matter of nursing support until the effects of the tablets wear off.

Overdoses with older tri-cyclic anti-depressants, like amitriptyline and imipramine, can cause potentially fatal heart rhythm disturbances and these patients need close monitoring in the first 24 hours. Newer anti-depressants are safer in overdose and are being used increasingly because of that reason. (See also **depression**, page 278.)

> *As few as twenty paracetamol tablets can cause liver damage, while death from liver failure is possible from just thirty tablets. Vigorous early treatment brings the patient round, but sadly liver damage may take three to four days to appear. To be most effective treatment has to begin within eight hours of overdose. Paracetamol overdoses account for 150 deaths a year and result in half of all referrals for liver transplantation.*

Aspirin overdose can cause convulsions, coma and swelling of the brain, together with rapid breathing, heavy sweating and ringing in the ears. This can occur after taking sixty or more tablets.

Many other substances are used in overdose, for each of which advice on management is established by a poisons information unit.

Psychiatric Assessment

Where the attempt is seriously intended a psychiatric assessment is essential. More controversial is the value in cases where a suicide attempt appears to be a spontaneous act; few people under these circumstances have any true psychiatric disturbance and many resent seeing a psychiatrist. Nevertheless, 1 to 2 per cent of such 'para-suicides' will go on to successful suicide in the next year, so an effort should be made to see if there are underlying drug, alcohol and relationship problems for which help can be offered.

Alternative Treatment

There are all manner of helpful counselling groups for those feeling depressed or stressed to the point of suicide. Many people clearly prefer to be able to speak to an anonymous lay person rather than authority figures such as doctors or social workers.

Following a suicide attempt, self-image and physical health and well-being may be improved through the use of alternative therapies. A registered practitioner in homoeopathy, herbalism, acupuncture or a number of other popular and increasingly respected therapies will be able to work out an individual plan.

Prevention

Suicide is seen as a logical next step by significant numbers of ill, elderly, isolated people each year. If someone in such circumstances threatens suicide it should be taken very seriously and they should be offered psychiatric assessment.

More clear-cut is the prevention of suicide in those who have a treatable depressive illness or who make impulsive use of agents which they think are harmless, such as paracetamol, but which can be dangerous.

PRACTICAL MEASURES

These include reducing the carbon monoxide content in domestic gas, wrapping medication individually to make it more difficult to swallow a lot at one time. Barbiturate tranquillizers, lethal in overdose, are now virtually unobtainable, being replaced by the benzodiazepine drugs which are safe in overdose.

- It is possible to produce paracetamol in a tablet combined with an antidote. It is not at all clear why this is not more widely available.
- Those judged to be at risk of suicide but who need potentially dangerous drugs, especially anti-depressants, should have them prescribed in small quantities only.

SOCIAL AND PSYCHIATRIC SUPPORT

People with severe depression and other psychiatric problems should be offered support, especially if they have mentioned suicide, have attempted it in the past and are isolated or elderly. It is very hard to know what can be offered to those young people for whom a suicide attempt is an impulsive act with unforeseen consequences, other than to try to publicize the helping agencies to whom the distressed can turn in crises and to emphasize the risks of overdosing on everyday drugs such as paracetamol or aspirin.

HELPLINES

The best known of these are the Samaritans; they offer a sympathetic, anonymous listening ear. It seems evident that this should help, although it is actually hard to prove the extent. Perhaps the very fact that so many unhappy people ring them is a measure of their value.

SOCIETY

There are wide international variations in the rate of suicide. The UK is quite low on the international scale; Hungary has the highest rate in Europe at forty suicides per 100,000 population per annum, some five times more than in the UK. This suggests that cultural factors are involved in suicide, though what these are is a matter of debate.

Self-Help

Samaritans
10 The Grove, Slough SL1 1PQ
Tel: 01753 532713

Diagnostic and Investigative Techniques and Treatment Tools

***

Allergy Testing

This is most commonly done by applying patches on the skin of the back. Each patch contains an extract from a different substance to which an individual might be allergic; e.g., grasses, lanolin, zinc. The patches are removed after a couple of days and the reaction is noted. A raised red area of skin confirms allergy. Allergies can also be tested by giving an injection of the suspected substance and seeing the reaction of the skin. Where people believe they are allergic to things in their food, allergy testing is difficult to do reliably. Ideally the individual would eat a very simple diet and then introduce the food to which they suspect they are allergic, while keeping a note of any reactions by way of diarrhoea, rashes etc.

Amniocentesis

The sampling of cells from the unborn baby by drawing off some of the fluid in which the baby floats within the womb and into which it sheds cells; this is the amniotic fluid. Done by passing a needle through the wall of the abdomen. The cells can be analyzed for chromosomal problems. Most commonly used to detect Down's syndrome.

Angiography

This means photographing the flow of blood through an artery. A thin tube (a catheter) is passed into an artery, usually in the groin and guided to the artery to be studied – commonly the heart. A dye is then injected into the bloodstream and a film is taken of how that dye flows, thus showing up blockages, narrowings and leaks. Widely used to see whether the arteries to the heart (the coronary arteries) are blocked or whether the large arteries down the legs are narrowed.

Arthroscopy

Looking inside a joint by passing a thin optical tube inside the joint. The surgeon can inspect the joint and remove debris. A great advance in the understanding and treatment of joint problems.

Barium Enema

Barium is a substance which shows up white on X-ray. Liquid barium is pumped into the bowel via the anus (back passage) and the patient is then tilted and turned to allow the barium to run back through the large intestine. The resulting X-rays show up ulcers, abnormal narrowings and possible tumours. Anything suspicious would be followed up by **colonoscopy** (see page 298).

Barium Meal

A means of investigating the gullet, stomach and small intestine, using liquid barium as above. The patient drinks the barium; a series of X-rays follows the path of the barium. It shows up ulcers, growths and narrowings. However, increasingly barium meals are being replaced by **endoscopy** (see page 299), which allows more precise diagnosis.

Biopsy

This involves taking a small sample of the body for analysis. Common examples are a biopsy of a breast lump, a mole, an unusual rash, enlarged glands, a stomach ulcer. It allows precise diagnosis to decide whether a larger operation is called for.

Blood Culture

A technique used to see whether germs are growing in the bloodstream, as in the very serious disease called septicaemia. Germs are frequently found in the bloodstream in the course of other infections such as pneumonia. The test involves taking a number of samples of blood and transferring them into bottles which contain the right ingredients to allow germs to grow. Thus the infection can be identified and the correct antibiotic selected to kill it.

Blood Tests

The body is a chemical factory. Blood tests measure the levels of the myriad chemicals found in the blood stream, so checking that the main functions of the body are normal. Common tests monitor kidney, liver, thyroid function, blood sugar and cholesterol. A blood count is a little different: this looks at the numbers and types of red cells (which carry oxygen); white cells (which fight infection); and platelets (which stop bleeding).

Chemotherapy

Cancerous cells grow at a faster rate than normal cells. Chemotherapy uses chemicals which destroy cells but which the fast-growing cancer cells absorb more than normal cells. Chemotherapy commonly causes side-effects such as hair loss and diarrhoea but cures certain types of leukaemia and cures or controls many other cancers, like breast, bowel and skin cancer.

Chromosome Studies

Chromosomes are the blueprints of life. They are made up of DNA, which carries the information for making all of the chemicals essential for life. Many conditions are caused by abnormalities within the chromosomes. Examples are Down's syndrome, cystic fibrosis, intersex. More common conditions are being increasingly shown to have a genetic element, such as diabetes, breast cancer, heart disease. It is possible to sample cells from the unborn baby to see whether it is carrying a chromosome abnormality (see **amniocentesis**, page 297).

Colonoscopy

A form of **endoscopy** (see page 299) in which a flexible tube is passed through the anus and is guided round the large intestine – up to 2 metres. Used to investigate unusual bleeding, chronic diarrhoea or to allow biopsies from the whole length of the large intestine.

Colposcopy

A technique using a specially adapted microscope in order to see the cervix (neck of the womb) under high magnification. The operator can select areas of the cervix which look suspicious, so as to take biopsies or to give treatment.

CT Scan (Computerised Tomography)

A series of X-rays is taken from a number of angles. By performing a computer analysis of the X-rays it is possible to construct a 'picture' of a cross section of the part of the body which was scanned. Unlike ordinary X-rays, which mainly show bones, this cross section also reveals soft tissues, like the brain or liver. CT scans revolutionized the investigation of brain and abdominal disorders, although they are now being overtaken by **MRI scans** (see page 300).

Cystogram

Measuring the rate and quantity of the flow of urine. Increasingly used to decide on the value of surgery for prostate problems or to investigate urinary incontinence in men and women.

Cystoscopy

Passing a narrow tube into the bladder via the urethra (outlet from the bladder). Used in the investigation of bleeding in the urine and recurrent infection of the urine.

Doppler Scanning

The Doppler effect means that a sound coming from something travelling towards you is higher in pitch than that same sound coming from something travelling away from you – think how the sound of a car alters as it passes you. This phenomenon is used to detect flows of liquid within the body, using a small probe which is just held against the skin. It is a reliable way of checking the baby's heart rate during pregnancy and for checking how well blood is flowing through the small arteries in the feet.

ECG (Electro-cardiogram)

A recording of the electrical activity of the heart, done by placing a number of small electrodes across the chest. ECGs are essential in diagnosing abnormalities of heart rate and rhythm. Useful in detecting a heart attack (see also **treadmill test**, see page 301).

Echocardiogram

Ultrasound waves (see **ultrasound**, page 301) are focussed on the walls and valves of the heart and bounce off to detectors (hence echo). Ultrasound is a quick, painless and harmless way of showing whether valves in the heart are leaking and showing how well the muscle of the heart is working. It has made the diagnosis of heart failure much more accurate.

EEG (Electro-encephalogram)

A recording of the electrical activity of the brain, shown as a series of waves on paper. Used mainly in diagnosing epilepsy.

Endoscopy

The term means 'looking inside the body'. It is done using a flexible tube carrying fibre optic cables and tiny instruments for taking biopsies and for performing simple procedures. Specialized forms are **gastroscopy, colonoscopy** and **ERCP** (see pages 300, 298 and below).

ERCP (Endoscopic Retrograde Cholangio-Pancreatography)

A means of showing up the drainage system from the gall-bladder and from the pancreas. This is important when trying to diagnose cancer of the pancreas or stones blocking the flow of bile from the gall bladder. It is done by passing an **endoscope** (see above) through to the duodenum and then manoeuvring a tiny tube into the outlet from the gall-bladder. By injecting a dye into the outlet the operator can outline abnormalities in the drainage system and in the pancreas.

ESR (Erythrocyte Sedimentation Rate)

A blood test which gives an idea of whether there is infection in the body, inflammation or certain blood disorders. It does not provide a diagnosis on its own, but a high ESR suggests that something serious is going on which calls for further investigation. It is used to monitor the level of control of chronic diseases such as rheumatoid arthritis.

Gastroscopy

Means looking inside the stomach, using a specially adapted endoscopic tube. It is done under light sedation. It allows the surgeon to inspect the lining of the stomach carefully and to take a biopsy from any ulcers. Gastroscopy gives more information than a **barium meal** (see page 297).

Glucose Tolerance Test

A blood test done to confirm the diagnosis of diabetes. The patient swallows a very sweet drink. Their blood and urine are sampled at regular intervals for the next two hours to see how high their blood sugar goes and whether any sugar appears in their urine. This test helps decide whether someone with sugar in their urine is truly diabetic or whether instead their kidneys are just a little leaky for sugar.

Immunoglobulins

These are complex chemicals which make up part of the body's defences against disease. They are substances which latch onto invading germs and immobilize them. In certain diseases the body's natural immunity declines and it is possible to give injections of immunoglobulins to provide some degree of protection against infection.

Kidney Function Tests

These are blood tests which check the levels of chemicals called urea and creatinine. These are breakdown products from the body's metabolism; high levels mean that the kidneys are not filtering the blood properly. More sophisticated tests can check the actual flow of urine from the kidneys.

Laparoscopy

A means of looking inside the abdomen using a tube passed through the wall of the belly. The operator can inspect the internal organs and perform operations. Female sterilization has been done this way for many years; the technique is increasingly being used for more ambitious procedures such as removal of gall-bladders and to repair hernias (key-hole surgery).

Lung Scan

A radioactive marker is injected into the bloodstream. Detectors display how the marker spreads through the lungs, thus showing if disease has blocked the flow of blood through the lungs. Useful in confirming pulmonary embolism.

Micro-discectomy

A way of dealing with a 'slipped disc' without a major operation. An instrument is passed through the back and guided to the slipped disc. The disc is cut away in small fragments Individuals can be back on their feet within a day or two.

MRI Scan (Magnetic Resonance Imaging)

A relatively recent advance in scanning the soft structures of the body. The procedure is similar to a CT scan but instead of X-rays, an MRI scanner sends powerful magnetic fields through the body. Detectors pick up how the body responds to those magnetic fields and sophisticated computer analysis generates a 'picture' of the body. The resulting images are astonishing; we see the living brain, inside joints and inside the spinal cord almost as if looking with the naked eye. Very expensive equipment needed.

Ophthalmoscope

A device for examining the eye. It is a very bright light plus a system of lenses which allows examination of the various structures of the eye and the back of the eye (the retina).

Radiotherapy

A mainstay of the treatment of cancer. It focuses X-rays on to cancerous growths, aiming to destroy the abnormal cells. It is often combined with **chemotherapy** (see page 298).

Sigmoidoscopy

Looking into the rectum using a rigid tube called a sigmoidoscope, passed up through the anus. Essential in the investigation of bleeding from the back passage or other symptoms suggesting inflammation or cancer of the lower bowel.

Skin Tests

By injecting a tiny amount of liquid into the skin it is possible to see whether someone has a reaction to that substance. A vigorous reaction means either a natural allergy or that the individual has met that substance before. This is the basis of the tuberculin test.

Thallium Scan

Thallium is a radioactive marker which can be injected into the blood stream. Detectors show how it spreads through the heart and this is a sensitive way of finding out whether the blood flow to the heart is poor.

Treadmill Test

An **ECG** (see page 299) of the heart, taken during exercise. The appearance of the tracing shows whether there is poor blood flow to the heart, before the stage is reached when blood flow is bad enough to cause chest pain.

Ultrasound

A harmless technique that uses sound waves to display internal organs. It is widely used in obstetrics to check on the growth of the baby and to detect abnormalities. It is also a safe, fast, inexpensive and straightforward way to investigate gallstones, the kidneys, the liver and the ovaries.

Venogram

A means of showing blood flow through the veins. Most often used in diagnosing a venous thrombosis; i.e., a blood clot within a vein. It involves injecting a dye into the veins and taking X-rays to show whether the dye flows normally through the veins.

X-Irradiation

The use of high energy X-rays in the treatment of cancer.

X-Rays

These are electrical waves similar to radio waves but which are much shorter and penetrate the body. Just as ordinary light casts shadows, so X-rays cast shadows of the dense structures they hit, especially bone. These shadows show up on photographic film. X-rays were discovered in 1895 by Roentgen, for which he received the Nobel Prize. Even after a century X-rays are still important diagnostic tools for investigating bone and chest problems.

INDEX